Northwest Vista College
Learning Resource Center
3535 North Ellison Drive
San Antonio, Texas 78251

NORTHWEST VISTA COLLEGE

R
853
.C55

Design and analysis of quality of life

DESIGN and ANALYSIS of QUALITY of LIFE STUDIES in CLINICAL TRIALS

CHAPMAN & HALL/CRC
Interdisciplinary Statistics Series

Series editors: N Keiding, B Morgan, T Speed, P van der Heijden.

AN INVARIANT APPROACH TO STATISTICAL ANALYSIS OF SHAPES	S. Lele and J. Richtsmeier
ASTROSTATISTICS	G. Babu and E. Feigelson
CLINICAL TRIALS IN ONCOLOGY	J. Crowley, S. Green, and J. Benedetti
DYNAMICAL SEARCH	L. Pronzato, H. Wynn, and A. Zhigljavsky
GRAPHICAL ANALYSIS OF MULTI-RESPONSE DATA	K. Basford and J. Tukey
INTRODUCTION TO COMPUTATIONAL BIOLOGY: MAPS SEQUENCES AND GENOMES	M. Waterman
MARKOV CHAIN MONTE CARLO IN PRACTICE	W. Gilks, S. Richardson, and D. Spiegelhalter
STATISTICS FOR ENVIRONMENTAL BIOLOGY AND TOXICOLOGY	A. Bailer and W. Piegorsch
DESIGN AND ANALYSIS OF QUALITY LIFE STUDIES IN CLINICAL TRIALS	Diane L. Fairclough

DESIGN and ANALYSIS of QUALITY of LIFE STUDIES in CLINICAL TRIALS

Interdisciplinary Statistics

Diane L. Fairclough

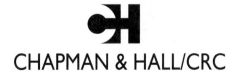

CHAPMAN & HALL/CRC

A CRC Press Company
Boca Raton   London   New York   Washington, D.C.

Library of Congress Cataloging-in-Publication Data

Fairclough, Diane Lynn.
  Design and analysis of quality of life studies in clinical trials / Diane L. Fairclough.
      p. cm. − (Interdisciplinary statistics series)
  Includes bibliographical references and index.
  ISBN 1-58488-263-8 (alk. paper)
    1. Clinical trials−Longitudinal studies. 2. Clinical trials−Statistical methods. 3. Quality of life−Research−Methodology. I. Title.
  II. Interdisciplinary statistics

R853.C55 .F355 2002
615.5′07′24−dc21   2002017479

This book contains information obtained from authentic and highly regarded sources. Reprinted material is quoted with permission, and sources are indicated. A wide variety of references are listed. Reasonable efforts have been made to publish reliable data and information, but the authors and the publisher cannot assume responsibility for the validity of all materials or for the consequences of their use.

Neither this book nor any part may be reproduced or transmitted in any form or by any means, electronic or mechanical, including photocopying, microfilming, and recording, or by any information storage or retrieval system, without prior permission in writing from the publisher.

The consent of CRC Press LLC does not extend to copying for general distribution, for promotion, for creating new works, or for resale. Specific permission must be obtained in writing from CRC Press LLC for such copying.

Direct all inquiries to CRC Press LLC, 2000 N.W. Corporate Blvd., Boca Raton, Florida 33431.

Trademark Notice: Product or corporate names may be trademarks or registered trademarks, and are used only for identification and explanation, without intent to infringe.

Visit the CRC Press Web site at www.crcpress.com

© 2002 by Chapman & Hall/CRC

No claim to original U.S. Government works
International Standard Book Number 1-58488-263-8
Library of Congress Card Number 2002017479
Printed in the United States of America 2 3 4 5 6 7 8 9 0
Printed on acid-free paper

Contents

Preface		xv
Acknowledgments		xix
1	**Introduction**	**1**
1.1	Health-related quality of life	1
1.2	Measuring health-related quality of life	2
	Characteristics of various measures	2
	Health status vs. patient preferences	2
	Objective vs. subjective	4
	Generic vs. disease-specific instruments	4
	Global index vs. profile of domain-specific measures	4
	Response format	6
	Period of recall	6
1.3	Example 1: Adjuvant breast cancer trial	7
	Patient selection	7
	Treatment	7
	Quality of life measure	8
	Timing of HRQoL assessments	8
	Questionnaire completion/missing data	10
1.4	Example 2: Advanced non-small-cell lung cancer (NSCLC)	10
	Treatment	12
	Quality of life measure	12
	Timing of assessments	13
	Questionnaire completion/missing data	13
1.5	Example 3: Renal cell carcinoma trial	15
	Patient selection	15
	Treatment	15
	Quality of life measure	15
	Timing of HRQoL assessments	16
	Questionnaire completion/missing data	17
1.6	Summary	18
2	**Study Design and Protocol Development**	**19**
2.1	Introduction	19
2.2	Background and rationale	19
2.3	Research objectives	20
	Domains of interest	21
	Pragmatic vs. explanatory inference	21

	2.4	Selection of subjects	22
	2.5	Longitudinal designs	23
		Event- or condition-driven designs	23
		Time-driven designs	24
		Timing of the initial HRQoL assessment	24
		Timing of the follow-up HRQoL assessments	24
		Timing of HRQoL assessments when therapy is cyclic	25
		Trials with different schedules of therapy	25
		Frequency of evaluations	25
		Duration of HRQoL assessment	26
		Assessment after discontinuation of therapy	27
	2.6	Selection of a quality of life measure	27
		Trial objectives	28
		Validity and reliability	29
		Appropriateness	30
	2.7	Conduct	31
		Mode of administration	31
		Data collection and management	32
		Avoiding missing data	32
		Education	33
		Forms	34
		Explicit procedures for follow-up	34
		Scoring instruments	35
		Reverse coding	35
		Scoring multi-item scales	35
		Item nonresponse	37
		SAS example	38
	2.8	Summary	39
3	**Models for Longitudinal Studies**	**41**
	3.1	Introduction	41
		Repeated measures models	41
		Growth curve models	42
		Selection between models	42
		Adjuvant breast cancer study (Example 1)	42
		NSCLC study (Example 2)	43
		Renal cell carcinoma study (Example 3)	43
	3.2	Building the analytic models	43
		Statistics guiding model reduction	44
		Likelihood ratio tests	44
		Other statistics	46
	3.3	Building repeated measures models	46
		Mean structure	46
		SAS example of a cell means model	47
		Covariance structures	48

		Unstructured covariance	48
		Structured covariance	49
		SAS example of a repeated measures model	50
		Hypothesis testing	52
	3.4	Building growth curve models	54
		Model for means	54
		Polynomial models	54
		Piecewise linear regression	54
		Covariance structure	57
		Variance of random effects	57
		Variance of residual errors	58
		SAS example of a polynomial growth curve model	59
		Fully parameterized model for the means	59
		Covariance structure	59
		Model reduction	63
		Estimation	63
		Hypothesis testing	64
		SAS example of a piecewise linear regression model	65
		Fully parameterized model for the means	65
		Covariance structure	65
		Model reduction	66
		Estimation	66
		Testing	67
	3.5	Summary	68
4	**Missing Data**		**69**
	4.1	Introduction	69
		Terminology	69
		Why are missing data a problem?	69
		How much data can be missing?	70
		Similar patterns of dropout among intervention arms	71
		Prevention	71
	4.2	Patterns of missing data	71
		Example: NSCLC study	72
	4.3	Mechanisms of missing data	72
		Notation	72
		Example	73
		The concept	74
		MCAR: Missing completely at random	75
		The concept	75
		Covariate-dependent dropout	75
		Identifying covariate-dependent missingness	76
		Example: NSCLC study	76
		Analytic methods	77
		MAR: Missing at random	77
		The concept	77

		Identification of dependence on observed data (Y_i^{obs})	78
		Analytic methods	80
		A test of MCAR vs. MAR for multivariate normal data	81
		Notation	81
		Test statistic	81
		NSCLC example	81
		Implementing in SAS	82
		MNAR: Missing not at random	84
		The concept	84
		Analytic methods	84
		Identification of dependence on unobserved data, Y_i^{mis}	85
		Example: NSCLC study	85
	4.4	Renal cell carcinoma study	87
		Plotting outcome by dropout	89
	4.5	Summary	90

5 Analytic Methods for Ignorable Missing Data 93
  5.1 Introduction 93
      Hypothetical example 93
  5.2 Repeated univariate analyses 94
      NSCLC example 96
  5.3 Multivariate methods 96
      Complete case analysis (MANOVA) 97
      NSCLC example 98
      Maximum likelihood estimation with all available data 101
      NSCLC example 102
      Further comments 104
      Exclusion of subjects 104
      Exclusion of observations 105
  5.4 Baseline assessment as a covariate 105
      NSCLC example 107
  5.5 Change from baseline 108
      NSCLC example 109
  5.6 Adding other baseline covariates 110
      NSCLC example 111
  5.7 Empirical Bayes estimates 112
  5.8 Summary 114

6 Simple Imputation 115
  6.1 Introduction 115
      Limitations of simple imputation 116
      NSCLC example 116
  6.2 Mean value substitution 117
  6.3 Explicit regression models 118

		Identification of the imputation model	119
		Simple univariate regression	120
		Conditional predicted values	123
	6.4	Last value carried forward	125
		δ-Adjustments	126
		Arbitrary high or low value	127
	6.5	Underestimation of variance	128
	6.6	Sensitivity analysis	130
	6.7	Summary	130

7 Multiple Imputation — 131

	7.1	Introduction	131
	7.2	Overview of multiple imputation	131
		Step 1: Selection of the imputation procedure	131
		Step 2: Generation of M imputed data sets	132
		Step 3: Analysis of M data sets	132
		Step 4: Combining results of M analyses	132
	7.3	Explicit univariate regression	133
		Identification of the imputation model	133
		Computation of imputed values	134
		Practical considerations	135
		Extensions to longitudinal studies	135
		Assumptions	135
		NSCLC example	136
	7.4	Closest neighbor and predictive mean matching	140
		Closest neighbor	142
		Predictive mean matching	142
	7.5	Approximate Bayesian bootstrap	142
		The basic procedure	143
		Extensions to longitudinal studies	144
		Propensity scores	144
		Practical issues	144
		The assumptions	145
		Nonignorable missing data	145
	7.6	Multivariate procedures for nonmonotone missing data	146
		NSCLC example	146
	7.7	Combining the M analyses	147
		SAS example	148
	7.8	Sensitivity analyses	150
	7.9	Imputation vs. analytic models	151
	7.10	Implications for design	152
	7.11	Summary	152

8 Pattern Mixture Models — 153

	8.1	Introduction	153
		NSCLC example	154

	8.2	Bivariate data (two repeated measures)	155
		NSCLC example	156
		Complete-case missing variable (CCMV) restriction	156
		NSCLC example	158
		Brown's protective restrictions	158
		NSCLC example	159
		Sensitivity analyses with intermediate restrictions	160
		Large-sample inferences for μ_2	160
		NSCLC example	161
	8.3	Monotone dropout	161
		NSCLC study	162
		Complete-case missing value restriction	162
		Available case missing value restriction	164
		Neighboring case missing value restriction	164
		Comparison of CCMV, ACMV, and NCMV estimates	167
	8.4	Parametric models	167
		Linear trends	168
		Variance estimation	172
		SAS example of a pattern mixture model	174
		Step 1: Estimates of π_h^P	174
		Step 2: Estimates of β_h^P	174
		Step 3: Pooling estimates and computing variance	175
		Step 4: Hypothesis testing	177
	8.5	Additional reading	178
		Extensions of bivariate case	178
		Extensions of the sensitivity analysis	178
		Nonparametric analyses	178
	8.6	Algebraic details	178
		Simple linear regression of Y on X	178
		Complete-case missing variable restriction	179
		Equation 8.9	179
		Equation 8.11	179
		Brown's protective restriction	179
		Equation 8.17	179
		Equation 8.19	180
		Other	180
	8.7	Summary	181
9	**Random-Effects Mixture, Shared-Parameter, and Selection Models**		**183**
	9.1	Introduction	183
		Mixture models	183
		Selection models	184
		Overview	184
	9.2	Conditional linear model	185

		Testing MAR vs. MNAR under assumptions	
		of conditional linear model	187
		NSCLC example	187
		Estimation of the standard errors	192
		Assumptions	192
		Random-coefficient mixture model	192
	9.3	Joint mixed-effects and time to dropout	193
		Testing MAR vs. MNAR under the assumptions	
		of the joint model	194
		Selection or mixture model?	195
		NSCLC example	195
		Initial estimates	197
		Extension to more complex mixed-effects models	198
		Renal cell carcinoma example	198
	9.4	Selection model for monotone dropout	198
		Outcome-dependent selection model	201
		NSCLC example	201
		Oswald program	206
		Longitudinal model	206
		Dropout model	208
		Oswald warnings	210
	9.5	Advanced readings	210
		Intermittent missing data	210
		More selection models	210
		Heckman probit stochastic dropout model	210
		Wu and Carroll	210
		Mori	210
		Nonparametric analyses	211
	9.6	Summary	211
10	**Summary Measures**		**213**
	10.1	Introduction	213
		Addressing multiplicity of endpoints	213
		Summary measures vs. summary statistics	213
		Strengths and weaknesses	215
		Easier interpretation	215
		Increased power	215
		Weakness	215
	10.2	Choosing a summary measure	215
	10.3	Constructing summary measures	217
		Notation	220
		Missing data	220
		Average rate of change (slopes)	222
		NSCLC example	222
		Missing data	222
		Area under the curve	225

		Missing data	225
		Differences at baseline	227
		Average of ranks	227
		Missing data	227
		Univariate analysis of summary measures	228
		Stratified analysis of summary measures	228
		NSCLC example	229
	10.4	Summary statistics across time	231
		Notation	231
		Area under the curve	231
		Repeated measures	231
		Growth curve models	232
	10.5	Summarizing across HRQoL domains or subscales	235
		Summary measures	235
		Weighting proportional to the number of questions	236
		Factor analytic weights	236
		Patient weights	237
		Statistically derived weights: Inverse correlation	238
		Summary statistics	239
	10.6	Advanced notes	240
		Nonparametric procedures	240
		Combining HRQoL and time to event	240
		Area under the curve	240
		Latent variable models	241
	10.7	Summary	241
11	**Multiple Endpoints**		**243**
	11.1	Introduction	243
		Limiting the number of confirmatory tests	243
		Summary measures and statistics	244
		Multiple comparison procedures	244
	11.2	Background concepts and definitions	245
		Univariate vs. multivariate test statistics	245
		Familywise and experimentwise error rates	245
		Global vs. individual tests	246
	11.3	Multivariate statistics	246
		Global tests	246
		Closed multivariate testing procedures	246
		Limitations	248
	11.4	Univariate statistics	249
		NSCLC example	249
		Alpha adjustments for K univariate tests	249
		Bonferroni adjustment	249
		Rüger's inequality	252
		Simes' global test	252

		Sequential rejective Bonferroni procedure	253
		p-value adjustments	253
	11.5	Resampling techniques	254
	11.6	Summary	255

12 Design: Analysis Plans — 257

	12.1	Introduction	257
	12.2	General analysis plan—Who is included?	258
	12.3	Models for longitudinal data	259
		Ignorable missing data	259
		Nonignorable missing data	259
		Event-driven designs and repeated measures models	259
		Time-driven designs and growth curve models	260
		Modification of analysis plan	260
	12.4	Multiplicity of endpoints	260
		Primary vs. secondary endpoints	260
		Summary measures	261
		Multiple comparison procedures	261
	12.5	Sample size and power	262
		Simple linear combinations of β	262
		Basic assumptions	264
		Incomplete designs	264
		Example 1: Repeated measures	266
		Example 2: Growth curve model	268
		Other considerations	270
		Intermittent missing data patterns and time-varying covariates	270
		Unequal allocations of subjects to treatment groups	270
		Multivariate tests	271
		Small sample size approximations	272
		Restricted maximum likelihood estimation	272
	12.6	Reporting results	272
	12.7	Summary	274

Appendix I	**Abbreviations**	**275**
Appendix II	**Notation**	**277**
Appendix III	**Formal Definitions for Missing Data**	**281**
References		**285**
Index		**295**

Preface

For almost 20 years I have been engaged by the challenges of design and analysis of longitudinal assessment of health outcomes in children and adults. Most of my research has been on the psychosocial outcomes for pediatric cancer survivors and health-related quality of life (HRQoL) of adult cancer patients, but it has included other diagnoses. As I have designed and analyzed these studies, many of the same themes continued to occur. This was irrespective of whether the studies were undertaken by the large cooperative groups, the pharmaceutical industry, or single institutions. The most common issues concerned missing or mistimed observations in longitudinal studies. The other issue is that of multiple comparisons. Five years ago, I began giving workshops three or four times a year on the design and analysis of HRQoL studies. My intent was to summarize that experience in this book; little did I realize how much more I would learn during the 2 years that I have been writing.

Numerous books discuss the wide range of topics that need to be addressed in the evaluation of quality of life. For example, Spilker [142] edited a comprehensive book published in 1996 with 1259 pages that includes chapters on general concepts; developing, choosing, and administering instruments; special populations; and cross-cultural aspects. Only 2 of the 127 chapters address analysis. Two years later, Staquet et al. [146] edited another book focusing on methods in clinical trials. Of the 18 chapters, 4 are devoted to design and analysis. Fayers and Machin [45] more recently published a text that focuses on assessment (questionnaire development and testing), analysis, and interpretation. Three chapters are devoted to analysis of longitudinal studies and three address design issues in clinical trials.

There still seemed to be a need for a book that addresses design and analysis in enough detail to enable readers to apply the methods to their own studies. To achieve that goal, I have limited the focus of the book to longitudinal studies of quality of life in clinical trials. Three clinical trials are used throughout the book to illustrate practical implementation of strategies and analytic methods. Finally, examples of SAS and S-Plus programs are included in the book. The intent is that readers, by following the examples in the book, will be able to follow the steps outlined with their own studies.

Intended Readers

My primary audience for this book is the researcher who is directly involved in the design and analysis of HRQoL studies. However, the book will also be useful to those who are expected to evaluate the design and interpret the results of HRQoL research.

More than any other research that I have been involved with, HRQoL research draws investigators from all fields of study with a wide range of training. This has included epidemiologists, psychologists, sociologists, behavioral and health researchers, clinicians, and nurses from all specialties, as well as statisticians. I expect that most readers will have had some graduate-level training in statistical methods including multivariate regression and multivariate analysis of variance. However, that training may have been some time ago and prior to some of the more recent advances in statistical methods. With that in mind, I have organized most chapters so that the concepts are discussed in the beginning of the chapters and sections. When possible, the technical details appear later in the chapters. Finally, each chapter ends with a summary of the important points.

Contents

Chapter 1 describes the general concept of HRQoL and characteristics of instruments used to assess HRQoL. Then the three clinical trials that are used throughout the book are described in detail.

I consider the careful and explicit definition of the research question to be the most important and critical step in the entire research process. All other decisions about the design and analysis follow. The principles of design will be considered throughout the book. In addition, Chapter 2 focuses on protocol development for longitudinal studies with HRQoL as an endpoint. Chapter 12 concludes the book with the development of analytic plans.

Because longitudinal studies of free-living subjects are subject to missing data, a major proportion of this book is devoted to that topic. Measurement of HRQoL and other patient-reported outcomes is particularly vulnerable to missing data in studies of patients who are experiencing morbidity or mortality due to their diseases or their treatments. Chapter 3 describes two general approaches to modeling longitudinal data, repeated measures and growth curve models, with a strategy for choosing between them. This will be a review for analysts who are regularly presented with longitudinal data. Chapter 4 defines patterns and mechanisms for missing data and then illustrates how one might determine which mechanisms apply in a particular clinical trial. This guides the selection of the appropriate analytic methods that are discussed in Chapters 5 through 9.

The greatest analytic challenge occurs when observations are missing because the patient is currently experiencing poorer (or better) HRQoL. If the data are missing for reasons related to toxicity of therapy or progression of disease, clinical experience suggests that the HRQoL at those time points where the patient was unable to complete the assessment is likely to be poorer than that at the time points where the patient completes the assessment. It is likely that no single approach is the best in all settings. Chapter 5 describes several widely used methods of analysis of longitudinal studies including repeated

PREFACE   xvii

univariate analyses, MANOVA, and mixed effects models. Chapter 6 discusses simple imputation of missing data. Most of the concepts in these two chapters are basic, but I am motivated to include this basic discussion because of common mistakes that I frequently observe. Chapters 7 through 9 discuss the more challenging methods for studies with non-ignorable (nonrandom) missing data. Analytic strategies such as multiple imputation (Chapter 7), pattern mixture models (Chapter 8), and shared parameter and selection models (Chapter 9) allow us to examine the sensitivity of the results to different assumptions about the missing data mechanism.

Typically, clinical trials measure multiple aspects of HRQoL or patient-reported outcomes repeatedly over time. As a result there are multiple scales with longitudinal assessment. To address the issues raised by this, Chapter 10 proposes the use of summary measures to facilitate interpretation and to increase the power of studies to detect meaningful changes in HRQoL. In Chapter 11, I discuss and illustrate the use of multiple comparison procedures to reduce the Type I error rates associated with hypothesis testing of multiple endpoints.

The Future

It was very difficult to stop writing this book. I would like to explore many topics that are not covered, new developments, and yet undiscovered old developments. One of the most obvious omissions is the development, translation, cultural adaptation, and validation of HRQoL instruments. If done well, instrument development requires considerable time and resources. This effort is often not appreciated by researchers who have never been involved in the process. I have chosen not to address this subject, as there are a large number of books already devoted to instrument development, including Schuman and Presser [143], Converse and Presser [25], Floyd and Fowler [50], DeVellis [33], Streiner and Norman [147], Juniper et al. [142, chapter 6], Frank-Stromborg and Olsen [52], Staquet et al. [146, part IV], and Fayers and Machin [45, chapters 2 through 7]. I am also sure that I will discover new ideas even before this book is published, but that is for the future.

                                                                              Diane L. Fairclough

Acknowledgments

I would like to thank all my friends and colleagues for their support and help. I would specifically like to thank Pam Wolfe, Mirium Dickenson, Melanie Bell, and Kathe Bjork for their careful proofreading of the material and Doris Borchert for finding all the journal articles that I requested.

CHAPTER 1

Introduction

1.1 Health-related quality of life

Traditionally, clinical trials have focused on endpoints that are physical or laboratory measures of response. For example, therapies for cancer are evaluated on the basis of disease progression and survival. The efficacy of a treatment for anemia is evaluated by hemoglobin levels or number of transfusions required. Although traditional biomedical measures are often the primary endpoints in clinical trials, they do not reflect how the patient feels and functions in daily activities, yet these perceptions reflect whether or not the patient believes he or she has benefited from the treatment. In certain diseases, the patient's perception of his or her well-being may be the most important health outcome [144]. More recently, clinical trials are including endpoints that reflect the patient's perception of his or her well-being and satisfaction with therapy. Sometimes clinical investigators assume that a certain change in therapy or a traditional biomedical outcome will improve the patient's quality of life. While in many cases this may be true, sometimes surprising results are obtained when the patient is asked directly. One classic example of this occurred with a study by Sugarbaker et al. [148] comparing two therapeutic approaches for soft-tissue sarcoma. The initial study compared two therapeutic options. The first was limb-sparing surgery followed by radiation therapy. The second treatment approach was full amputation of the affected limb. The investigator hypothesized, "Sparing a limb, as opposed to amputating it, offers a quality of life advantage." As a result of the study, the hypothesis was rejected; subjects receiving the limb-sparing procedures reported limitations in mobility and sexual functioning. These observations were confirmed with physical assessments of mobility and endocrine function. Radiation therapy was modified and physical rehabilitation was added to the limb-sparing therapeutic approach [65].

The World Health Organization (WHO) defined *health* in 1948 [164, 165] as a "state of complete physical, mental and social well-being and not merely the absence of infirmity and disease." This definition reflects the focus on a broader picture of health. Wilson and Cleary [163] propose a conceptual model of the relationships among health outcomes (Figure 1.1). Five levels of outcomes progress from biomedical outcomes to quality of life. The biological and physiological outcomes include the results of laboratory tests, radiological scans, and physical examination as well as diagnoses. Symptom status is defined as "a patient's perception of an abnormal physical, emotional or cognitive state." Functional status includes four dimensions: physical, physiological,

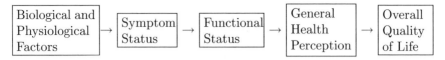

Figure 1.1. Five progressive levels of outcomes from Wilson and Cleary's conceptual model of the relationship among health outcomes.

social, and role. General health perceptions include the patient's evaluation of past and current health, his or her future outlook, and concerns about health.

The term *quality of life* has been used in many ways. Although the exact definitions vary among authors, there is general agreement that it is a multidimensional concept that focuses on the *impact* of disease and its treatment on the well-being of an individual.

In the broadest definition, the quality of our lives is influenced by our physical and social environment as well as our emotional and existential reactions to that environment. Kaplan and Bust [77] proposed the use of the term *health-related quality of life* (HRQoL) to distinguish health effects from other factors influencing the subjects' perceptions, including job satisfaction and environmental factors. In most clinical research, we limit the scope to focus on the measurement of HRQoL. Cella and Bonomi [16] state, "Health-related quality of life refers to the extent to which one's usual or expected physical, emotional and social well-being are *affected* by a medical condition or its treatment." In some settings, we may also include other aspects like economic and existential well-being. Patrick and Erickson [112] propose a more inclusive definition, which combines quality and quantity: "The value assigned to duration of life as modified by the impairments, functional states, perceptions and social opportunities that are influenced by disease, injury, treatment or policy." It is important to note that an individual's well-being or health status cannot be directly measured. We are only able to make inferences from measurable indicators of symptoms and reported perceptions.

Often the term *quality of life* is used when any *patient-reported outcome* is measured. Side effects are not equivalent to quality of life. Solely assessing symptoms is a simple, convenient way of avoiding the more complex task of assessing HRQoL. Symptoms do impact HRQoL and are part of the assessment of HRQoL.

1.2 Measuring health-related quality of life

Characteristics of various measures

Health status vs. patient preferences

There are two general types of HRQoL measures, health status assessment and patient preference assessment [169]. These two forms of assessment have developed as a result of the differences between the perspectives of two different disciplines: psychometrics and econometrics. In the health status assessment measures, multiple aspects of the patient's perceived well-being are self-assessed and a score is derived from the responses on a series of questions. This score reflects the patient's relative HRQoL as compared to other patients and to the HRQoL of the same patient at other times. The assessments range from a single global question asking patients to rate their current quality of life to a series of questions about specific aspects of their daily life during a recent period of time. These instruments generally take 5 to 10 min to complete. Examples include the Functional Living Index—Cancer (FLIC) [130], European Organization for Research and Treatment of Cancer EORTC QLQ-C30 [1], and the Functional Assessment of Cancer Therapy (FACT) [13]. Among these health status measures, there is considerable range in the context of the questions, with some measures focusing more on the perceived impact of the disease and therapy (How much are you bothered by hair loss?) and other measures focusing on the frequency and severity of symptoms (How often do you experience pain?). These measures are primarily designed to compare groups of patients receiving different treatments or to identify change over time within groups of patients. As a result, these measures have most often been used in clinical trials to facilitate the comparisons of therapeutic regimens.

Quality of life measures in patient preference assessments are influenced strongly by the concept of *utility*, borrowed from econometrics, that reflects individual decision making under uncertainty. These preference assessment measures are primarily used to evaluate the tradeoff between the quality and quantity of life. Values of utilities are always between 0 and 1, with 0 generally associated with death and 1 with perfect health. Examples include time tradeoffs [98], standard gamble [150], and multiattribute assessment measures such as the Health Utility Index (HUI) [46] and the Q-Tility index [159]. Time tradeoff utilities are measured by asking respondents how much time in their current health state they would give up for a specified period of time in perfect health. If, for example, a patient responded that he would give up 1 year in his current health for 5 years of perfect health, the resulting utility is 0.8. Standard gamble utilities are measured by asking respondents to identify the point at which they become indifferent to the choices between two hypothetical situations. For example, one option is a radical surgical procedure with no chance of relapse but significant impact on HRQoL and the other option is watchful waiting, with a chance of relapse and death. The chance of relapse and death is raised or lowered until the respondent considers the two options to be equivalent. Assessment of time tradeoff and standard gamble utilities requires the presence of a trained interviewer or specialized computer program. Because of the resource needs, these approaches are generally too time- and resource-intensive to use in a large clinical trial. Multiattribute assessment measures combine the advantages of self-assessment with the conceptual advantages of utility scores. Their use is limited by the need to develop and validate the methods by which the multiattribute assessment scores are converted to utility scores for each of the possible health states defined by the multiattribute assessments. For example, if a measure assesses five domains of HRQoL, with three possible levels for each domain, there will be 243 possible health states with a corresponding utility score. Utilities have traditionally been used in the calculation of quality-adjusted life years for cost-effectiveness analyses and in analytic approaches such as Q-TWiST [56, 58].

Objective vs. subjective

Health status measures differ in the extent to which they assess observable phenomena or require the respondent to make inferences. On the one hand, these measures will assess symptoms or functional benchmarks. In these instruments, subjects are asked about the frequency and severity of symptoms or whether they can perform certain tasks such as walking a mile. At the other end of the scale, the impact of symptoms or conditions is assessed. In these instruments, subjects are asked how much symptoms *bother* them or *interfere* with their usual activities. Many instruments provide a combination. The value of each will depend on the research objectives: Is the focus to identify the intervention with the least severity of symptoms or to assess the impact of the disease and its treatment?

There may exist a misconception that objective assessments are more valid. This is generally based on the observation that patient ratings do not agree with ratings of trained professionals. If we take objective assessments to be more valid, we are assuming that the ratings of the professionals constitute the *gold standard*, when in fact they have more limited information than the patient about how the patient views his or her health and quality of life. Further, many of the biomedical endpoints that we consider objective include a high degree of measurement error (e.g., blood pressure), are misclassified among experts, or have poor predictive and prognostic validity (e.g., pulmonary function tests) [162].

Generic vs. disease-specific instruments

There are two basic types of instruments—generic and disease-specific. The generic instrument is designed to assess HRQoL in individuals with and without active disease. The MOS SF-36 is a classic example of a generic instrument. This broad basis of a generic test is an advantage when comparing vastly different groups of subjects or following subjects for extended periods after treatment has ended. Disease-specific instruments narrow the scope of assessment and address in a more detailed manner the impact of a particular disease or treatment. As a result, they are more sensitive to smaller but clinically significant changes induced by treatment.

Global index vs. profile of domain-specific measures

Some HRQoL instruments are designed to provide a single global *index* of HRQoL. Others are designed to provide a *profile* of the dimensions such as the physical, emotional, functional, and social well-being of patients. Many instruments attempt to assess both but often in different ways. The index and the profile represent two different approaches to the use of the HRQoL

Table 1.1. Questions assessing *global quality of life* in the EORTC QLQ-30.

How would you rate your overall *health* during the past week?
  1   2   3   4   5   6   7
Very poor   Excellent

How would you rate your overall *quality of life* during the past week?
  1   2   3   4   5   6   7
Very poor   Excellent

measure. The advantage of a single index is that it provides a straightforward approach to decision making. Indexes that are in the form of utilities are very useful in cost-effectiveness analyses performed in pharmacoeconomic research. Health profiles are useful when the objective is to measure potentially different effects on the multiple dimensions of HRQoL.

When a construct is quite simple, a single question may be adequate to provide a reliable measure.* As the construct becomes more complex, more aspects of the construct need to be incorporated into the measure, creating a demand for multiple items. However, at some point the construct becomes so complex that a single question is used, allowing the subject to integrate the complex aspects into one response. At this point there is no way to identify all of the various aspects that are relevant.

Two widely used instruments designed for patients with cancer, FACT and EORTC QLQ-30, use summated scores from multiple questions to create domain-specific measures, but they take very different approaches to obtain global measures. For the FACT measures [14, 15], the overall score is the summated score from all items in the questionnaire. In Version 4 of the FACT, this consists of seven questions, each measuring physical, functional, and social well-being; six questions measuring emotional well-being; and a variable number addressing disease-specific concerns. In the EORTC QLQ-30, Aaronson et al. [1] do not propose adding the subscale scores to form an overall score, arguing that a profile of the various domains more accurately reflects the multidimensional character of quality of life. The global score is instead constructed from two questions that are distinct from those used to measure specific domains (Table 1.1).

A global measure of HRQoL has the obvious attraction of the simplicity of a single indicator. Unfortunately, it is difficult, if not impossible, to construct a single score that aggregates the multiple dimensions of HRQoL that is valid in all contexts. There is also a potential for the loss of information in a single measure. It is possible that a particular intervention may produce benefits in one dimension and deficits in another which cancel each other and are thus not observed.

---

* In general, scales constructed from multiple items have better reliability than single items, as the random measurement errors tend to cancel.

Table 1.2. Example of a Likert and visual analog scale.

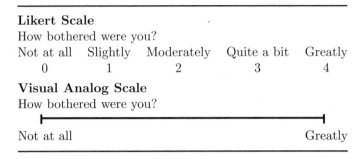

Response format

Questionnaires may also differ in their response format. Two of the most widely used formats are the Likert and visual analog scales (VAS) (Table 1.2). The Likert scale contains a limited number of ordered responses that have a descriptive label associated with each level. Individuals can discriminate at most seven to ten ordered categories [101, 147, p. 35], and reliability and the ability to detect change drop off at five or fewer levels. It is likely that as patients become more ill, the number of response levels they can easily respond to drops.

The VAS consists of a line with descriptive anchors at each end of the line. The respondent is instructed to place a mark on the line. Often the length of the line is 10 cm. The concept behind the VAS is that the measure is continuous and can potentially discriminate more effectively than a Likert scale. This has not generally been true in validation studies where both formats have been used. The VAS format has several limitations. First, it requires a level of eye–hand coordination that may be unrealistic for anyone with a neurological condition and for elderly people. Second, it requires an additional data management step in which the position of the mark is measured. If forms are copied, rather than printed, the full length of the line may vary, requiring two measurements and additional calculations. Third, VAS precludes telephone assessment and interview formats.

Period of recall

HRQoL scales often request subjects to base their evaluations on the last 7 days or 4 weeks. The selection of the appropriate time frame is a balance between being able to detect differences between treatments and to minimize short-term fluctuations (noise) that do not represent real change [102]. Scales specific to diseases or treatments where there can be rapid changes will have a shorter recall duration. Two widely used instruments for cancer patients, the Functional Assessment of Cancer Therapy (FACT) and the European Organization for Research and Treatment of Cancer scale (EORTC QLQ-C30) use 7 days. HRQoL instruments designed for assessment of general populations will often have a longer recall duration. For example, the Medical Outcomes Study SF-36 uses a 4-week window for most of its questions.

1.3 Example 1: Adjuvant breast cancer trial

Increasing dose intensity and scheduling drugs more effectively are two strategies for improving the effectiveness of breast cancer adjuvant chemotherapy. Although these strategies have advanced cancer therapy, the increased toxicity with more aggressive regimens is a concern, especially if there are modest improvements in survival. If more aggressive regimens produce comparable disease control and survival benefits, then the selection of optimum therapy should include not only the assessment of toxicity but also the impact of treatment on HRQoL.

In this trial, a 16-week dose-intensive therapy was compared to a conventional 24-week therapy (CAF*) in patients with breast cancer [47].** The primary hypothesis of the study was that disease-free and overall survival is superior on the more aggressive 16-week regimen. However, the 16-week regimen is a more dose-intense therapy than the 24-week CAF regimen and, in addition to potentially increasing physical symptoms, the inconvenience of the treatment and expected fatigue may have a greater impact on the psychosocial aspect of patients' lives. Thus, it was hypothesized that HRQoL during CAF therapy is superior to that during the 16-week regimen. This discrepancy in expectations creates a need to reconcile competing outcomes if they indeed occur.

Patient selection

The patients eligible for the treatment trial had hormone receptor-negative, node-positive breast cancer. Enrollment in the HRQoL substudy started after the initiation of the treatment trial. Patients registered on the treatment trial who had not yet started therapy were eligible for the quality of life study. Patients were also required to be able to read and understand English to be eligible. Consent was obtained separately for the treatment trial and the HRQoL substudy.

Treatment

Patients were randomized to receive either 24 weeks of a three-drug (CAF) regimen or a shorter, more intense 16-week multidrug regimen [48]. The CAF regimen consisted of 28-day cycles with 14 days of oral therapy and 2 days of intravenous therapy (days 1 and 8). Thus, patients on this regimen had

---

* CAF = cyclophosphamide, doxirubicin, and 5-flurouracil.
** Eastern Cooperative Oncology Group funded by the National Cancer Institute Grant CA-23318.

a 2-week break every 4 weeks. In contrast, the 16-week regimen consisted of weekly therapy. During odd-numbered weeks patients received 7 days of oral therapy plus 2 days of intravenous therapy. During even-numbered weeks, patients received 2 days of intravenous therapy.

Quality of life measure

The Breast Chemotherapy Questionnaire (BCQ) was selected among available validated HRQoL instruments that were suitable for cooperative group trials [102] and also suited to the goals of this study. The BCQ was developed to evaluate treatment-related problems identified by patients and clinicians as most important to HRQoL during breast cancer adjuvant chemotherapy [86]. It is a self-administered questionnaire of 30 questions about the past 2 weeks, answered on a 1- to 7-point scale (Table 1.3). Seven domains were identified: consequences of hair loss, positive well-being, physical symptoms, trouble and inconvenience, fatigue, emotional dysfunction, and nausea.

The overall raw score (R) is calculated as the mean of answers to the 30 questions; higher scores indicate better HRQoL, with a range of possible scores from 1 to 7. The raw score is then rescaled ($S = 10 * (R-1)/6$) so that the range of possible BCQ scores (S) is from 0 to 10 points [86]. Similarly, the subscale score for each of the seven domains is the mean of the responses to the questions for that domain rescaled in the same manner. If any of the items are skipped, the overall and subscale scores are calculated using the mean of the completed items.

Timing of HRQoL assessments

The BCQ assessments were limited to one assessment before, during, and after treatment. The assessment prior to therapy was scheduled to be within 14 days of start of chemotherapy. The assessment during treatment was scheduled on day 85 of treatment. This was halfway through the CAF therapy (day 1 of cycle 4) and three quarters of the way through the 16-week regimen (day 1 of week 13). By day 85 it was expected that patients would be experiencing the cumulative effects of both regimens without yet experiencing the psychological lift that occurs at the end of treatment. The third assessment following therapy was scheduled 4 months after the completion of therapy. Since the duration of therapy differed between the two treatment regimens (16 vs. 24 weeks), the third assessment occurred at different points in time for patients on the different regimens but at comparable periods relative to the completion of therapy. Additional variability in the timing of the third assessment was introduced for women who discontinued therapy earlier than planned or for those whose times to complete treatment may have been extended or delayed as a result of toxicity. The exact timing of the assessments is illustrated in Figure 1.2.

Table 1.3. Sample questions from the Breast Chemotherapy Questionnaire.

1. How often during the past 2 weeks have you felt worried or upset as a result of thinning or loss of your hair?
   - (1) All of the time
   - (2) Most of the time
   - (3) A good bit of the time
   - (4) Some of the time
   - (5) A little of the time
   - (6) Hardly any of the time
   - (7) None of the time
2. How often during the past 2 weeks have you felt optimistic or positive regarding the future?
   - (1) None of the time
   - (2) A little of the time
   - (3) Some of the time
   - ⋮
   - (7) All of the time
3. How often during the past 2 weeks have you felt your fingers were numb or falling asleep?
   - (1) All of the time
   - (2) Most of the time
   - (3) A good bit of the time
   - ⋮
   - (7) None of the time
4. How much trouble or inconvenience have you had during the last 2 weeks as a result of having to come to or stay at the clinic or hospital for medical care?
   - (1) A great deal of trouble or inconvenience
   - (2) A lot of trouble or inconvenience
   - (3) A fair bit of trouble or inconvenience
   - ⋮
   - (7) No trouble or inconvenience
5. How often during the past 2 weeks have you felt low in energy?
   - (1) All of the time
   - (2) Most of the time
   - (3) A good bit of the time
   - ⋮
   - (7) None of the time

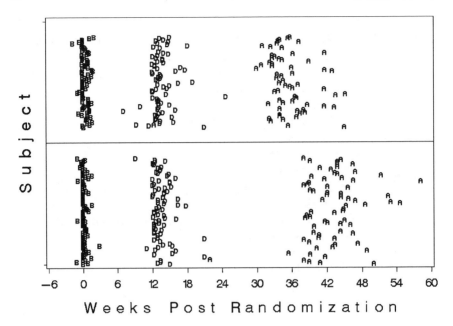

Figure 1.2. Timing of observations in a study with an event-driven design with assessments before (B), during (D), and 4 months after (A) therapy. Data are from the adjuvant breast cancer study [41]. Each row corresponds to a randomized subject. Subjects randomized to the 16-week regimen appear in the upper half of the figure and subjects randomized to the CAF regimen are in the lower half of the figure.

Questionnaire completion/missing data

There were 163 eligible patients registered on the HRQoL study. Assessments were completed by 157 (96%) patients prior to therapy, by 149 (91%) of the patients during therapy, and by 141 patients (87%) following therapy (Table 1.4). In an exploratory analysis (Table 1.5), women under 50 years of age were less likely to complete the assessment prior to therapy. Missing assessments during therapy were associated with early discontinuation of therapy (regardless of reason), concurrent chronic disease, and four or more positive nodes at diagnosis. Assessments were more likely to be missing following therapy in women who went off therapy early or who had four or more positive nodes at diagnosis. The association of missing assessments with factors that are also associated with poorer outcomes suggests that these assessments may not be missing by chance. (We will develop this argument in Chapter 4.)

1.4 Example 2: Advanced non-small-cell lung cancer (NSCLC)

To evaluate therapeutic effectiveness of new strategies for NSCLC, a multicenter phase III clinical trial* was activated to compare two new paclitaxel–cisplatin regimens with a traditional etoposide–cisplatin regimen for the

---

* Eastern Cooperative Oncology Group funded by the National Cancer Institute Grant CA-23318.

Table 1.4. Documentation of HRQoL assessments in the adjuvant breast cancer study (Example 1).

	Before therapy		During therapy		After therapy	
Status/reason	N	(%)	N	(%)	N	(%)
Completed	157	(96)	149	(91)	141	(87)
Too late for baseline[a]	4	(2)				
No longer receiving therapy[b]			2	(1)		
Patient refused	1	(1)	1	(1)	5	(3)
Staff oversight	0	(0)	4	(2)	3	(2)
Patient too ill	0	(0)	0	(0)	4	(2)
Other, Early off therapy	0	(0)	7	(4)	5	(3)
Other, Not specified	1	(1)	0	(0)	4	(2)
Not documented	0	(0)	0	(0)	1	(1)
Total expected	163		163		163	

[a] First assessment occurred after therapy began, excluded from analysis.
[b] Second assessment occurred after therapy ended, excluded from analysis.

Table 1.5. Patient characteristics associated with missing assessments (Example 1).

Time of assessment	Characteristic[b]	Odds ratio (95% CI)	
Before therapy	Age(<50 vs. ≥50)	(93 vs. 100%)[a]	
During therapy	Off therapy early	202	(24, 999)
	Concurrent disease	7.9	(1.3, 47)
	4+ positive nodes	15.3	(1.4, 166)
Following therapy	Off therapy early	9.6	(2.8, 34)
	4+ positive nodes	6.2	(1.2, 32)

[a] Odds ratio could not be estimated because of division by zero. CI = confidence interval.

[b] Other potential explanatory variables include minority race, initial performance status, treatment arm, the presence and severity of selected toxicity including vomiting, diarrhea, alopecia, and weight loss, and early discontinuation of therapy specifically related to toxicity, relapse, or patient preference.

treatment of stage IIIB–IV non-small-cell lung cancer (NSCLC) [7]. In addition to traditional endpoints, such as time to disease progression and survival, HRQoL was included in this trial. The stated objective of the HRQoL component of this study was "to compare quality of life for the three treatment arms and correlate quality of life to toxicity."

Table 1.6. Sample questions from the Functional Assessment of Cancer Therapy (FACT)-Lung (Version 2) Questionnaire.

Please indicate how true each statement has been for you *during the past 7 days*

Additional concerns		Not at all	A little bit	Some-what	Quite a bit	Very much
34.	I have been short of breath	0	1	2	3	4
35.	I am losing weight	0	1	2	3	4
36.	My thinking is clear	0	1	2	3	4
37.	I have been coughing	0	1	2	3	4
38.	I have been bothered by hair loss	0	1	2	3	4
39.	I have a good appetite	0	1	2	3	4
40.	I feel tightness in my chest	0	1	2	3	4
41.	Breathing is easy for me	0	1	2	3	4
	If you ever smoked, please answer 42:					
42.	I regret my smoking	0	1	2	3	4

Treatment

All three treatment arms included cisplatin at the same dose. The traditional treatment arm contained VP-16 with the cisplatin. The other two arms contained low-dose paclitaxel or high-dose paclitaxel with G-CSF. The planned length of each cycle was 3 weeks. Treatment was continued until disease progression or excessive toxicity. In all, 332 patients (58%) started four or more cycles of therapy and 210 (36%) started six or more cycles.

Quality of life measure

The Functional Assessment of Cancer Therapy, Lung Cancer Version 2 (FACT-L) was used to measure HRQoL in this trial [7]. It is a self-administered 43-item questionnaire, 33 items of which are general questions relevant to all cancer patients and 10 of which are items relevant to lung cancer (Table 1.6). It provides reliable scores for physical well-being, social/family well-being, emotional well-being, functional well-being, and lung cancer symptoms [7, 15]. In addition to the five major subscales, a number of summary scales can be constructed, including the FACT-Lung Trial Outcome Index (FACT-Lung TOI), which is the sum of the physical well-being, functional well-being, and lung cancer symptom scores. Higher scores imply better quality of life. Details of scoring the FACT are presented in Chapter 2. For easier interpretation of the presentations in this book, all subscales were rescaled to have a possible range of 0 to 100 with higher scores indicating better outcomes.

EXAMPLE 2: ADVANCED NON-SMALL-CELL LUNG CANCER (NSCLC)

Timing of assessments

Four HRQoL assessments were scheduled for each patient. The assessment times were carefully selected after balancing a number of considerations:

1. Concern for excessive burden to this often debilitated group of patients
2. The relatively short median time to both progressive growth of the tumor and death expected in these patients
3. Practical matters related to feasibility of the study at multiple clinical treatment sites.

These issues contributed to the decision to have relatively few assessments (four) over a fairly brief period of time (6 months from initiation of treatment). Standard community oncology practice for metastatic lung cancer very often involves the administration of two cycles of cytotoxic chemotherapy with reevaluation at the end of the second cycle (6 weeks) before moving on to further chemotherapy. Because the investigators were particularly interested in obtaining data from this study that would be useful to the community practitioner, they selected cycle 3, day 1 as the first clinically relevant assessment after baseline. The third assessment, which occurred at the end of the fourth cycle (cycle 5, day 1), was selected because it represented the same interval of time (6 weeks) and we believed it possible that patients' experience with therapy would enable them to tolerate it better over time. The final assessment at 6 months was selected as the best long-term follow-up in this population because it was several months before the expected median survival, which ensured that a sufficient number of patients could be studied. Thus, the four assessments were scheduled to be prior to the start of treatment, before the start of the third and fifth courses of chemotherapy, and at 6 months (week 26). If patients discontinued the protocol therapy, then the second and third assessments were to be scheduled 6 and 12 weeks after the initiation of therapy.

The actual timing of the HRQoL assessments showed much more variability than the plan would suggest (Figure 1.3). Some of the variation was to be expected. For example, when courses of therapy were delayed because of toxicity, the second and third assessments were delayed. Some variation in the 6-month assessment was also expected, as the HRQoL assessment was linked to clinic visits that might be more loosely scheduled at the convenience of the patient and medical staff. There was also an allowed window of 2 weeks prior to the start of therapy for the baseline assessment.

Questionnaire completion/missing data

A total of 1402 HRQoL assessments were obtained in this study. This represents 94, 72, 60, and 50% of the expected assessments in surviving patients at each of the four planned assessment times (Table 1.7). The most commonly documented reasons for missing assessments are patient refusal (8%) and "staff oversight" (8%). A detailed listing is presented in Table 1.7. A more extensive exploration of the missing data will follow in Chapter 4.

Table 1.7. Documentation of FACT-Lung assessments (Example 2).

Status/reason missing	Baseline N (%)	6 weeks N (%)	12 weeks N (%)	6 months N (%)
Completed[a]	538 (94)	382 (72)	290 (60)	192 (50)
Refusal	9 (2)	40 (8)	53 (11)	69 (18)
Language	0 (0)	2 (0)	0 (0)	0 (0)
Staff unavailable	0 (0)	5 (1)	2 (0)	1 (0)
Staff oversight	9 (2)	35 (7)	66 (14)	57 (15)
Patient feels too ill	0 (0)	4 (1)	3 (1)	3 (1)
Staff felt patient too ill	1 (0)	19 (4)	15 (3)	11 (3)
Other	9 (2)	12 (2)	23 (5)	19 (5)
Unknown	9 (2)	30 (6)	28 (6)	32 (8)
Total expected	575	529	480	384
Patients expired[b]	0 (0)	46 (8)	95 (17)	191 (33)
Total patients	575	575	575	575

[a] Percent of expected assessments (e.g., patient still alive).
[b] Percent of all possible assessments.

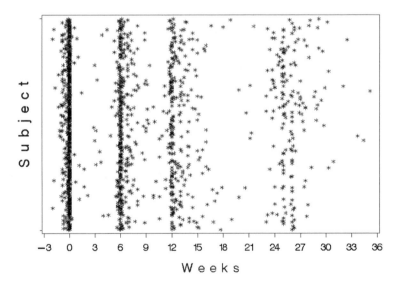

Figure 1.3. Timing of observations in a time-driven design with four planned assessments. Data are from the NSCLC study (Example 2). Each row corresponds to a randomized patient in this study. Symbols represent the actual timing of the HRQoL assessments relative to the date the patient was randomized.

1.5 Example 3: Renal cell carcinoma trial

Both exploration and sensitivity analysis will suggest that dropout in this study was likely to be nonrandom [42]. Consequently, methods of analysis described in Chapters 7 through 9 must be considered for this study.

1.5 Example 3: Renal cell carcinoma trial

A multicenter randomized phase III trial was conducted to determine whether combination therapy with 13-*cis*-retinoic acid (13-CRA) plus interferon alpha-2a (IFNα2a) was superior therapy to IFNα2a alone in patients with advanced renal cell carcinoma.[*] The influence of cytokine treatment on quality of life was considered to be an important aspect of the management of advanced renal cell carcinoma. No difference was found for the clinical endpoints [104]. This population experiences considerable morbidity and mortality, with a median survival of approximately 15 months.

Patient selection

Between April 1994 and July 1996, 284 patients were entered into the randomized trial. Eligibility requirements included histological confirmation of renal cell carcinoma, Karnofsky performance status (KPS) ≥ 70, and estimated life expectancy of more than 3 months. Patients enrolled after February 1995 were asked to complete HRQoL assessments.

Treatment

Patients were randomized to receive either daily treatment with IFNα2a plus 13-CRA or IFNα2a alone. IFNα2a was given as a single subcutaneous injection and the 13-CRA was given orally. Doses were adjusted in response to symptoms of toxicity. Treatment was continued until progression of disease, complete response, or development of excessive toxicity.

Quality of life measure

The trial utilized the Functional Assessment of Cancer Therapy Version 3 (FACT-G) as the tool for HRQoL assessment. Since the effect of biologic response modifiers (BRM) has not been adequately studied, 17 disease-specific questions were appended to the core questionnaire to measure the expected symptoms of 13-CRA and IFNα2a (Table 1.8). Validation of the disease-specific questions was undertaken to assess whether these questions are a reliable measure of HRQoL. Using factor analysis and internal consistency coefficients on the 2-week and baseline assessments, the original pool of 17 questions was reduced to a 13-item measure [2]. The factor analysis suggested that two definable dimensions were being measured by this set of questions. Examination of item content of the first dimension or subscale (factor 1) suggests it could be labeled as a *BRM-Physical* component. The second factor

---

[*] Memorial Sloan-Kettering Cancer Center and Eastern Cooperative Oncology Group funded by the National Cancer Institute Grant CA-05826.

Table 1.8. Sample questions from the Functional Assessment of Cancer Therapy— Biologic Response Modifiers including CRA (FACT-BRM/CRA Version 3) questionnaire.

Please indicate how true each statement has been for you *during the past 7 days*

Additional concerns	Not at all	A little bit	Some- what	Quite a bit	Very much
35. I get tired easily	0	1	2	3	4
36. I feel weak all over	0	1	2	3	4
37. I have trouble concentrating	0	1	2	3	4
38. I have trouble remembering things	0	1	2	3	4
39. My thinking is clear	0	1	2	3	4
40. I have a good appetite	0	1	2	3	4
41. I have pain in my joints	0	1	2	3	4
42. I am bothered by the chills	0	1	2	3	4
43. I am bothered by fevers	0	1	2	3	4
44. I am bothered by dry skin	0	1	2	3	4
45. I am bothered by dry mouth	0	1	2	3	4
46. I am bothered by dry eyes	0	1	2	3	4
47. I get depressed easily	0	1	2	3	4
48. I get annoyed easily	0	1	2	3	4
49. I have emotional ups and downs	0	1	2	3	4
50. I feel motivated to do things	0	1	2	3	4
51. I am bothered by sweating	0	1	2	3	4

included items related to mental or emotional symptoms/side effects (*BRM-Mental*). The initial BRM-Physical subscale included three items that were specific to dryness (skin, mouth, eyes), which were specific to the effects of CRA. This subscale was subsequently modified to reflect a more generic class of biologic response–modifying therapies. Coefficients of reliability (internal consistency) range from 0.61 to 0.92 for the baseline assessments and from 0.64 to 0.94 for the week 2 assessments. The Trial Outcome Index (FACT-BRM TOI), calculated by adding the physical and functional well-being scores and the two BRM subscale scores, was used as a summary measure of HRQoL. Details for scoring the FACT scales are presented in Chapter 2. In the examples presented in this book, the original 0- to 108-point scale was rescaled to have a 0- to 100-point range.

Timing of HRQoL assessments

At the time the study was designed, knowledge about the impact of therapy on the HRQoL of patients with renal cell carcinoma was extremely limited. Six assessments were scheduled. The first was to be obtained in a 2-week period

EXAMPLE 3: RENAL CELL CARCINOMA TRIAL

Table 1.9. Renal cell carcinoma trial: Summary of missing HRQoL assessments over time among 213 patients with at least one HRQoL assessment; 17 patients did not complete any assessments.

Schedule (weeks)	0	2	8	17	34	52
Surviving patients	213	212	201	176	142	118
TOI completed	190	163	123	75	55	27
% of surviving patients	89	77	61	43	39	23
% of total patients	89	77	57	35	26	13

Windows defined as <7 days, 1 to <6 weeks, 6 to <15 weeks, 15 to <30 weeks, 30 to <48 weeks, 48 to 65 weeks.

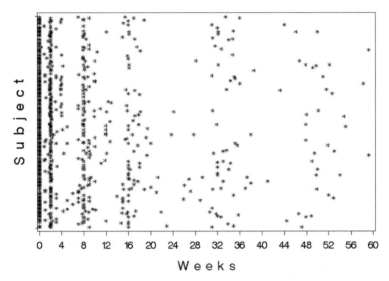

Figure 1.4. Timing of observations in a time-driven design with increasing numbers of mistimed observations. Data are from the renal cell carcinoma study [3]. Each row represents a subject.

prior to initiating therapy. The second was scheduled 2 weeks after initiation of therapy to assess acute toxicity. The remaining assessments were to occur at 2, 4, 8, and 12 months (8, 17, 34, and 52 weeks) to assess chronic toxicity. This schedule was to be continued for patients who discontinued the protocol therapy as a result of toxicity or disease progression to assess the continued impact of the disease and toxicity. The exact timing of the assessments became more variable with time (Figure 1.4).

Questionnaire completion/missing data

At least one questionnaire was received from 213 patients, with a total of 735 questionnaires. The compliance rates among the 213 patients for the six assessments were 89, 77, 61, 43, 39, and 23%, respectively (Table 1.9).

Early dropout from the HRQoL study was characterized by poorer prognosis (Kendall's $\tau_b = -0.25$), lower initial FACT-Lung TOI scores ($\tau_b = 0.27$), lower final FACT-Lung TOI score ($\tau_b = 0.22$), and early death ($\tau_b = 0.48$), but not with treatment ($\tau_b = -0.01$). A more extensive exploration of the missing data will follow in Chapter 4. As in the NSCLC study, this suggests that dropout in this study was likely to be nonrandom. Consequently, methods of analysis described in Chapters 7 through 9 must be considered for this study.

1.6 Summary

- Health-related quality of life
  1. HRQoL represents the impact of disease and treatment on a patient's daily living; it does not represent aspiration or satisfaction.
  2. HRQoL is multidimensional.
  3. HRQoL is subjective.
- Example 1: Adjuvant breast cancer study
  1. Simple design with one assessment before, during, and after therapy.
  2. Minimal (<5%) missing data.
- Example 2: Advanced non-small-cell lung cancer study
  1. Four planned assessments: one assessment before therapy and three during or after therapy.
  2. Extensive missing data as a result of death and other reasons probably related to HRQoL. More than 50% missing at time of last assessment.
- Example 3: Advanced renal cell carcinoma study
  1. Six planned assessments: one assessment before therapy and five during or after therapy.
  2. Extensive missing data as a result of both death and other reasons probably related to HRQoL. More than 50% missing at time of last assessment.
  3. Timing of assessments became more variable as the study progressed.

CHAPTER 2

Study Design and Protocol Development

2.1 Introduction

> Implicit in the use of measures of HRQoL, in clinical trials and in effectiveness research, is the concept that clinical interventions such as pharmacologic therapies, can affect parameters such as physical function, social function, or mental health. (Wilson and Cleary, 1995 [163])

Development of *a priori* objectives and an analytic plan are essential to both good trial design and subsequent scientific review. This chapter will focus on design and protocol development, with the exception of the statistical considerations such as sample size and analysis plans (see Chapter 12). Table 2.1 is a checklist for protocol development. All principles of good clinical trial methodology are applicable [49, 53, 99, 113, 141], but there are additional requirements specific to HRQoL. These include selection of an appropriate measure of HRQoL and the conduct of the assessment to minimize any bias. Because of the multidimensional nature of HRQoL and repeated assessments over time, objectives need to be explicitly specified and a strategy developed for handling multiple endpoints.

2.2 Background and rationale

Providing sufficient background and rationale to justify the resources required for an investigation of HRQoL will contribute to the success of the investigation. The rationale should provide answers to such questions as: How exactly might the results affect the clinical management of patients? How will the HRQoL results be used when determining the effectiveness of the treatment arms? The justification should include a motivation for the particular aspects of HRQoL that will be measured in the trial (e.g., physical, functional, or emotional) as they relate to the disease and its treatment.

The same demands for a rationale should be applied to all information collected in any clinical trial. However, investigators already have a habit of collecting laboratory and radiological tests so that minimal motivation is required to implement this data collection. The same is not necessarily true for the collection of data that requires patient self-assessment, and greater motivation may be necessary. Writing a rationale for HRQoL assessments also facilitates the development of well-defined research objectives.

Table 2.1. Checklist for protocol development.

- Rationale for studying HRQoL
- Explicit research objectives
- Strategies for limiting the exclusion of subjects from the HRQoL study
- Rationale for timing of assessments and off-study rules
- Rationale for instrument selection
- Details for conducting HRQoL assessments that minimize bias and missing data
- Analytic plan (Chapter 12)

Table 2.2. Checklist for developing well-defined objectives.

- Which dimensions of HRQoL are relevant?
- What is the population of interest (inference)?
- What is the time frame of interest?
- Is the intent confirmatory or exploratory?
- Is the intent to demonstrate superiority or equivalence?

2.3 Research objectives

The most critical component of any clinical trial is a list of explicit research objectives; Table 2.2 is a checklist. It is only when the research objectives provide sufficient detail to guide the design, conduct, and analysis of the study that the success of the trial is ensured. If no further thought is given to the specific research questions, it is likely that there will be neither rhyme nor reason to the design, conduct, and analysis of the HRQoL assessments. Then, because of either poor design or the lack of a definite question, the analyst will ask questions such as: What is the question? Why did you collect the data this way? Why didn't you collect data at this time? There is a real concern that the lack of meaningful results from poorly focused and thus potentially poorly designed and analyzed trials will create the impression that HRQoL research is not worthwhile.

General objectives state the obvious. Regardless of whether HRQoL is considered to be a secondary or primary outcome, a stated HRQoL objective such as *To compare the quality of life between treatment A and B* is too nonspecific. When the outcome is a univariate measure such as survival, it is reasonable to state the objective simply. Unlike the event of death, which occurs at a single point in time, HRQoL is experienced over time. The assessment of HRQoL also involves the various aspects of HRQoL, including physical, functional, emotional, and social well-being. A vague objective is insufficient.

Further, the detail of the objectives includes identifying (1) relevant dimensions of HRQoL, (2) population of interest, and (3) the time frame. Hypotheses should be clear whether the intent is to demonstrate superiority or equivalence and whether the objective is confirmatory or entirely exploratory.

Consider a hypothetical example in which two analgesics (Pain-Free and Relief) are compared for a painful condition. Both drugs require a period of titration in which the dose is slowly increased to a maintenance level. Assessments are obtained during the titration phase and the maintenance phase of the trial. An objective such as *To compare the quality of life in subjects receiving* Pain-Free *vs.* Relief does not provide any guidance. If the condition is permanent and the drugs are intended for extended use, the objective could be restated as *To compare the quality of life while on a maintenance dose of* Pain-Free *vs.* Relief. Alternatively, if the pain associated with the condition was brief, the drug that provided earlier relief would be preferable and the objective could be stated as *To compare the time to **20% improvement** in quality of life with* Pain-Free *vs.* Relief. These objectives now provide more guidance. In the first situation, assessments during maintenance are important, and in the second the earlier assessments are the basis of defining the outcome and should be frequent enough to detect differences between the two regimens. The same logic should be applied to the different dimensions of HRQoL.

Domains of interest

If HRQoL is defined as a primary endpoint, it implies that the demonstration of efficacy of intervention is based on some or all of the dimensions of HRQoL and other primary endpoints. Secondary endpoints are supportive of primary endpoints. In this case, HRQoL may measure a more distant outcome of therapy. For example, in the treatment of anemia, the primary endpoints are the expected biological changes (increased hemoglobin levels) and the secondary endpoints are consequences of the physiological changes (reduction in transfusions, less fatigue, improved HRQoL). Finally, when HRQoL is considered to be a tertiary outcome, the analysis is intended to be descriptive. Tertiary outcomes often address safety rather than efficacy measures. In HRQoL, tertiary measures are typically subscales that are not expected to be affected by the intervention.

Pragmatic vs. explanatory inference

The objectives should clarify to whom the inferences will apply: all study subjects, subjects who complete therapy, or only subjects alive at the end of the study? A useful terminology for characterizing the trial objectives is described by Schwartz et al. [63, 136]. They distinguish between *pragmatic* and *explanatory* investigational aims. The investigational aims for HRQoL will typically be pragmatic rather than explanatory. The distinction becomes important when the investigators make decisions about the study design and analysis.

Pragmatic objectives are closely related to the *intent-to-treat* analytic strategies. In these trials, the objective is to compare the relative impact of each intervention on HRQoL under practical and realistic conditions. For example, it may not be desirable for all subjects to complete the entire course of intended therapy exactly as specified because of toxicity or lack of efficacy. Some individuals may need to be given additional therapy. Others may be noncompliant for a variety of reasons. In a study with a pragmatic aim, the intent is to make inferences about all subjects for the entire period of assessment. Thus, assessment of HRQoL should be continued regardless of whether the patient continues to receive the intervention as specified in the protocol. HRQoL assessments should not stop when the patient goes *off study*.

In contrast, with an explanatory aim, we compare the HRQoL impact of treatments given in a manner that is carefully specified in the protocol. This is sometimes described as the analysis of the *per-protocol* subgroup. In this setting, HRQoL assessments may be discontinued when subjects are no longer compliant with the treatment plan. The analysis of these studies appears simple on the surface, but there is a real chance of selection bias. The analyst can no longer rely on the principle of randomization where unmeasured patient characteristics that confound the results are unbalanced across the treatment arms.

2.4 Selection of subjects

Ideally, the subjects who are involved in the HRQoL assessments are the same subjects who are evaluated for all of the study endpoints. This is recommended for several reasons [59]. The first is practical. It is much easier to implement a study if all patients require the same assessments. The second is scientific. The credibility and interpretation of a study is increased when all subjects are evaluable for all endpoints.

In practice, there may be some limitations. Physical, cognitive, or language barriers may make self-assessment infeasible. If the exclusions constitute a small proportion of the subjects, it is unlikely to compromise the validity of the results. However, if the investigation involves a substantial proportion of subjects either initially or eventually unable to complete self-assessments, a strategy must be developed to deal with the issue. For example, in a study where progressive cognitive impairment is expected, a design option is to start with concurrent subject and proxy assessments, continuing the proxy assessments when the patient is no longer able to provide assessments. The value of this design will be discussed in later chapters.

In some cases, the number of subjects required to detect a clinically meaningful difference in the HRQoL endpoints is substantially smaller than that required for the other endpoints. If the resource savings are substantial enough to warrant the logistical difficulties of obtaining HRQoL assessment on a subset of patients, the selection must be done in a completely random manner. It is not acceptable to allow selection of the subjects by the researchers or even by the patient's accessibility to telephone interview, as these methods are likely to introduce a selection bias.

Care should be taken when defining which subjects are excluded from an analysis. It is not uncommon to read a protocol where the analysis is limited to subjects with at least two HRQoL assessments (baseline and one follow-up). This criterion may change the population to which the results can be generalized by excluding all patients who drop out of the trial early. If this is a very small proportion of patients, it will not matter. But if a substantial number of subjects on one or more arms of the trial drop out before the second HRQoL assessment, this rule could have a substantial impact on the results.

2.5 Longitudinal designs

Longitudinal data arise in most HRQoL investigations because we are interested in how a disease or an intervention affects an individual's well-being over time. The optimal timing of HRQoL assessments depends on the disease, its treatment, and the scientific question. The number and timing of HRQoL assessments are influenced by both the objectives and practical considerations such as when the investigators have access to the subjects. Some studies have event- or condition-driven designs. Other studies have periodic evaluations based on the time elapsed since the beginning of treatment or the onset of the disease. Some studies incorporate a mixture of these two designs. The timing of assessments influence how we approach the analysis of each study (see Chapter 3).

Event- or condition-driven designs

When the objective of the study is to compare HRQoL in subjects experiencing the same condition, assessments are planned to occur at the time of clinically relevant events or to correspond to specific phases of the intervention. These designs are more common when the intervention or therapy is of limited duration. For example, one might consider a simple design with a pre- and postintervention assessment when comparing the HRQoL after two surgical procedures. The adjuvant breast cancer study (Example 1) provides a second example in which therapy is of limited duration. The design includes one assessment to measure HRQoL during each of the three phases: prior to, during, and after therapy. Many variations are possible. For example, there may be reason to believe that differences in HRQoL may exist during only the early or later periods of therapy. In this case, the design would include a minimum of two assessments during therapy. Studies with a limited number of phases of interest in the scientific investigation, where HRQoL is expected to be constant during those phases, are amenable to an event-driven design.

Time-driven designs

When the scientific questions involve a more extended period of time or the phases of the disease or its treatment are not distinct, the longitudinal designs are based on time. These designs are appropriate for chronic conditions where therapies are given over extended periods of time. In the NSCLC study (Example 2) and the renal cell carcinoma study (Example 3), therapy was to be given until there was evidence that it was ineffective or that it occasioned unacceptable toxicity. Thus, the duration of therapy was indeterminate at the onset of the study. More obvious examples would include treatment of chronic conditions such as diabetes and arthritis. Timing in these designs is based on regularly spaced intervals (e.g., every 3 months), sometimes more frequent initially (e.g., every month for 3 months and then every 3 months).

Timing of the initial HRQoL assessment

It is critical that the initial assessment occur prior to randomization. Because the measurement of HRQoL is generally based on self-evaluation, there is a potential that the knowledge of treatment assignment will influence a subject's responses [9]. This is especially true when the patient is aware that one of the interventions is new, possibly more effective than standard therapy, and exciting to his or her physician. The possible exception occurs if the intervention is double-blinded and treatment starts within a reasonable period of time of randomization. In this case, it is allowable to obtain initial assessment prior to the beginning of treatment but after randomization.

Timing of the follow-up HRQoL assessments

Similar attention should be paid to the timing of follow-up assessments. Assessments should be made consistently across treatment arms. Attention should be paid to the timing of diagnostic procedures. Especially with life-threatening diseases, the choices are not particularly easy. Prior to the testing, patients are likely to be experiencing stress in anticipation of the yet unknown results. After the procedure, the patients will be experiencing either great relief or anxiety.

The period of accurate recall is between 1 and 4 weeks, with better recall of major events and more recent experiences. Schipper [131] notes that the side effects of chemotherapy in patients with cancer may have a less adverse effect on a patient's HRQoL than similar side effects attributable to the disease. This observation may be true in other disease conditions as well. Testing immediately after toxicity occurs will emphasize that experience and deemphasize the benefits of treatment and disease symptoms. It is important not to pick a particular timing that will automatically bias the results against one treatment arm. In studies where the timing and length of treatment differ across arms, this may be challenging if not impossible.

Timing of HRQoL assessments when therapy is cyclic

Treatment for some conditions is cyclic, with administration of therapy only during the initial part of the cycle. This is characteristic of most chemotherapy regimens for the treatment of cancer. Typically, intense and toxic therapy is given for 1 to 2 weeks, with a hiatus for another 1 or 2 weeks to allow for recovery from the toxic effects of the treatment. Thus, it may not be possible to identify a time when the HRQoL is typical. For very practical reasons, HRQoL assessments have traditionally been scheduled to occur just prior to the beginning of the next cycle. Patients return to the clinic at this time for laboratory tests and other clinical evaluations; thus, they are consistently available for HRQoL assessment. As a result, there is potential for the measurement obtained just prior to the next cycle to overestimate the HRQoL over the entire cycle. More frequent assessment would solve this problem, but it must be weighed against increased patient burden and logistical issues of obtaining HRQoL assessments between patient visits.

Trials with different schedules of therapy

Another example is the timing of assessments when the impact of the therapy may differ by treatment arm. The timing of HRQoL assessments may, either by design or by chance, favor one of the treatment arms. The adjuvant breast cancer study (Example 1) provides a good example of how different treatment schedules can make the timing of HRQoL assessment a difficult choice. In this study, patients on one of the regimens receive some type of therapy on a weekly basis. On the other arm, therapy is cyclic with the patients receiving treatment during the first 2 weeks and then being free from treatment for the next 2 weeks. The HRQoL tool used in this trial asked the patient to respond relative to the last 2 weeks. The HRQoL assessments were scheduled to occur just prior to the beginning of a new cycle of therapy. Thus, in one arm the period of evaluation included the time when the patient was receiving therapy and in the other arm it did not. One possible solution might have been to change the time of the HRQoL assessment to the middle of the CAF treatment cycle, but this would have required an additional patient visit.

Frequency of evaluations

The frequency of the assessments should correspond appropriately to the natural history of the disease and the likelihood of changes in HRQoL within that period. Other considerations are a practical follow-up schedule and the timing of therapeutic and diagnostic interventions (Table 2.3). The assessments should be frequent enough to capture meaningful change but not so frequent as to be burdensome to the patient or incongruent with the assessment tool. If rapid change is expected during the early part of the study, more frequent early assessments are needed. In the renal cell carcinoma study (Example 3),

Table 2.3. Timing of HRQoL assessments relative to clinical and laboratory assessments.

	Design 1: HRQoL less frequent								
Clinical/Labs	X		X		X		X		X
HRQoL	Q				Q				Q
	Design 2: HRQoL linked with clinical								
Clinical	X		X		X		X		X
Labs	L	L	L	L	L	L	L	L	L
HRQoL	Q		Q		Q		Q		Q
	Design 3: HRQoL linked with labs								
Clinical	X		X		X		X		X
Labs	L	L	L	L	L	L	L	L	L
HRQoL	Q	Q	Q	Q	Q	Q	Q	Q	Q
	Design 4: HRQoL more frequent								
Clinical/Labs	X		X		X		X		X
HRQoL	Q	Q	Q	Q	Q	Q	Q	Q	Q

assessments were planned more frequently during the early phase of the study than toward the end. However, in retrospect, even more assessments during the early phase of therapy would have been informative, as HRQoL changed very rapidly during the early weeks of the treatment.

Assessments should not be more frequent than the period of recall defined for the instrument. The quality of the patient's life does not generally change on an hourly or daily basis as one would expect for symptoms. Thus, HRQoL scales often request the subjects to base their evaluations on the last 7 days or 4 weeks. Scales specific to diseases or treatments where there can be rapid changes generally have a shorter recall duration. Thus, if the HRQoL instrument is based on recall over the previous month, assessments should not be weekly or daily.

Duration of HRQoL assessment

First, it is important that the assessment is of sufficient duration to observe changes in HRQoL. Physiological responses to a therapy may occur more rapidly than changes in HRQoL. This is especially true for chronic diseases that have associated physical or functional disabilities.

For practical reasons it is wise to define a specific limit to the duration of assessment, specifically avoiding statements such as "and every 6 months thereafter." This is another situation that illustrates the need to have a well-defined objective. For example, are the investigators interested in the HRQoL of subjects while on a therapy that is of limited duration or is it especially important to understand the long-term impact of the treatment on HRQoL? If the former is the case, the additional information that can be obtained from continued assessments may diminish after some point either because there is little or no change or because the number of subjects with assessments is too small to analyze. If none of the objectives of the study requires continued assessment, then follow-up beyond that point is unwarranted.

Assessment after discontinuation of therapy

A very clear policy needs to be developed for following patients who cannot follow the treatment protocol. There are two major considerations when developing this policy. The first is scientific and depends on the research question. For example, if the discontinuation of treatment limits any future therapy to more intensive and toxic treatments or eliminates treatment options altogether as the disease progresses, the failure to continue HRQoL assessment can lead to overoptimistic bias. A treatment arm with a high rate of dropout may appear artificially beneficial because only the healthiest of the patients remain on the treatment.

On the other hand, discontinuation of assessment may make scientific sense in other disease settings. If HRQoL assessment is continued, the off-therapy assessments can be excluded if later deemed uninformative with respect to the research question. The opposite is not true; one can never retrospectively obtain the off-therapy assessments at a later date if they are determined to be of interest. The second aspect is practical; the off-treatment assessments are often difficult to obtain, especially if the patient no longer remains under the care of the same physician.

2.6 Selection of a quality of life measure

Guyatt et al. [62] define an *instrument* to include the questionnaire, the method of administration, instructions for administration, the method of scoring, and analysis and interpretation for a health status measure. All these aspects are important when evaluating the suitability of an instrument for a clinical trial; Table 2.4 is a checklist. Many of the steps in the selection of the HRQoL instruments for a trial can be accomplished by examining the literature and the questions posed in the instrument. However, empirical data are also valuable, especially with diseases or treatments that have not been previously studied. Bouchet et al. [8] describe a pilot study in which they evaluated three possible measures for a primary prevention trial. Included in the evaluation were ceiling effects, convergent validity, known discrimination, reproducibility among individuals reporting no change, and responsiveness among individuals reporting change.

Selecting a previously validated instrument is vastly preferable to the use of a new, unvalidated instrument. Developing a new instrument is expensive, is time consuming, and should be undertaken only when existing instruments

Table 2.4. Checklist for the selection of HRQoL instruments for a clinical trial.

- Does the instrument measure what it proposes to measure?
- Is the information relevant to the research question?
    How well does the instrument cover the important aspects of what is to be measured?
    Is a generic or disease-specific instrument more appropriate?
    Heath profile (rating scale) vs. patient preference (utility)?
- Will the instrument discriminate among subjects in the study and will it detect change?
- How well does the instrument predict related outcomes?
- Are the questions appropriate for the subjects across time?
- Are the format and mode of administration appropriate to the subjects and the trial?
- Has the instrument been previously validated in the target or similar population? If not, what are the plans to do so for current study?
- If using new instrument or items, the rationale and reasons for new items are indispensable.

are clearly unsuitable. Clinical researchers who have never undertaken this task severely underestimate the time and effort required. Instrument development is not limited to the generation of a list of questions and use in a single clinical trial. Development involves numerous steps of item generation (expert panels, focus groups), cognitive interviews evaluating comprehension of questionnaire wording (pilot tests with probing questions), data collection in a wide range of patients receiving the entire range of treatment options, item reduction, validation studies, translation, and cultural adaptation. Development of a new instrument can easily require 3 years and often more. The final limitation is that new instruments or questions may not be accepted as primary HRQoL endpoints in regulatory settings.

Trial objectives

Ware et al. [156] suggests:

> When searching for measures of health status, one first needs a clear understanding of the reasons for studying health status. A second requirement is a clear statement of the aspect of health being studied.

It is important to be clear on which of the different dimensions (physical, cognitive, emotional, and social) are relevant to the specific research questions and verify that all relevant domains are included. If the objective is to provide data for economic evaluations, a utility measure will facilitate the calculation of quality-adjusted life years. If the objective is to compare the impact of two therapies for the same condition on specific domains of disease-specific HRQoL, a disease-specific instrument is the most suitable.

Validity and reliability

There are numerous aspects and terms for the various components of reliability and validity of an instrument. For a formal presentation, the reader is referred to one of the numerous textbooks presenting these definitions. A partial list specific to HRQoL includes Streiner and Norman [147], McDowell and Newell [95, chapters 1 and 2], Juniper et al. [in 142, chapter 6], Naughton et al. [in 142, chapter 15], Frank-Stromborg and Olsen [52], Staquet et al. [146, part IV], and Fayers and Machin [45, chapters 3 through 7].

The validity of a measure in a particular setting is the most important and the most difficult aspect to establish. This is primarily because there are no gold standards against which the empirical measures of validity can be compared. In establishing the validity of measures of HRQoL, we compare the measures to other potentially flawed measures of HRQoL. Nonetheless, we can learn a good deal about an instrument by examining the instrument itself and the empirical information that has been collected.

The first questions about the content of an instrument—Does the instrument measure what it proposes to measure? Are the questions comprehensible and without ambiguity?—are referred to as *face validity*. Note that across instruments the same label or descriptor is sometimes given to groups of questions that measure different constructs. The wording of the questions should be examined to establish whether the content of the questions is relevant to the population of subjects and the research question. Although expert opinion (physicians, nurses) may make this evaluation, it is wise to check with patients, as they may have a different perspective.

Criterion validity is the strength of a relationship between the scale and a gold-standard measure of the same construct. As there is no gold standard for the dimensions of quality of life, we rely on the demonstration of *construct validity*. This is the evidence that the instrument behaves as expected and shows similar relationships (*convergent validity*) and the lack of relationships (*divergent validity*) with other reliable measures for related and unrelated characteristics.

The next question—Would a subject give the same response at another time if he was experiencing the same HRQoL?—is referred to as *reliability*. If there is a lot of variation (noise) in responses for subjects experiencing the same level of HRQoL, then it is difficult to discriminate between subjects who are experiencing different levels of HRQoL or change in HRQoL over time. Finally, we ask: Does the instrument discriminate among subjects who are experiencing different levels of HRQoL? Is the instrument sensitive to changes that are considered important to the patient? These characteristics are referred to as *discriminant validity* and *responsiveness*.

Although all the above characteristics are necessary, responsiveness is the most important in a clinical trial, as it directly affects the ability to detect changes that occur as the result of an intervention. One of the obvious factors that can affect responsiveness is the *floor and ceiling effect*. If responses are clustered at either end of the scale, it may not be possible to detect change due to the intervention.

Appropriateness

Will the instrument discriminate among subjects in the study and will it detect change in the target population? Ware et al. [156] suggest two general principles:

1. When studying general populations, consider using positively defined measures. Only some 15% of general population samples will have chronic physical limitations and some 10 to 20% will have substantial psychiatric impairment. Relying on negative definitions of health tells little or nothing about the health of the remaining 70 to 80% of the general population.
2. By contrast, when studying severely ill populations, the best strategy may be to emphasize measures of the negative end of the health status continuum.

Are the questions appropriate and unambiguous for subjects? One cannot always assume that a questionnaire that works well in one setting will work well in all settings. For example, questions about the ability to perform the tasks of daily living, which make sense to individuals who are living in their own homes, may be confusing when administered to a patient who has been in the hospital for the past week. Similarly, questions about the amount of time spent in bed provide excellent discrimination for nonhospitalized subjects but not for a hospitalized patient.

Are the questions appropriate for the subjects across time? In cases where the population is experiencing very different HRQoL over the length of the study, very careful attention must be paid to the selection of the instrument or instruments. Some studies will require difficult choices between the ability to discriminate among subjects during different phases of their diseases and treatments. In the adjuvant breast cancer study, the subjects were free of any symptoms or detectable disease. At the time of the pre- and post-treatment assessments, they were much like the general population. During therapy, they were likely to be feeling ill from the side effects of the treatment. In the example, at the time that the study was planned there were very few choices of HRQoL instruments. The compromise was the selection of the Breast Chemotherapy Questionnaire (BCQ), which was very sensitive on chemotherapy side effects but may have been insensitive to any post-treatment differences.

If an international trial, has the instrument been validated in other languages and cultures? Simple backward and forward translations are unlikely to be adequate for HRQoL instruments. There are numerous examples where investigators have found problems with certain questions as questionnaires were validated in different languages and cultures. Cognitive testing with subjects describing verbally what they are thinking as they form their responses has been very valuable when adapting a questionnaire to a new language or culture. This should be followed by formal validation studies.

2.7 Conduct

In many clinical trials, the decision to include HRQoL assessments was made at the end of the planning phase. Often, a questionnaire was added to the data collection without any appreciation of the amount of staff time required and with no allocation of additional resources. This generally resulted in overly ambitious assessment schedules and large amounts of missing data, which made analysis difficult and any results open to criticism. Although this behavior has decreased over time, there are still too many trials in which the details of how the HRQoL assessments are to be obtained are missing from the protocol and training materials.

Hopwood et al. [71] surveyed 29 centers participating in one or more of three randomized trials for lung and head and neck cancer. They observed that there was a very high proportion of preventable missing data. The three most commonly reported problems were that staff were not available, questionnaires were not available, and the staff considered the patient to be too ill. Preplanning and budgeting have the potential to fix the first two problems. Education is needed to address the third.

Mode of administration

Methods of administration that have been used successfully in clinical trials include paper-and-pencil self-report, in-clinic face-to-face assessments with trained interviewers, and centralized telephone administration with trained interviewers. Paper-and-pencil self-report is the most economical but requires that the patients be available on a regular basis. Interviewer administration is useful when the population has low literacy (children, immigrant populations), physical difficulty exists with pen-and-pencil forms (advanced neurological conditions, hospice patients), or the questionnaire involves complex skip patterns (standard gamble assessments).

Schipper [131] cautions against administration of an instrument designed for self-administration by a third party, noting several issues. There is evidence that self-report data differ from interview-generated data in ways that cannot be predicted. This is particularly true when there is the potential for the influence of social desirability on the responses. Great care must be taken to ensure that patients do not feel the need to please the clinical investigator with their answers. Similarly, patients may feel reluctant to answer the questions honestly in the presence of family and friends. Answering the questionnaire at home may result in different responses than in a hospital/clinic environment [162].

Regardless of what mode of administration is selected, it is preferable to use the same mode throughout the study unless it has been shown that responses are not affected by mode of administration. This advice is balanced by considerations of greater bias that can be introduced if this policy results in more nonresponse among selected groups of patients (e.g., those who are sicker). Often a compromise is required to balance feasibility and resources with ideal research conditions. Whatever procedures are selected, they should be carefully documented in the protocol and emphasized during training.

Data collection and management

First, it should be absolutely clear who is the key person at each clinical site responsible for administering the HRQoL. This will include, in addition to the usual responsibilities associated with the clinical trial, ensuring that there is someone who knows when the patient will arrive, will make sure the patient receives the questionnaire prior to undergoing diagnostic or therapeutic procedures and has a quiet place to complete the assessment, and is responsible for implementing follow-up procedures when the patient is not available as expected. At the time of the first assessment, this key person should emphasize the importance to the investigators of obtaining the patient's perspective, review the instructions with the subjects, emphasize that there are no correct or incorrect responses, encourage the subjects to provide the best answer they can to every question, and remind the subjects that they will be asked to repeat the assessment at later dates (if applicable). This person may have the responsibility of reviewing the forms for missing responses, but care needs to be taken to balance confidentiality with the need to minimize missing data. If the assessment consists of an interview, it requires sufficient trained personnel to schedule and conduct the interview.

Second, there needs to be a system that identifies when patients are due for assessments. This may include preprinted orders in the patient's chart that identify which HRQoL assessments should be administered at each clinic visit. This process may be assisted by support from a central data management office where calendars and expectation notices are generated. Stickers on the patient's chart identifying him or her as part of a study may also be helpful. Other options include flow sheets, study calendars, and patient tracking cards [102].

Avoiding missing data

Although analytic strategies exist for missing data, their use is much less satisfactory than initial prevention. Some missing data, such as that due to death, is not preventable. However, both primary and secondary prevention are desirable. In terms of primary prevention, missing data should be minimized at both the design and implementation stages of a clinical trial [37, 171]. In most studies, a nurse or research coordinator is responsible for giving the HRQoL questionnaire to the patient. Among these individuals, the reasons for missing data include lack of time and perceived lack of physician support, inadequate protocols, lack of knowledge on justification and rationale for collecting HRQoL data, lack of reminders, and lack of adequate sites for questionnaire completion [171]. Thus, clearly specified procedures in the protocol for collecting HRQoL are the first step in minimizing missing data. This should include information of collection procedure if treatment schedule is disrupted and procedures for completion of the questionnaire when the patient requires assistance. Provide a system for prompting nurses and research personnel that a HRQoL assessment is due. Consider alternative methods to obtain follow-up data when patients do not complete questionnaires. Educate patients, research assistants, and primary investigators about the importance of collecting these assessments on all patients willing to complete the questionnaire. Point out that reluctance to approach all patients on all occasions will lead to selection bias. The timing and duration of assessment should also be reasonable. Be practical about how often and how long you can follow patients.

Secondary prevention consists of gathering information that is useful in the analysis and interpretation of the results. This includes collection of data on factors that may contribute to missing assessments and data that are likely to predict the missing HRQoL measures. Thus, one should prospectively document reasons for missing data. The classifications that are used should be specified in a manner that helps the analyst decide whether the reason is related to the individual's HRQoL. For example, "Patient refusal" does not clarify this, but reasons such as "Patient refusal due to poor health" and "Patient refusal unrelated to health" will be useful. Other strategies for secondary prevention may include gathering concurrent data on toxicity, evaluations of health status by the clinical staff, or HRQoL assessments from a caretaker. Uses of this type of data are discussed in later chapters.

Education

Education can be an important part of minimizing missing data. It must start at the investigator level and include research assistants (often nurses) as well the patient. Vehicles for education include the protocol (with strong justifications for the HRQoL assessments), symposia, videos, and written materials. Videos may be valuable as training vehicles for both research staff and patients. Although there are often face-to-face training sessions at the initiation of a study, research personnel can change over time. Training tapes directed toward research personnel can deal with procedures in more detail than is possible in the protocol. Examples include how to handle a patient who is not able to fill in the questionnaire and not letting family or friends assist with the completion of the questionnaire. Training tapes are especially useful for providing positive ways of approaching the patient. For example, instead of referring to participation as burdensome (e.g., "We have a lot of forms that you'll need to fill out"), the HRQoL assessment can be placed in a positive light [13]:

> We want to know more about the quality of life of people as they go through this treatment and the only way to know is to ask you. In order to do this, we ask that you complete this brief questionnaire. It usually takes about (X) minutes ...

Hopwood et al. [71] noted that, in three trials for lung and head and neck cancer, staff's considering the patient to be too ill to complete the HRQoL assessments was the most commonly cited problem affecting the distribution of questionnaires. However, patient refusal was the least-cited problem. It is understandable that study personnel are reluctant to approach patients when they appear to be feeling particularly ill, but to minimize the bias from selecting out these patients, all should be asked to complete the questionnaire. There may be ways of encouraging ill patients, specifically by providing conditions that make it as easy as possible for them to complete the questionnaire. When a patient refuses, of course, that refusal must be respected.

Patient information sheets, which explain to the patient the rationale behind the HRQoL assessments, will minimize missing data. These sheets can contain messages about the importance of the patient's perspective, notes that there are no "correct" answers to the questions, and the reasons it is important to respond to every question and to complete the follow-up questionnaires. In addition to the persuasive information, the fact that patients can refuse the questionnaire without affecting their treatment or their relationship with their doctor should be included.

Forms

The data collection forms should be attractive and professional in appearance, using fonts that are large enough to ensure readability (e.g., 12-point characters or greater). Do not use two-sided forms! Patients will often not look at the back of the page, and if forms are copied at the sites, there is a high probability that only the front side will be copied.

Explicit procedures for follow-up

A practical schedule with HRQoL assessments linked to planned treatment or follow-up visits can decrease the number of missing HRQoL assessments. When possible, it is wise to link HRQoL assessments with other clinical assessments (Designs 2 and 3 in Table 2.3). This has several advantages. The availability of the patient increases the likelihood that the HRQoL assessment will be completed. Staff may be more likely to remember when the HRQoL assessment is scheduled if the timing is linked to clinical or laboratory follow-up. Finally, it is possible to link clinical events and laboratory values to the HRQoL assessments. Less frequent assessment of HRQoL (Design 1) decreases patient burden slightly but may introduce confusion about the schedule and thus lead to missed assessments. If more frequent assessments of HRQoL (Design 4) are specified in the design, strategies for obtaining the additional assessments must be identified. If the duration of HRQoL assessment continues after therapy is discontinued, this should be clearly stated and protocol flowcharts for treatment and assessment schedules should clearly reflect the difference.

The protocol and training materials should include specific procedures to minimize missing data. It should be clear what the allowable windows are for each assessment. The protocol should specify whether or not follow-up by telephone or mail is acceptable. Finally, since missing data will occur, it is important to document the reasons for the missing assessment. When constructing the set of possible reasons, the responses should differentiate whether the nonresponse was likely to be related to the patient's HRQoL. Documentation of the reasons for missing assessments can be combined with other questions

Table 2.5. Reverse coding procedure of subtracting response from sum of the lowest and highest possible responses to obtained reversed score.

Original responses	0	1	2	3	4
Calculation	4–0	4–1	4–2	4–3	4–4
Reversed score	4	3	2	1	0
Original responses	1	2	3	4	5
Calculation	6–1	6–2	6–3	6–4	6–5
Reversed score	5	4	3	2	1

When possible responses range from 0 to 4, sum is 4. When responses range from 1 to 5, sum is 6.

about the conditions under which the HRQoL was administered. For example: What was the site and mode of administration? Was any assistance given and, if so, by whom?

Scoring instruments

Protocols should include explicit instructions or references to the instructions for creating summary or subscale scores for the HRQoL instruments. References to methodology should be accessible and not in hard-to-obtain manuals or personal communications. If the scoring procedure does not include a strategy for handling missing items, there is the potential for a substantial number of subjects to have missing scores, even when they completed the assessment. If there are any proposed variations in the scoring procedure, they also should be specified in the protocol.

Reverse coding

The FACT scales are typical of many HRQoL health status measures. The first step is to reverse the scoring of negatively worded questions (Table 2.5). Notice that, in contrast to most of the questions in the Social/Family Wellbeing section of the FACT (Table 2.6), a higher score is associated with a negative outcome for questions 9 (distant from friends) and 13 (communication is poor). A quick trick to reverse the coding is to add the lowest and highest possible scores for the questions and subtract the response from that sum (see Table 2.5). For example, when the range of scores is 0 to 4, the sum is 4. If the responses to questions 9 and 13 are 2 and 3, respectively, the reverse scores are $4 - 2 = 2$ and $4 - 3 = 1$.

Scoring multi-item scales

Most HRQoL instruments combine the responses from multiple questions to derive summated scores for the relevant dimensions of HRQoL. The motivation is to increase the reliability of the scores and to facilitate interpretation. The most widely used method of combining responses is the method of *summated*

Table 2.6. Sample questions from the Social/Family Well-being subscale of the Functional Assessment of Cancer Therapy (FACT) questionnaire (version 3).

Below is a list of statements that other people with your illness have said are important. **By circling one number per line, please indicate how true each statement has been for you** *during the past 7 days.*

	Social/family well-being	Not at all	A little bit	Some-what	Quite a bit	Very much
9.	I feel distant from my friends	0	1	2	3	4
10.	I get emotional support from my family	0	1	2	3	4
11.	I get support from my friends and neighbors	0	1	2	3	4
12.	My family has accepted my illness	0	1	2	3	4
13.	Family communications about my illness is poor	0	1	2	3	4
14.	I feel close to my partner (or person who is my main support)	0	1	2	3	4
15.	Have you been sexually active during the past year? No __ Yes __ If yes: I am satisfied with my sex life	0	1	2	3	4

ratings or *Likert summated scales* [45]. The total score is obtained by adding the responses from all items. For a scale containing k items, each scored from 0 to r, the summated score will range from 0 to $k \times r$. If the scale is scored from 1 to r, the summated score will range from k to $k \times r$.

Because different scales (and even subscales within the same instrument) have a different number of items and a different range of responses, the range of these summated scores will have different ranges, making interpretation more difficult. For example, the emotional well-being score of the FACT (version 2) has a range of 0 to 20; the functional well-being, physical well-being, and family social well-being scores have a range of 0 to 28; and the total score has a range of 0 to 140. It is common practice to standardize the summated scores to range from 0 to 100. This is done by subtracting the lowest possible summated score ($S_{\min}$) from each score (S_i) and then multiplying the result by $100/(S_{\max} - S_{\min})$.

A much smaller number of HRQoL instruments use factor-analytic weights to construct scales. The source of these weights should be very carefully examined before accepting them. The weights need to be established in very large representative samples of subjects that include all levels of disease (or lack of disease) and expected types of treatment. Fayers and Hand [44] point out how sensitive the factor structure and resulting weights are to the population from which they were derived. Weights derived from another clinical

Table 2.7. Selected physical function questions from the SF-36 Health Survey that have a roughly hierarchical structure.

The following items are about activities you might do during a typical day. **Does your health now limit you in these activities?** If so, how much?

	Yes, limited a lot	Yes, limited a little	No, not limited at all
a. Vigorous activities, such as running, lifting heavy objects, participating in strenuous sports	0	1	2
b. Moderate activities, such as moving a table, pushing a vacuum cleaner, bowling, or playing golf	0	1	2
c. Lifting or carrying groceries	0	1	2
d. Climbing several flights of stairs	0	1	2
e. Climbing one flight of stairs	0	1	2
f. Bending, kneeling, or stooping	0	1	2
g. Walking more than a mile	0	1	2
h. Walking several blocks	0	1	2
i. Walking one block	0	1	2
j. Bathing or dressing yourself	0	1	2

---

trial or a selected population are likely to reflect the side effects of the specific treatments in that trial rather than the underlying construct.

Item nonresponse

It is not uncommon to have a small proportion (1 to 2%) of the items skipped. The frequency of missing items has been observed to be higher among elderly individuals [81] and those that are more ill. If the responses from selected patients are excluded from analysis because of missing items, there is a danger of biasing the results. Sometimes skipping an item is inadvertent, but it may also occur because a question is not applicable for that subject. Question 13 of the Social/Family Well-being is a good example of a question that is skipped by some subjects. To avoid missing subscale scores because of one or two missing responses, most scales specify exactly how to score the question in the presence of missing items. When a strategy is specified for a particular instrument, that strategy should be used for scoring when reporting the results of a clinical trial unless the new strategy was specified in the protocol as an alternative scoring system.

The most typical strategy, sometimes referred to as the *half rule*, is to substitute the mean of the answered questions for that specific subscale for the missing responses as long as at least half the questions were answered. This strategy works well for scales where there is no particular ordering of the *difficulty* of the questions, as in the FACT [38], and the difficulty of the question does not have a wide range across the subscale items. It should be used cautiously (or not at all) when the questions have a hierarchy,* as when functional well-being is assessed through the ability to do certain activities (Table 2.7). The physical functioning scale of the SF-36 is a good example of a scale where the individual items have a wide range of difficulty. If individuals are *limited a lot* in moderate activities, it is clear that they are also limited a lot in strenuous activities. Similarly, if subjects respond that they can walk a mile without limitations, they will also be able to walk several blocks. Special strategies may need to be specified for these types of questions [81].

SAS example

Both reverse coding and scoring can be accomplished in a few lines of code using macros rather than separate statements for every item and scale. This minimizes the possibility of typographical errors. The responses to the items are ITEM1, ITEM2,..., ITEMK, etc. where missing values are coded as SAS missing values. The first step is to reverse-code questions that are negatively worded. The second step is to create a scoring macro that (1) checks whether the number of completed responses (N(of &ITEMS(*))) is greater than half the possible responses (DIM(of &ITEMS(*))), (2) calculates the summated score in the presence of missing items, and (3) standardizes the summated score to have a range of 0 to 100. Arrays are then constructed with the items specific to each subscale included, and the macro is invoked to calculate the subscales.

```
DATA WORK.SCORES;
  SET WORK.ITEMS;

  *** Reverse Code Selected Items Coded 0-4 ***;
  *** REV is the list of questions that are reverse coded ***;
  ARRAY REV ITEM1 ITEM7 ITEM13 ... ITEM31;
  DO I=1 to DIM{REV};
    REV[I]=4-REV[I];
  END;

  *** Define Scoring Macro                                  ***;
  *** ITEM is the name of an array of items                 ***;
  *** MIN is the lowest possible response to a question     ***;
  *** MAX is the highest possible response to a question    ***;
  *** SUMSCORE is the name of the summated score            ***;
  *** STDSCORE is the name of the standardized score        ***;

  %MACRO SCORE(ITEMS,MIN,MAX,SUMSCORE,STDSCORE);
    N_SCALE=DIM(&ITEMS);         * # items in subscale *;
```

* When questions have a strict hierarchy, the scale is referred to as a Guttman scale.

```
    IF N(of &ITEMS(*)) GE N_SCALE/2 THEN
        &SUMSCORE=MEAN(of &ITEMS(*))*N_SCALE;
    &STDSCORE=(&SUBSCORE-(&MIN*N_SCALE))
            *100/((&MAX-&MIN)*N_SCALE);
%MEND SCORE;

*** Array items for each subscale ***;
ARRAY PWB ITEM1 ITEM2 ITEM3 ITEM4 ITEM5 ITEM6 ITEM7;
ARRAY EWB ITEM20 ITEM21 ITEM22 ITEM23 ITEM24;

*** Compute summated scores and standardized scores ***;
%SCORE(PWB,0,4,PWB_SUM,PWB_STD);
%SCORE(EWB,0,4,EWB_SUM,EWB_STD);
```

2.8 Summary

- It is critical to establish explicit research objectives during protocol development. Details should include (1) domains, (2) population, and (3) time frame relevant to the research questions.
- The HRQoL instruments should be selected carefully, ensuring that they are appropriate to the research question and the population under study. New instruments and questions should be considered only if all other options have been eliminated.
- The frequency and duration of HRQoL assessments should reflect the research objectives and the disease and treatment under study.
- The protocol should include explicit instructions for the conduct of the study to avoid bias and missing data. Educational materials for research staff and patients will be useful.

CHAPTER 3

Models for Longitudinal Studies

3.1 Introduction

This chapter addresses the analysis of longitudinal studies in the context of HRQoL investigations. In the previous chapter, event- or condition-driven and time-driven designs were described. These designs have corresponding analytic models: a repeated measures model and a growth curve model. In a repeated measures model, *time* is conceptualized as a categorical variable. Each assessment must be assigned to one category. In the NSCLC study (Example 2), these categories are "Pre-therapy," "6 weeks," "12 weeks," and "6 months." In a growth curve model, *time* is conceptualized as a continuous variable. In the NSCLC study, the variable is days since randomization.

In some trials, either analytic design is appropriate, and in other cases there will be clear reasons for preferring one or the other of these approaches. Although the schedule for HRQoL assessments is often constrained by practical considerations such as the timing of patient visits, the research question and the analytic methods appropriate for that question should be the primary consideration.

Repeated measures models

Repeated measures models are used in longitudinal studies with event-driven designs where there is a strong conceptual identity for each assessment. A good example is the adjuvant breast cancer study (Example 1) where assessments occurred during the three phases of the study: prior to therapy, while on therapy, and 4 months after the end of therapy. Repeated measures models may also be useful in some studies with a limited number (two to four) of assessments. If the timing of the longitudinal assessments occurs within predefined windows of time, then it is feasible to classify each of the assessments uniquely as one of the repeated measures.

Assignment of assessments to a planned assessment time (landmark) may become difficult in studies with more frequent assessments. These studies typically have more mistimed* observations with increasing rates of dropout. The process of defining windows of time for each assessment becomes increasingly difficult. If the windows are wide, an individual may have more than one observation within the window. This will require the analyst to discard all but one of the observations occurring within that window. Not only will

---

* The term *mistimed* does not necessarily refer to design (protocol) violations but rather indicates that the interval between observations may vary across subjects.

this reduce the statistical power of the study, but it may also lead to biased estimates, depending on how the observations are selected for discard. For example, bias may occur if discarded assessments were delayed when individuals were experiencing toxicity. Using narrow intervals may lead to fewer subjects with data at each landmark. This creates instability of the estimation of both the means and the covariance. In summary, one of the restrictions associated with the choice of a repeated measures model for the analysis of the trial is the necessity of identifying each assessment with each landmark.

Growth curve models

The term *growth curve models* comes from early applications to describe changes in height and weight as a function of age. Typically, these measurements were taken at different ages for each child in a study. Curves were fit to the data to estimate the typical height or weight for a child as a function of age. The same concept is relevant when we want to describe changes in HRQoL as a function of time. The curves can be defined in many ways, but they are most often described by polynomial functions or piecewise linear regressions. The simplest example of a growth curve model is a straight line.

Growth curve models are useful in several settings. The first is when the timing of assessments differs widely among individuals. Growth curve models are also useful in studies with a large number of HRQoL assessments, where it is feasible to model changes over time with a smaller number of parameters than is required for a repeated measures model. Finally, there may be analytic approaches where a mixed-effects model is necessary to model HRQoL in the presence of dropout. Two of the models described in Chapter 9 will utilize a mixed-effects model.

Selection between models

Adjuvant breast cancer study (Example 1)

In the adjuvant breast cancer study, the design requires the use of a repeated measures model. Each of the three assessments was planned to measure HRQoL at a different phase of the study. Because of different durations of therapy, the final assessments, scheduled 4 months after the completion of therapy, did not occur as scheduled for all subjects but at approximately 32 and 40 weeks after the beginning of the study (see Figure 1.2). Some post-therapy observations also occurred earlier when a patient discontinued therapy early. However, the intent of the design was to compare HRQoL when subjects had been off therapy long enough to recover from the effects of acute toxicity. Thus, the exact timing of the HRQoL assessment relative to the time they started therapy was not relevant.

BUILDING THE ANALYTIC MODELS 43

NSCLC study (Example 2)

With only four assessments that were widely spaced in time, either a repeated measures or a growth curve model can be justified. Figure 1.3 displays the actual timing of the assessments, which were clustered around the planned time of the assessment but became more variable as the study progressed. As previously mentioned, one restriction associated with a repeated measures model is the necessity of identifying each assessment with a landmark time. In this example, this was not too difficult because of the limited number of assessments and the wide spacing between them. There were no cases where an individual had more than four assessments, and there were only a few cases where there was some question about whether an assessment was closer to the 12- or 26-week target (see Figure 1.3). If this study had been designed to continue past 26 weeks or if there had been more frequent assessments, such as at 18 weeks, it would have been more difficult to classify each assessment uniquely, as required in a repeated measures model.

A growth curve model could also be considered for the NSCLC study. Although the assessments are based on the schedule of chemotherapy cycles, the changes in HRQoL can be easily modeled as a function of calendar time. Further, the assessments are not directly linked to an event or condition. The chemotherapy was given in 3-week cycles, but cycles could be delayed as a result of toxicity. With recognition of the potential for delays in therapy, the second and third HRQoL assessments were specified to occur on the first day (prior to therapy) of the third and fifth cycle of therapy, at approximately 6 and 12 weeks. The final assessment was planned for 26 weeks.

Renal cell carcinoma study (Example 3)

In the renal cell carcinoma study, only a growth curve model is feasible. This is because of the large number of potential observations where the timing relative to randomization becomes more varied as time progresses (see Figure 1.4). Thus, it becomes increasingly difficult to assign each observation to a landmark time. Forcing this study into a repeated measures design will also produce unstable estimates of covariance parameters during the later follow-up periods.

3.2 Building the analytic models

Consider a longitudinal study where n assessments of HRQoL are planned for each subject over the course of the study. We will consistently use h to indicate the hth group, i to designate each unique individual, and j to indicate the jth assessment of the ith subject. Thus, Y_{hij} indicates the jth observation of HRQoL on the ith individual in the hth group. The indicator of group (h) will often be dropped to simplify notation when it is not necessary to distinguish between groups.

A general linear model for the HRQoL outcomes can be expressed as

$$Y_{ij} = X_{ij}\beta + \epsilon_{ij} \qquad (3.1)$$

or in matrix notation as

$$Y_i = X_i\beta + \epsilon_i, \qquad (3.2)$$

where
Y_i = the *complete data* vector of n planned observations of the outcome for the ith individual, which includes both the *observed data* Y_i^{obs} and *missing data* Y_i^{mis}
X_i = the design matrix of fixed covariates corresponding to the *complete data* (Y_i)
β = the corresponding vector of fixed-effects parameters
ϵ_i = the vector of residual errors
Σ_i = the covariance of the *complete data* (Y_i), which is a known function of the vector of unknown variance parameters, τ: $\Sigma_i = f(\tau)$

This general linear model can be formed as either a repeated measures model or a growth curve model.

The recommended model building process [33, 150] starts by defining a fully parameterized model for the means $(X_i\beta)$, then identifying the structure of Σ_i, and finally simplifying the mean structure. This procedure is described in the remainder of this chapter.

Statistics guiding model reduction

Likelihood ratio tests

Two models, one nested within the other, can be compared with a maximum likelihood (ML) ratio test [75] or restricted maximum likelihood (REML) ratio test [87, p. 278]. The statistics are constructed by subtracting the values of -2 times the log likelihood and comparing the statistic with a χ^2 distribution with degrees of freedom equal to the difference in the number of parameters in the two covariance structures. Tests based on the REML are valid as long as the fixed effects are the same. Thus, either ML or REML ratio tests are valid when comparing nested covariance structures. However, likelihood tests for nested fixed-effects models must be limited to the use of ML (`METHOD=ML`) because the restricted likelihood adjustment depends upon the fixed-effects design matrix [87, pp. 298, 502].

To identify nesting, consider whether a set of restrictions on the parameters in one model can be used to define the other model. Typical restrictions are constraining a parameter to be zero or two parameters to be equal to each other. For example, the restriction $\rho_1 = \rho_2 = \rho_3$ on the *Toplitz* structure defines the *Compound Symmetry* structure (see Table 3.1). The homogeneous structures are all nested within their respective heterogeneous structure, $\sigma_1 = \sigma_2 = \sigma_3 = \sigma_4$. Most structured covariance matrices are nested within the

Table 3.1. Examples of covariance structures for three repeated measures. Examples progress from the least structured at the top of the table to the most structured at the bottom of the table.

	No. of parameters	Structure			
Unstructured TYPE=UN	10	σ_1^2	σ_{12} σ_2^2	σ_{13} σ_{23} σ_3^2	σ_{14} σ_{24} σ_{34} σ_4^2
Heterogeneous Toplitz TYPE=TOEPH	7	σ_1^2	$\sigma_1\sigma_2\rho_1$ σ_2^2	$\sigma_1\sigma_3\rho_2$ $\sigma_2\sigma_3\rho_1$ σ_3^2	$\sigma_1\sigma_4\rho_3$ $\sigma_2\sigma_4\rho_2$ $\sigma_3\sigma_4\rho_1$ σ_4^2
Heterogeneous Compound Symmetry TYPE=CSH	5	σ_1^2	$\sigma_1\sigma_2\rho$ σ_2^2	$\sigma_1\sigma_3\rho$ $\sigma_2\sigma_3\rho$ σ_3^2	$\sigma_1\sigma_4\rho$ $\sigma_2\sigma_4\rho$ $\sigma_3\sigma_4\rho$ σ_4^2
Heterogeneous Autoregressive [AR(1)] TYPE=ARH(1)	5	σ_1^2	$\sigma_1\sigma_2\rho$ σ_2^2	$\sigma_1\sigma_3\rho^2$ $\sigma_2\sigma_3\rho$ σ_3^2	$\sigma_1\sigma_4\rho^3$ $\sigma_2\sigma_4\rho^2$ $\sigma_3\sigma_4\rho$ σ_4^2
Toplitz TYPE=TOEP	4	σ^2	$\sigma^2\rho_1$ σ^2	$\sigma^2\rho_2$ $\sigma^2\rho_1$ σ^2	$\sigma^2\rho_3$ $\sigma^2\rho_2$ $\sigma^2\rho_1$ σ^2
First-order Autoregressive moving Average [ARMA(1,1)] TYPE=ARMA(1,1)	3	σ^2	$\sigma^2\lambda$ σ^2	$\sigma^2\lambda\rho$ $\sigma^2\lambda$ σ^2	$\sigma^2\lambda\rho^2$ $\sigma^2\lambda\rho$ $\sigma^2\lambda$ σ^2
Compound Symmetry TYPE=CS	2	σ^2	$\sigma^2\rho$ σ^2	$\sigma^2\rho$ $\sigma^2\rho$ σ^2	$\sigma^2\rho$ $\sigma^2\rho$ $\sigma^2\rho$ σ^2
First-order Autoregressive [AR(1)] TYPE=AR(1)	2	σ^2	$\sigma^2\rho$ σ^2	$\sigma^2\rho^2$ $\sigma^2\rho$ σ^2	$\sigma^2\rho^3$ $\sigma^2\rho^2$ $\sigma^2\rho$ σ^2

unstructured matrix, but structures such as the Toplitz and AR(1) models cannot be directly compared.

Other statistics

Criteria such as Akaike's Information Criterion (AIC) and the Bayesian Information Criterion (BIC) are also useful. These are the -2 log likelihood values penalized for the number of parameters estimated. The BIC imposes a greater penalty than the AIC.

3.3 Building repeated measures models

Mean structure

Repeated measures models for the HRQoL can be conceptualized several ways that are analytically equivalent. The most straightforward model is referred to as a *cell means model*. The parameters (usually means) from the repeated measures models are interpreted in the same way that parameters are interpreted in simple regression and analysis of variance (ANOVA) models. If we think of two-factor design with treatment arm and time as the factors, each cell represents one point in time within a specific treatment arm (Table 3.2). The equation for the model is

$$Y_{hij} = \mu_{hj} + \epsilon_{hij}, \tag{3.3}$$

where μ_{hj} is the average HRQoL score for the jth measurement of the hth group.

For example, in the adjuvant breast cancer study we have two treatments and three assessments over time. The simplest model for this study is a two-factor (treatment and time) design with the mean HRQoL score estimated for

Table 3.2. Adjuvant breast cancer example: Repeated measures cell means model with two factors, treatment (h) and time (j).

Model	$Y_{hij} = \mu_{hj} + \epsilon_{hij}$		
Treatment arm	Before therapy	During therapy	After therapy
Cell Means (μ_{hj})			
CAF	μ_{11}	μ_{12}	μ_{13}
16-week	μ_{21}	μ_{22}	μ_{23}
Estimates			
CAF ($\hat{\mu}_{1j}$)	7.6	6.8	8.0
16-week ($\hat{\mu}_{2j}$)	7.7	6.3	8.1
Difference ($\hat{\mu}_{2j} - \hat{\mu}_{1j}$)	-0.18	0.51	-0.09

Table 3.3. Adjuvant breast cancer example: Repeated measures model with two discrete factors (treatment and time) and a continuous covariate (age).

Model	$Y_{hij} = \mu_{hj} + \beta_{\text{age}} X_i(\text{age}) + \epsilon_{hij}$		
Treatment arm	Before therapy	During therapy	After therapy
Cell Means			
CAF	$\mu_{11} + \beta_{\text{age}} X_i(\text{age})$	$\mu_{12} + \beta_{\text{age}} X_i(\text{age})$	$\mu_{13} + \beta_{\text{age}} X_i(\text{age})$
16-week	$\mu_{21} + \beta_{\text{age}} X_i(\text{age})$	$\mu_{22} + \beta_{\text{age}} X_i(\text{age})$	$\mu_{23} + \beta_{\text{age}} X_i(\text{age})$

each of the two treatments prior to therapy, during therapy, and after therapy (Table 3.2).

Covariates can be added to the model when needed. For example, if the effect of age is independent of treatment and time, we can add age at the time of diagnosis (without interactions) to the model (Table 3.3). The equation for the model is

$$Y_{hij} = \mu_{hj} + \beta_{\text{age}} X_i(\text{age}) + \epsilon_{hij}, \tag{3.4}$$

where $X_i(\text{age})$ = age in years at diagnosis -50. The interpretation of the means (μ_{hj}) will change with the addition of these covariates. To facilitate the interpretation, it is advisable to center continuous covariates at a meaningful point. In this example, the average age at diagnosis is approximately 50 years, so the covariate is centered at that point. The interpretation of μ_{hj} is the expected (or average) HRQoL score for the jth measurement of the hth group for a woman who is 50 years of age. Without this centering process, estimates of μ_{hj} may be outside the range of possible values and the interpretation of each parameter is difficult. Using the age example without centering, we are estimating the mean HRQoL for a woman who is 0 years of age.

More covariates can be added to the model as needed, including those in which there are interactions with treatment, time, or both. Indiscriminate addition of covariates with missing values can create analytic problems because of the deletion of cases from the study.

SAS example of a cell means model

In the adjuvant breast cancer study, the datafile EXAMPLE1 has a unique record for each HRQoL assessment. CASEID identifies the patient. FUNO identifies the time of the assessment with values of 1, 2, and 3. TRTM identifies the treatment arm. The first part of the MIXED procedure for a cell means model might appear as

```
PROC MIXED DATA=EXAMPLE1;
  * Cell Means Model *;
  CLASS FUNO TRTM;
  MODEL BCQ=FUNO*TRTM/NOINT SOLUTION;
```

The CLASS statement identifies TRTM and FUNO as categorical variables with two levels of treatment and three levels of time. The term FUNO*TRTM in the MODEL statement creates a design matrix corresponding to the cell means model previously displayed in Table 3.2. The intercept term is suppressed by the NOINT option. The estimates of the means for each treatment by time combination are generated by the SOLUTION option in the MODEL statement:

```
                    Solution for Fixed Effects

  Effect      FUNO              TRTM      Estimate        Std Error

  FUNO*TRTM   Pre- Treatment     A        7.56837973      0.12785128
  FUNO*TRTM   Pre- Treatment     B        7.75274306      0.13857029
  FUNO*TRTM   During Treatment   A        6.82574053      0.16542708
  FUNO*TRTM   During Treatment   B        6.31521676      0.17716578
  FUNO*TRTM   4 months Post-Tx   A        8.00584072      0.12788503
  FUNO*TRTM   4 months Post-Tx   B        8.09419911      0.13935828
```

With addition of the age covariate AGE_EVAL, the MIXED statements become

```
PROC MIXED DATA=EXAMPLE1;
  * Cell Means Model *;
  CLASS FUNO TRTM;
  MODEL BCQ=FUNO*TRTM AGE_EVAL/NOINT SOLUTION;
```

In this example, none of the baseline covariates was associated with the outcome and none is included in the remainder of the analysis.

Covariance structures

The major difference between a univariate regression model for independent observations and a multivariate model for repeated measures is that the assessments for each individual are assumed to be correlated over time, $\text{Var}[Y_i] = \Sigma_i$. Examples of covariance structures include unstructured, Toplitz, compound symmetry (exchangeable), and autoregressive (Table 3.1).

Unstructured covariance

The unstructured covariance is the least restrictive and generally the best choice when the number of repeated measures is small. With only three assessments, this structure has six variance parameters. First, the variance of the HRQoL measure at each time point $(\sigma_1^2, \sigma_2^2, \sigma_3^2)$ is allowed to be different. The need for this type of flexible structure is illustrated in the adjuvant breast cancer study (see Table 3.4) where there is more variation in the HRQoL measure while the subjects are on therapy ($\sigma_2^2 = 2.28$) than before or after therapy ($\sigma_1^2 = 1.43, \sigma_3^2 = 1.32$). Further, the covariance of each pair of HRQoL measures ($\sigma_{12}, \sigma_{13}, \sigma_{23}$) is allowed to be different. It is not uncommon for HRQoL assessments occurring during therapy to be more strongly correlated with each other than with the initial pretherapy assessment.

Table 3.4. Estimated covariance and correlation for the adjuvant breast cancer study (Example 1).

Structure	r	AIC	BIC	Covariance			Correlation		
Unstructured TYPE=UN	6	1370.9	1408.0	1.43	1.11 2.28	0.75 1.12 1.32	1.00	0.62 1.00	0.54 0.64 1.00
Heterogeneous Toplitz TYPE=TOEPH	5	1369.1	1403.1	1.44	1.14 2.28	0.75 1.09 1.31	1.00	0.63 1.00	0.54 0.63 1.00
Heterogeneous Compound Symmetry TYPE=CSH	4	1370.1	1401.0	1.45	1.08 2.23	0.84 1.04 1.34	1.00	0.60 1.00	0.60 0.60 1.00
Heterogeneous Autoregressive TYPE=ARH(1)	4	1375.1	1406.0	1.44	1.13 2.28	0.53 1.07 1.29	1.00	0.63 1.00	0.39 0.63 1.00
Homogeneous Toplitz TYPE=TOEP	4	1386.4	1414.2	1.64	0.98 1.64	0.95 0.98 1.64	1.00	0.59 1.00	0.58 0.59 1.00

r = Number of unique parameters in covariance structure; AIC = Akaike's Information Criterion, smaller values are better; BIC = Bayesian Information Criterion, smaller values are better.

When the number of repeated measures increases, the number of parameters in the unstructured covariance matrix increases dramatically. For example, as the number increases from three to six repeated measures, the number of parameters increases from 6 to 21 (Table 3.5). In large data sets with nearly complete follow-up, estimation of the covariance parameters is not a problem. As the dropout increases, especially in smaller studies, it becomes more difficult to obtain stable estimates of the covariance parameters. In these settings it may be advisable to place restrictions on the covariance structure.

Structured covariance

If the correlation between measures is roughly equal regardless of how far apart in time the observations are taken, then compound symmetry is a possible candidate. This covariance structure is typically observed when the profile of each subject's HRQoL is roughly parallel over time. This structure is typical of measures that are unaffected by the disease or its treatment during the course of the study or when all subjects are equally affected.

When HRQoL observations are taken closely in time, the correlation of the residual errors is likely to be strongest for observations that are close in

Table 3.5. Number of parameters required to model covariance for two to seven repeated measures.

	No. of repeated measures					
Covariance structure	2	3	4	5	6	7
Unstructured	3	6	10	15	21	28
Heterogeneous Toplitz	3	5	7	9	11	13
Heterogeneous autoregressive	3	4	5	6	7	8
Heterogeneous compound	3	4	5	6	7	8
Toplitz	3	3	4	5	6	7
ARMA(1,1)	2	3	3	3	3	3
Compound symmetry	2	2	2	2	2	2
Autoregressive	2	2	2	2	2	2

Note that the number of parameters increases more rapidly for the least-structured covariance matrices.

time and weakest for observations that are the furthest apart. The Toplitz, autoregressive moving average (ARMA(1,1)) and autoregressive structures (AR(1)) allow observations that are further apart to be less strongly correlated. The autoregressive is the most restrictive of these structures. The correlation between two observations is a function of the separation between the observations.* The covariance decays exponentially as a function of the time lag. It is rare that the correlation of HRQoL measures declines this rapidly, even when the observations are far apart in time. The Toplitz and (ARMA(1,1)) provide more flexible structures that more closely fit the correlation typical of HRQoL measures.

There are numerous other possible covariance structures that are variations of these. One option is to allow the variance to be heterogeneous but retain the correlation structures. Additional options for covariance structures are described in detail in other sources, including Jennrich and Schluchter [75], chapters 3 and 6 of Jones [76], chapter 3 of Verbeke and Molenberghs [154], and in the SAS Proc Mixed documentation [115].

SAS example of a repeated measures model

In the adjuvant breast cancer example, there are only three repeated measures and enough observations to reliably estimate an unstructured covariance (Table 3.4). The unstructured covariance of the repeated measures is defined by the REPEATED statement with TYPE=UN. METHOD=ML is added to the PROC statement to facilitate comparisons between different models. The expanded

---

* The autoregressive structure shown in Table 3.1 assumes the observations are equally spaced. Further discussion of covariance structures for unequally spaced observations can be found in Jones [76, chapters 3 and 6].

MIXED procedure assuming an unstructured covariance would appear as

```
PROC MIXED DATA=EXAMPLE1 METHOD=ML;
  * Cell Means Model *;
  CLASS FUNO TRTM;
  MODEL BCQ=FUNO*TRTM/NOINT;
  * Unstructured Covariance *;
  REPEATED FUNO/SUBJECT=CASEID TYPE=UN R RCORR;
```

Other TYPE= options specifying the covariance structure are displayed in Table 3.4. The estimates of the covariance parameters appear as follows:

Covariance Parameter Estimates

Cov Parm	Subject	Estimate
UN(1,1)	CASE	1.4112
UN(2,1)	CASE	1.0963
UN(2,2)	CASE	2.2496
UN(3,1)	CASE	0.7389
UN(3,2)	CASE	1.1037
UN(3,3)	CASE	1.3052

The R and RCORR options request the output of the covariance and correlation matrices for the first subject in the more familiar format. (R=2 would request the covariance matrix for the second subject.)

Estimated R Matrix for Subject 1

Row	Col1	Col2	Col3
1	1.4112	1.0963	0.7389
2	1.0963	2.2496	1.1037
3	0.7389	1.1037	1.3052

Estimated R Correlation Matrix for Subject 1

Row	Col1	Col2	Col3
1	1.0000	0.6153	0.5445
2	0.6153	1.0000	0.6441
3	0.5445	0.6441	1.0000

The procedure generates statistics that can be used to guide the model selection.

Fit Statistics

-2 Log Likelihood	1346.9
AIC (smaller is better)	1370.9
AICC (smaller is better)	1371.6
BIC (smaller is better)	1408.0

The correlations estimated for the unstructured covariance range from 0.54 to 0.64, with the correlation the lowest between the two observations furthest apart in time. This suggests that the correlation would possibly fit the Toplitz structure. The increase in variation during the second assessment (during chemotherapy) suggests heterogeneity along the main diagonal.

More than one covariance structure is likely to provide a reasonable fit to the data. Unless the sample size for the study is very large, it is difficult to choose definitively among the various covariance structures. The information criteria can be used to provide guidance. For example, although the heterogeneous Toplitz structure provides the "best" fit as indicated by AIC, this structure only reduces the number of parameters by one. Similarly, the heterogeneous compound symmetry is suggested by the BIC. More critically, the estimates of all three covariance structures are very similar and the differences are unlikely to affect the results of the primary analyses.

Hypothesis testing

Although the *cell means model* generates estimates of the means for each treatment, we are usually interested in comparisons of these means. Any hypothesis that can be expressed as a linear combination of the estimated parameters (means) can be tested. For example, to test for differences at each time point the null hypotheses are

$$H_0: \mu_{21} = \mu_{11} \quad \text{vs.} \quad H_A: \mu_{21} \neq \mu_{11},$$
$$H_0: \mu_{22} = \mu_{12} \quad \text{vs.} \quad H_A: \mu_{22} \neq \mu_{12},$$
$$H_0: \mu_{23} = \mu_{13} \quad \text{vs.} \quad H_A: \mu_{23} \neq \mu_{13}.$$

These equations can be rewritten, placing all parameters on one side of the equality:

$$H_0: \mu_{21} - \mu_{11} = 0 \quad \text{vs.} \quad H_A: \mu_{21} - \mu_{11} \neq 0,$$
$$H_0: \mu_{22} - \mu_{12} = 0 \quad \text{vs.} \quad H_A: \mu_{22} - \mu_{12} \neq 0,$$
$$H_0: \mu_{23} - \mu_{13} = 0 \quad \text{vs.} \quad H_A: \mu_{23} - \mu_{13} \neq 0.$$

Putting the parameters in exactly the same order as they appear in the Solution for Fixed Effects displayed above,

$$H_0: -1\,\mu_{11} + 1\,\mu_{21} + 0\,\mu_{12} + 0\,\mu_{22} + 0\,\mu_{13} + 0\,\mu_{23} = 0,$$
$$H_0: 0\,\mu_{11} + 0\,\mu_{21} - 1\,\mu_{12} + 1\,\mu_{22} + 0\,\mu_{13} + 0\,\mu_{23} = 0,$$
$$H_0: 0\,\mu_{11} + 0\,\mu_{21} + 0\,\mu_{12} + 0\,\mu_{22} - 1\,\mu_{13} + 1\,\mu_{23} = 0.$$

The estimates of these differences and the corresponding tests are generated by the ESTIMATE statements with the coefficients from the above equations following the FUNO*TRTM term:

```
* Estimates of Treatment Differences *;
ESTIMATE 'Pre-Therapy Diff'    FUNO*TRTM -1 1 0 0 0 0;
ESTIMATE 'During Therapy Diff' FUNO*TRTM 0 0 -1 1 0 0;
ESTIMATE 'Post-Therapy Diff'   FUNO*TRTM 0 0 0 0 -1 1;
```

The results appear in the output as

```
                   ESTIMATE Statement Results

Parameter           Estimate   Std Err   DF     t      Pr > |t|
Pre-Therapy Diff    -0.184     0.189     161    -0.98  0.3296
During Therapy Diff  0.511     0.242     151     2.11  0.0368
Post-Therapy Diff   -0.088     0.189     143    -0.47  0.6411
```

One might consider an alternative hypothesis that patients in both treatments experienced a significant decline in HRQoL during therapy. The null hypothesis is

$$H_0: \mu_{12} - \mu_{11} = 0 \quad \text{and} \quad \mu_{22} - \mu_{21} = 0.$$

The hypotheses can be tested separately with ESTIMATE statements or jointly with the CONTRAST statement.

```
* Estimates of Change from Pre-therapy to Post-therapy *;
ESTIMATE 'Change in CAF pts'    FUNO*TRTM -1 0 1 0 0 0;
ESTIMATE 'Change in 16wk pts'   FUNO*TRTM 0 -1 0 1 0 0;
* Test Change from from Pre-therapy to Post-therapy *;
CONTRAST 'During-Pre Change'    FUNO*TRTM -1 0 1 0 0 0,
                                FUNO*TRTM 0 -1 0 1 0 0;
```

Notice that the CONTRAST statement contains the same syntax for identifying the terms in the hypothesis as the two ESTIMATE statements, but the two elements are separated by a comma.

The estimates of change in the BCQ scores while on therapy in the CAF and 16-week arms represent declines of approximately 0.6 and 1.1 standard deviations[*]; for the BCQ measure, these are moderate and strong effects, respectively [18].

```
                  ESTIMATE Statement Results

Parameter           Estimate   Std Err   DF     t      Pr > |t|
Change in CAF pts   -0.743     0.136     145    -5.46  0.0001
Change in 16 wk pts -1.438     0.145     144     9.92  0.0001

                  CONTRAST Statement Results

Source              NDF   DDF      F     Pr > F
During-Pre Change    2    145    64.10   0.0001
```

In this example, the option DDFM=SATTERTH was added to the MODEL statement. This option calculates the degrees of freedom of test statistics based on the actual design rather than relying on the variable names in the MODEL statement. (See appendix A.4 of Verbeke and Molenberghs [154] and the SAS Proc Mixed documentation [115] for further explanation.)

---

[*] $-0.743/1.29$ and $-1.438/1.29$, where $1.29 = \sqrt{\hat{\sigma}^2}$ and $\hat{\sigma}^2$ is the average baseline variance.

3.4 Building growth curve models

Model for means

Polynomial models

The most commonly used method of fitting growth curves is to use a polynomial function to describe change:

$$Y_{hij}(t) = \beta_{h0} + \beta_{h1}t_{hij} + \beta_{h2}t_{hij}^2 \cdots + \varepsilon_{hij}.$$

The purpose of the polynomial model is to approximate a curve that fits the observed data. There is no biological or theoretical reason that growth of children or HRQoL would follow a such a model. However, polynomial functions can provide a good approximation of the average HRQoL. Figure 3.1A shows how a polynomial model might appear in the renal cell carcinoma example.

Without CRA:

$$\hat{Y}_{1ij}(t) = 87.0 - 11.2t + 2.92t^2 - 0.272t^3 + 0.0101t^4 - 0.000130t^5. \quad (3.5)$$

With CRA:

$$\hat{Y}_{2ij}(t) = 85.7 - 14.8t + 3.38t^2 - 0.279t^3 + 0.0095t^4 - 0.000114t^5. \quad (3.6)$$

The higher-order terms, such as quadratic (t^2) and cubic (t^3) terms, allow the curves to depart from linearity. However, when the model contains higher-order terms, interpretation of the corresponding coefficients is difficult. In theory, the maximum number of terms (including the intercept) is equal to the number of assessments. In the example, six is the maximum number of terms that can be included. But with extensive dropout and mistiming of the later observations, more parsimonious models may be necessary.

An overall test of postrandomization differences is straightforward; we compare the parameters across the H groups. But this test does not provide information about when the groups may be experiencing differences in HRQoL. Comparisons of the time-specific estimates are more useful. If, for example, in the renal cell carcinoma study, we were interested in comparisons of HRQoL shortly after beginning treatment (2 weeks or 0.46 months), well into treatment (2 months), and 6 months after treatment began, we might construct the estimates displayed in Table 3.6.

Piecewise linear regression

A useful alternative is a piecewise linear regression model. The change in HRQoL is modeled as a linear function over short intervals of time. As in the polynomial model, the model is not based on theory but the need to get a reasonable fit to the data. Thus, although we do not expect changes in HRQoL to be strictly linear, it is reasonable to assume that changes are approximately linear over short intervals of time. Figure 3.1B illustrates the use of a piecewise linear model for the renal cell carcinoma study. In this study, we could consider

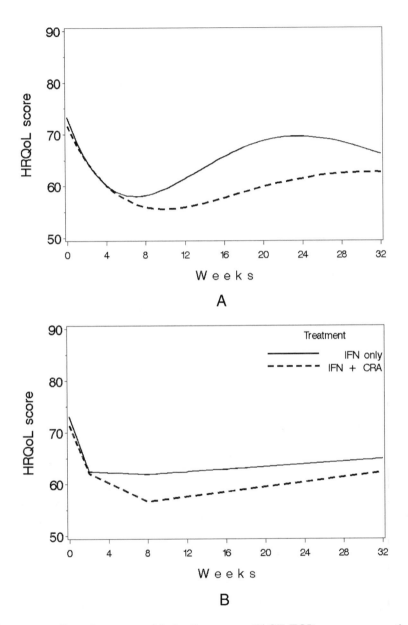

Figure 3.1. Growth curve models for the average FACT-TOI score among patients treated on the renal cell carcinoma study [3]. (A) Polynomial model, (B) piecewise linear regression.

Table 3.6. Renal cell carcinoma example: Polynomial growth curve model.

Treatment	Baseline	2-week mean	2-month mean	6-month mean
Model				
−CRA	β_{10}	$\sum_0^5 \beta_{1k} 0.46^k$	$\sum_0^5 \beta_{1k} 2^k$	$\sum_0^5 \beta_{1k} 6^k$
+CRA	β_{20}	$\sum_0^5 \beta_{2k} 0.46^k$	$\sum_0^5 \beta_{2k} 2^k$	$\sum_0^5 \beta_{2k} 6^k$
Estimates				
−CRA	90.3	78.3	72.3	81.3
+CRA	88.7	74.9	67.2	67.9
Difference	1.6	3.3	5.0	13.4

Table 3.7. Renal cell carcinoma example: Piecewise linear regression model with selected time-specific means.

Treatment	Baseline mean	2-week mean	2-month mean	6-month mean
Model				
−CRA	β_{10}	$\beta_{10} + \beta_{11} 2$	$\beta_{10} + \beta_{11} 8.67 + \beta_{12} 6.67 + \beta_{13} 0.67$	$\beta_{10} + \beta_{11} 26 + \beta_{12} 24 + \beta_{13} 18$
+CRA	β_{20}	$\beta_{20} + \beta_{21} 2$	$\beta_{20} + \beta_{21} 8.67 + \beta_{22} 6.67 + \beta_{32} 0.67$	$\beta_{20} + \beta_{21} 26 + \beta_{22} 24 + \beta_{23} 18$
Estimates				
−CRA	90.9	76.3	74.5	77.9
+CRA	89.0	73.3	66.0	72.0
Difference	1.8	2.8	8.5	5.9

terms that allow the slope to change at 2, 8, 17, and 34 weeks (Table 3.7).

$$Y_{hij}(t) = \beta_{h0} + \beta_{h1} t_{hij} + \beta_{h2} t_{hij}^{[2]} + \beta_{h3} t_{hij}^{[3]} + \beta_{h4} t_{hij}^{[4]} + \beta_{h5} t_{hij}^{[5]} + \varepsilon_{hij},$$

$$t_{hij}^{[c]} = \max(t_{hij} - T^{[c]}, 0),$$

$$T^{[1]} = 0, \quad T^{[2]} = 2, \quad T^{[3]} = 8, \quad T^{[4]} = 17, \quad T^{[5]} = 34.$$

The selected points of change should correspond to the times when changes in HRQoL might occur as the result of treatment or some other clinically relevant process. In practice, the points in time where observations are clustered will provide the most efficient estimates of change. Ideally, the study is designed so that the points of clinical interest correspond to data collection. Note that as with the polynomial model, we start with a maximum of six unknown parameters in each group.

After a model-fitting procedure, described in more detail in the next section, the piecewise regression model for the renal cell study is

without CRA:
$$\hat{Y}_{1ij}(t) = 90.9 - 7.30t + 7.03t^{[2]} + 0.44t^{[8]} \qquad (3.7)$$

and with CRA:
$$\hat{Y}_{2ij}(t) = 89.0 - 7.85t + 6.76t^{[2]} + 1.38t^{[8]}. \qquad (3.8)$$

This can be interpreted as follows: The two groups start with average scores of 91 and 89, respectively. There is a rapid decline during the first 2 weeks, which is slightly more rapid in the patients receiving CRA (-7.85 vs. -7.30 points/week). This initial rapid decline ceases around week 2, with estimated rates of decline between weeks 2 and 8 equal to -0.27^* and -1.09^{**} points per week in the two arms, respectively. After approximately 8 weeks, HRQoL begins to improve slightly in both arms ($+0.17^{***}$ and $+0.29\dagger$ points per week, respectively).

Covariance structure

Because there are multiple assessments on each subject, we expect the assessments for each individual to be correlated over time. The most typical approach for modeling the covariance structure uses a mixed-effects model. The term *mixed* refers to the mixture of *fixed* and *random* effects:

$$Y_{hi} = \underbrace{X_{hi}\beta_h}_{\text{Fixed effects}} + \underbrace{Z_{hi}d_{hi}}_{\text{Random effects}} + \underbrace{e_{hi}}_{\text{Residual error}}. \qquad (3.9)$$

In the context of growth curve models, the fixed effects ($X_i\beta$) model the *average* HRQoL, whereas the random effects ($Z_i d_i$) model the variation among individuals relative to the average. The *fixed effects* are also referred to as the *mean response*, the *marginal expectation* of the response [35], and the *average evolution* [154, 155]. The covariance of a mixed-effects model for Y_{hi} has the general structure:

$$\begin{aligned}\Sigma_{hi} = \text{Var}(Y_{hi}) &= \text{Var}(Z_{hi}d_{hi} + e_{hi}) \\ &= \text{Var}(Z_{hi}d_{hi}) + \text{Var}(e_{hi}) \\ &= Z_{hi}\mathcal{D}_h Z'_{hi} + \mathcal{R}_{hi}, \end{aligned} \qquad (3.10)$$

where $\mathcal{D}_h$ and $\mathcal{R}_{hi}$ can have a number of structures.

Variance of random effects

The simplest random-effects model ($Z_{hi}d_{hi}$) has a single random effect (d_{hi1}). This model has a random intercept for each individual ($Y_{hi} = X_{hi}\beta_h + d_{hi1} +$

---

* Slope between weeks 2 and 8 for patient without CRA $=\beta_{11}+\beta_{12}=-7.30+7.03-0.27$.
** Slope between weeks 2 and 8 for patient with CRA $=\beta_{21}+\beta_{22}=-7.85+6.76-1.09$.
*** Slope after 8 weeks for patient without CRA $=\beta_{11}+\beta_{12}+\beta_{13}=-7.30+7.03+0.44$.
† Slope after 8 weeks for patient without CRA $=\beta_{21}+\beta_{22}+\beta_{23}=-7.85+6.76+1.38$.

e_{hi}), where d_{hi1} can be interpreted roughly as the average difference between the individual's response and the mean response. This implies the variation between individuals does not change over time. Basically, the curves for each individual are parallel:

$$Z_{hi} = [1], \qquad \mathcal{D}_h = \text{Var}[d_{hi1}] = [\varsigma_{h1}^2]. \tag{3.11}$$

A more typical model for longitudinal studies has two random effects. The second random effect (d_{hi2}) allows variation in the rate of change over time among individuals. This model has a random intercept and random slope for each individual ($Y_{hi} = X_{hi}\beta_h + d_{hi1} + d_{hi2}\mathbf{t}_{hi} + e_{hi}$). In most examples, the two random effects are correlated:

$$Z_{hi} = \begin{bmatrix} 1 & \mathbf{t}_{hi} \end{bmatrix}, \qquad \mathcal{D}_h = \text{Var}\begin{bmatrix} d_{hi1} \\ d_{hi2} \end{bmatrix} = \begin{bmatrix} \varsigma_{h1}^2 & \varsigma_{h12} \\ \varsigma_{h21} & \varsigma_{h2}^2 \end{bmatrix}. \tag{3.12}$$

In theory we can keep adding random effects, but in most cases the addition of these two random effects is sufficient to obtain a good approximation of the covariance structure.

Variance of residual errors

The second part of the variance structure, $\mathcal{R}_{hi}$, can be as simple as $\sigma_h^2 \mathbf{I}$ or quite complex (Table 3.8). The most common alternative to the simple structure is a first-order autoregressive error structure (AR(1)). Although this structure is rarely suitable for the repeated measures setting, it can be useful when used to model the residual errors in combination with random effects [76].

Table 3.8. Useful covariance structures for $\mathcal{R}_{hi}$ in a mixed-effects model.

	No. of parameters	Structure
Simple ($\sigma^2 \mathbf{I}$) TYPE=SIMPLE	1	$\begin{matrix} \sigma^2 & 0 & 0 & 0 \\ & \sigma^2 & 0 & 0 \\ & & \sigma^2 & 0 \\ & & & \sigma^2 \end{matrix}$
Autoregressive Equal spacing TYPE=AR(1)	2	$\begin{matrix} \sigma^2 & \sigma^2\rho & \sigma^2\rho^2 & \sigma^2\rho^3 \\ & \sigma^2 & \sigma^2\rho & \sigma^2\rho^2 \\ & & \sigma^2 & \sigma^2\rho \\ & & & \sigma^2 \end{matrix}$
Autoregressive Unequal Spacing $\delta_{rc} = \lvert t_r - t_c \rvert$ TYPE=SP(POW)(*time_var*)	2	$\begin{matrix} \sigma^2 & \sigma^2\rho^{\delta_{12}} & \sigma^2\rho^{\delta_{13}} & \sigma^2\rho^{\delta_{14}} \\ & \sigma^2 & \sigma^2\rho^{\delta_{23}} & \sigma^2\rho^{\delta_{24}} \\ & & \sigma^2 & \sigma^2\rho^{\delta_{34}} \\ & & & \sigma^2 \end{matrix}$
Toplitz Equal Spacing TYPE=TOEP	4	$\begin{matrix} \sigma^2 & \sigma^2\rho_1 & \sigma^2\rho_2 & \sigma^2\rho_3 \\ & \sigma^2 & \sigma^2\rho_1 & \sigma^2\rho_2 \\ & & \sigma^2 & \sigma^2\rho_1 \\ & & & \sigma^2 \end{matrix}$

BUILDING GROWTH CURVE MODELS

Note that certain structures, such as compound symmetry, described in Table 3.1, cannot be used for modeling $\mathcal{R}_{hi}$. In the case of compound symmetry, one of the parameters in $\mathcal{D}$ can be rewritten as a linear combination of parameters in $\mathcal{R}$. In fact, when $Z_{hi} = [\mathbf{1}]$ and $\mathcal{R} = \sigma^2 I$, the covariance structure is the same as compound symmetry when the random effect is omitted.

Finally, the covariance structures may differ among the treatment arms. For example, there may be more variation in the rate of change of HRQoL among patients receiving an active treatment than a placebo treatment.

SAS example of a polynomial growth curve model

Fully parameterized model for the means

In the renal cell carcinoma study, the datafile EXAMPLE3 has a unique record for each HRQoL assessment. CASEID identifies the patient, TOI is the score for the FACT-TOI, MNTH identifies the time of the assessment relative to randomization, and TREAT identifies the treatment arm.* The CLASS statement identifies two levels of treatment. The terms in the MODEL statement create a design matrix corresponding to the polynomial model displayed in Table 3.6, with the default option for an intercept term suppressed by the NOINT option. As previously mentioned, the first step is to specify a fully parameterized model for the mean. The first part of the SAS program for this model might appear as:

```
PROC MIXED DATA=EXAMPLE3 COVTEST IC METHOD=ML;
  CLASS TREAT CASEID;
  * Polynomial Model *;
  MODEL TOI=TREAT
            TREAT*MNTH
            TREAT*MNTH*MNTH
            TREAT*MNTH*MNTH*MNTH
            TREAT*MNTH*MNTH*MNTH*MNTH
            TREAT*MNTH*MNTH*MNTH*MNTH*MNTH
       /NOINT SOLUTION PREDMEANS DDFM=SATTERTH;
```

Covariance structure

In the next step, we examine possible covariance structures. Table 3.9 illustrates some possible combinations of covariance structures for the random effects and residual errors. The random effects contribution to the covariance structure is defined by the RANDOM statement. For a model with a single random effect that is homogeneous across groups (Models 1 and 2, Table 3.9), the following statement defines Z_{hi} and $\mathbf{D}_h$:

```
* Single random effect (Equal across groups) *;
RANDOM INTERCEPT /SUBJECT=CASEID TYPE=UN;
```

---

* The choice of months rather than weeks as a measure of time is a practical consideration. By using the larger unit of time, we minimize the differences in the magnitude of the coefficients for higher-order terms. This does not affect any of the statistics but facilitates construction of tables reporting coefficients. In this example, we avoid reporting coefficients with seven zeros after the decimal place.

Table 3.9. Variance structures tested for growth curve models of the renal carcinoma study ($\Sigma_{hi} = Z_{hi}D_h Z'_{hi} + \mathcal{R}_{hi}$).

Variance model	Random effects (D_h)		Residual error ($\mathcal{R}_{hi}$)		Total var. parameters[a]
	No. of effects	Groups	Structure	Groups	
1	1	Equal[1]	Simple	Equal[3]	$1+1=2$
2	1	Equal[1]	AR(1)[b]	Equal	$1+2=3$
3	1	Unequal[2]	Simple	Equal	$2+1=3$
4	1	Unequal[2]	Simple	Unequal[4]	$2+2=4$
5	2	Equal[1]	Simple	Equal	$3+1=4$
6	2	Unequal[2]	Simple	Equal	$6+1=7$

[1] $D_1 = D_2$; [2] $D_1 \neq D_2$; [3] $\mathcal{R}_1 = \mathcal{R}_2$; [4] $\mathcal{R}_1 \neq \mathcal{R}_2$.
[a] # in $\mathcal{D}_h$ + # in $\mathcal{R}_h$ = Total.
[b] Autoregressive for unequal spacing of observations.

The term INTERCEPT defines $Z_{hi} = [1]$. Since $\mathbf{D}_h$ is a scalar, it is not necessary to specify the structure. With the TYPE=UN option, the estimate of ς_{h1}^2 is displayed as UN(1,1). In Model 1, the estimate of ς_{h1}^2 is 185.23.

The residual error contribution to the covariance structure is defined by the REPEATED statement. When there is no RANDOM statement, as in Model 1, a simple homogeneous structure is assumed ($\mathcal{R} = \sigma^2 \mathbf{I}$) and displayed as Residual. This is the specification for Models 1, 3, and 5 (see Table 3.9). In Model 1, the estimate of the diagonal elements of $\mathcal{R}$ is 116.13 and the off-diagonal elements are 0.

```
         Covariance Parameter Estimates - Model 1

                                   Standard        Z
Cov Parm     Subject    Estimate      Error    Value      Pr Z

UN(1,1)      CASEID       185.23    23.9908     7.72    <.0001
Residual                  116.13     8.1905    14.18    <.0001
```

An autoregressive error structure for unequal spacing of observations (Model 2) is specified using the term TYPE=SP(POW)(QSDAY), where QSDAY is the number of days since randomization. Note that QSDAY has a unique value for each HRQoL assessment within a particular patient.

```
* Autoregressive structure for unequal spacing of Observations *;
REPEATED /SUBJECT=CASEID TYPE=SP(POW)(QSDAY);
```

The estimate of the additional parameter ρ is displayed as SP(POW). Thus, the estimate of the diagonal elements of $\mathcal{R}$ are 122.13 and the off-diagonal elements (r, c) are $\sigma^2 \rho^{\delta_{rc}}$ or $122.13 * 0.8979^{\delta_{rc}}$, where δ_{rc} is the absolute difference in the number of days QSDAY between the rth and cth assessment.

BUILDING GROWTH CURVE MODELS

Table 3.10. Covariance structures tested for the renal carcinoma study.

Model	Variance Parameters	Polynomial −2 log L	Polynomial AIC	Piecewise −2 log L	Piecewise AIC
1	2	5162.4	5190.4	5154.2	5182.2
2	3	5159.7	**5189.7**	5148.3	**5178.3**
3	3	5162.3	5193.0	5154.1	5184.1
4	4	5162.1	5194.9	5154.0	5186.0
5	4	5160.4	5192.4	5152.2	5184.2
6	7	5157.9	5193.9	5150.5	5188.5

```
              Covariance Parameter Estimates - Model 2

                                       Standard        Z
Cov Parm     Subject     Estimate      Error         Value      Pr Z

UN(1,1)      CASEID       179.12       24.6260        7.27      <.0001
SP(POW)      CASEID         0.8978      0.03726      24.10      <.0001
Residual                  122.13       10.0471       12.16      <.0001
```

By adding GROUP=TREAT to the RANDOM statement, we request different estimates of $\mathbf{D}_h$ in each treatment arm (Models 3 and 4, Table 3.9).

```
* Single random effect (Unequal across groups) *;
RANDOM INTERCEPT/SUBJECT=CASEID TYPE=UN GROUP=TREAT;
```

In Model 3 we have separate estimates for ς_{h1}^2 in the two treatment groups, 195.85 and 176.90, respectively. If this model represented a significant improvement over Model 1, it would suggest that there is more variation among subjects in the IFNα + CRA group than in the IFNα-only group. The statistics displayed in Table 3.10 suggest this is not the case.

```
              Covariance Parameter Estimates - Model 3

                                              Standard       Z
Cov Parm  Subject  Group             Estimate Error       Value   Pr Z

UN(1,1)   CASEID   TREAT IFN + CRA    194.85  36.2256      5.38   <.0001
UN(1,1)   CASEID   TREAT IFN only     176.90  31.2410      5.66   <.0001
Residual                              116.03   8.1815     14.18   <.0001
```

Addition of GROUP=TREAT to the REPEATED statement specifies different estimates of the variance parameter in each treatment group ($R_{hi} = \sigma_h^2 \mathbf{I}$), as in Model 4.

```
* Simple uncorrelated random errors (Unequal across groups) *;
REPEATED/SUBJECT=CASEID TYPE=SIMPLE GROUP=TREAT;
```

The separate estimates of σ_{wh}^2 in the two groups are 119.80 and 112.41, respectively. Again, there is no evidence that there is more or less variation between the two groups (see Table 3.10).

Covariance Parameter Estimates - Model 4

Cov Parm	Subject	Group	Estimate	Standard Error	Z Value	Pr Z
UN(1,1)	CASEID	TREAT IFN + CRA	192.35	36.6248	5.25	<.0001
UN(1,1)	CASEID	TREAT IFN only	178.64	31.5004	5.67	<.0001
Residual	CASEID	TREAT IFN + CRA	119.80	12.0797	9.92	<.0001
Residual	CASEID	TREAT IFN only	112.41	11.0939	10.13	<.0001

A second random effect, allowing variation in the rate of change over time among subjects, can be added to the random-effects model. The following statement defines a model with two correlated random effects (Models 5 and 6, Table 3.9) as defined in Equation 3.12.

```
* Two correlated random effects *;
RANDOM INTERCEPT MNTH/SUBJECT=CASEID TYPE=UN;
```

The second random effect is added to the RANDOM statement, where MNTH defines $Z_{hi2} = t_{hi}$. TYPE=UN specifies an unstructured covariance of the random effects with three covariance parameters, UN(1,1), UN(1,2), and UN(2,2), which correspond to ς_1^2, $\varsigma_{1,2}$, and ς_2^2.

Covariance Parameter Estimates - Model 5

Cov Parm	Subject	Estimate	Standard Error	Z Value	Pr Z
UN(1,1)	CASEID	181.89	25.1413	7.23	<.0001
UN(2,1)	CASEID	1.2952	3.4955	0.37	0.7110
UN(2,2)	CASEID	0.3870	0.4216	0.92	0.1793
Residual		111.64	8.7304	12.79	<.0001

Finally, we attempt to allow these random effects to vary across the treatment groups by adding a GROUP=TREAT to the random statement. Note that the estimate of the variation in the slopes in the IFNα-only group UN(2,2) is close to zero and the algorithm fails to obtain an estimate.*

Covariance Parameter Estimates - Model 6

Cov Parm	Subject	Group	Estimate	Standard Error
UN(1,1)	CASEID	TREAT IFN + CRA	203.18	39.0561
UN(2,1)	CASEID	TREAT IFN + CRA	-3.5354	5.3937
UN(2,2)	CASEID	TREAT IFN + CRA	0.5752	0.5891
UN(1,1)	CASEID	TREAT IFN only	158.36	31.0568
UN(2,1)	CASEID	TREAT IFN only	6.9927	4.5872
UN(2,2)	CASEID	TREAT IFN only	0	.
Residual			112.71	8.2840

* An alternative parameterization TYPE=FA0(2) ensures that the estimates of the variance of the random effects is non-negative definite. This is particularly helpful when there is the possibility that one of the variance parameters is close to zero.

BUILDING GROWTH CURVE MODELS

Table 3.10 summarizes the results of testing the six covariance structures. Based on the AIC, Model 2 is the *best* model. However, there is very little difference between the AIC values for Models 1 and 2, and a formal test of the two additional parameters in Model 2 is nonsignificant. Either model will provide a good approximation of Σ_i.

Model reduction

The next step is to consider simplifying the model for the means. A portion of the SAS output from the fully parameterized model follows. Neither the estimates nor the test statistics suggest a strategy for model reduction. Elimination of the highest-order terms does not improve the model fit as measured by the AIC (5781.3 vs. 5770.6), so we will continue with the 5th degree model.

```
                    Solution for Fixed Effects

Effect                       TREAT  Estimate  Std Err    t      Pr > |t|
TREAT                          0     89.77     1.91    46.94    0.0001
TREAT                          1     87.95     1.93    45.39    0.0001
MNTH*TREAT                     0    -28.44     3.78    -7.51    0.0001
MNTH*TREAT                     1    -30.93     3.75    -8.24    0.0001
MNTH*MNTH*TREAT                0     13.85     2.58     5.36    0.0001
MNTH*MNTH*TREAT                1     14.73     2.62     5.62    0.0001
MNTH*MNTH*MNTH*TREAT           0     -2.50     0.64    -3.89    0.0001
MNTH*MNTH*MNTH*TREAT           1     -2.90     0.66    -4.40    0.0001
MNTH*MNT*MNT*MNT*TREAT         0      0.18     0.066    2.85    0.0047
MNTH*MNT*MNT*MNT*TREAT         1      0.25     0.068    3.70    0.0003
MNTH*MNT*MNT*MN*MN*TRE         0     -0.005    0.002   -2.11    0.0357
MNTH*MNT*MNT*MN*MN*TRE         1     -0.008    0.002   -3.25    0.0013

                    Tests of Fixed Effects

Source                             NDF   DDF   Type III F   Pr > F
TREAT                               2    280    2131.99    0.0001
MNTH*TREAT                          2    280      62.18    0.0001
MNTH*MNTH*TREAT                     2    280      30.14    0.0001
MNTH*MNTH*MNTH*TREAT                2    280      17.23    0.0001
MNTH*MNTH*MNTH*MNTH*TREAT           2    280      10.90    0.0001
MNTH*MNTH*MNTH*MNTH*MNTH*TREAT      2    280       7.50    0.0007
```

Estimation

As previously mentioned, it is difficult to interpret the polynomial terms directly. Estimating the means at specific points in time, as shown in Table 3.6, is often more informative.

$$\hat{\mu}_h(t) = \sum_{0}^{5} \hat{\beta}_{hk} t^k. \tag{3.13}$$

The estimates of the means for each treatment by time combination generated by the **ESTIMATE** statements is illustrated below:

```
* Group Specific Estimates at selected times *;
ESTIMATE '2 weeks -CRA'
        TREAT 1 0
        TREAT*MNTH 0.462 0
        TREAT*MNTH*MNTH   0.213 0
        TREAT*MNTH*MNTH*MNTH 0.0983 0
        TREAT*MNTH*MNTH*MNTH*MNTH 0.0454 0
        TREAT*MNTH*MNTH*MNTH*MNTH*MNTH 0.0209 0
        TREAT*MNTH*MNTH*MNTH*MNTH*MNTH*MNTH 0.00967 0;
```

Alternatives include the change from baseline

$$\hat{\mu}_h(t) - \hat{\mu}_h(t=0) = \sum_0^5 \hat{\beta}_{hk} t^k - \hat{\beta}_{h0} = \sum_1^5 \hat{\beta}_{hk} t^k. \tag{3.14}$$

```
* Group Specific Estimates at selected times *;
ESTIMATE '2 weeks change from baseline -CRA'
        TREAT*MNTH 0.462 0
        TREAT*MNTH*MNTH   0.213 0
        TREAT*MNTH*MNTH*MNTH 0.0983 0
        TREAT*MNTH*MNTH*MNTH*MNTH 0.0454 0
        TREAT*MNTH*MNTH*MNTH*MNTH*MNTH 0.0209 0
        TREAT*MNTH*MNTH*MNTH*MNTH*MNTH*MNTH 0.00967 0;
```

Hypothesis testing

An overall test of postrandomization treatment differences can be constructed using the CONTRAST statement illustrated below.

$$H_0: \beta_{1k} = \beta_{2k}, \quad k = 1, \ldots, 5. \tag{3.15}$$

```
*** Overall Post Baseline Treatment Effect ***;
CONTRAST 'Overall Diff'
        TREAT*MNTH 1 -1,
        TREAT*MNTH*MNTH 1 -1,
        TREAT*MNTH*MNTH*MNTH 1 -1,
        TREAT*MNTH*MNTH*MNTH*MNTH 1 -1,
        TREAT*MNTH*MNTH*MNTH*MNTH*MNTH 1 -1,
        TREAT*MNTH*MNTH*MNTH*MNTH*MNTH*MNTH 1 -1;
```

The results appear as follows:

```
                CONTRAST Statement Results
Source          NDF   DDF       F    Pr > F
Overall Diff     6    485    1.94    0.0732
```

Tests of differences between the groups at a specific time (t) can be constructed using an ESTIMATE statement:

$$H_0: \sum_0^5 \beta_{1k} t^k = \sum_0^5 \beta_{2k} t^k. \tag{3.16}$$

```
*** Test Differences at Specific Times ***;
ESTIMATE 'Baseline Diff' TREAT 1 -1;
ESTIMATE '2 weeks Diff'  TREAT 1 -1
```

```
            TREAT*MNTH 0.462 -0.462
            TREAT*MNTH*MNTH  0.213 -0.213
            TREAT*MNTH*MNTH*MNTH 0.0983 -0.0983
            TREAT*MNTH*MNTH*MNTH*MNTH 0.0454 -0.0454
            TREAT*MNTH*MNTH*MNTH*MNTH*MNTH 0.0209 -0.0209
            TREAT*MNTH*MNTH*MNTH*MNTH*MNTH*MNTH 0.00967 -0.00967;
```

Finally, contrasts of changes from baseline are tested. The intercept terms cancel (see Equation 3.14) and are dropped:

$$H_0: \sum_{1}^{5} \beta_{1k} t^k = \sum_{1}^{5} \beta_{2k} t^k. \tag{3.17}$$

```
*** Test Differences in Change from Baseline at Specific Times ***;
ESTIMATE '2 weeks change Diff'
            TREAT*MNTH 0.462 -0.462
            TREAT*MNTH*MNTH   0.213 -0.213
            TREAT*MNTH*MNTH*MNTH 0.0983 -0.0983
            TREAT*MNTH*MNTH*MNTH*MNTH 0.0454 -0.0454
            TREAT*MNTH*MNTH*MNTH*MNTH*MNTH 0.0209 -0.0209
            TREAT*MNTH*MNTH*MNTH*MNTH*MNTH*MNTH 0.00967 -0.00967;
```

SAS example of a piecewise linear regression model

Fully parameterized model for the means

In the same renal cell carcinoma study, we construct five new variables to model possible changes in the slope at 2, 8, 17, and 34 weeks.

```
DATA EXAMPLE3;
  SET EXAMPLE3;
  * Piecewise regression terms *;
  WEEKS2=MAX(WEEKS-2,0);
  WEEKS8=MAX(WEEKS-8,0);
  WEEKS17=MAX(WEEKS-17,0);
  WEEKS34=MAX(WEEKS-34,0);
RUN;
```

The first part of the SAS program for this model might appear as

```
PROC MIXED DATA=EXAMPLE3 COVTEST IC;
  CLASS TREAT CASEID;
  * Piecewise Regression Model *;
  MODEL TOI=TREAT TREAT*WEEKS TREAT*WEEKS2 TREAT*WEEKS8
            TREAT*WEEKS17 TREAT*WEEKS34
    /NOINT SOLUTION DDFM=SATTERTH;
```

Covariance structure

The procedure for examining the covariance structure is exactly the same as outlined for the polynomial model. The results for the piecewise regression model are summarized in Table 3.10 and are very similar to those found for the polynomial model.

Model reduction

In contrast to the polynomial model, the strategy for simplifying the piecewise regression model is straightforward. The following SAS output comes from the fully parameterized model. The results indicate that there is no evidence of a change in the slopes after 34 weeks ($\beta_{k5} = 0$) and that this term can be dropped. Notice that this model reduction is performed in a stepwise manner, as we are relying on Type III test statistics. Although the terms involving WEEKS17 appear to be nonsignificant, the test of the WEEKS17*TREAT is conditional on inclusion of WEEKS34*TREAT and the result may be quite different when these terms are removed.

Tests of Fixed Effects

Source	NDF	DDF	Type III F	Pr > F
TREAT	2	280	2088.76	0.0001
WEEKS*TREAT	2	280	61.28	0.0001
WEEKS2*TREAT	2	280	31.82	0.0001
WEEKS8*TREAT	2	280	3.37	0.0358
WEEKS17*TREAT	2	280	0.78	0.4585
WEEKS34*TREAT	2	280	0.11	0.8948

After refitting the model without the WEEKS34*TREAT terms, it is obvious that the WEEKS17*TREAT terms can also be dropped (AIC = 5757.5). The final model (See Figure 3.1B) allows the slope to change at 2 and 8 weeks (AIC = 5172.1).

Tests of Fixed Effects

Source	NDF	DDF	Type III F	Pr > F
TREAT	2	284	2086.56	0.0001
WEEKS*TREAT	2	284	61.00	0.0001
WEEKS2*TREAT	2	284	33.45	0.0001
WEEKS8*TREAT	2	284	6.58	0.0016

Estimation

The terms in the MODEL statement create a design matrix corresponding to the polynomial model displayed in Table 3.7. The estimates of the means for each treatment by time combination are generated by the ESTIMATE statements.

```
PROC MIXED DATA=WORK.EXAMPLE3;
 * Group Specific Estimates at selected times *;
 ESTIMATE '2 weeks  -CRA' TREAT 1 0
                         TREAT*WEEKS 2 0;
 ESTIMATE '2 months -CRA' TREAT 1 0
                         TREAT*WEEKS 8.67 0
                         TREAT*WEEKS2 6.67 0
                         TREAT*WEEKS8 0.67 0;
```

Testing

An overall test of postrandomization treatment differences can be constructed using a CONTRAST statement illustrated above.

$$H_0: \beta_{1k} = \beta_{2k}, \quad k = 1, \ldots, 3. \tag{3.18}$$

```
*** Overall Post Baseline Treatment Effect ***;
CONTRAST 'Overall Diff'   TREAT*WEEKS    1 -1,
                          TREAT*WEEKS2   1 -1,
                          TREAT*WEEKS8   1 -1;

         CONTRAST Statement Results

Source              NDF    DDF      F   Pr > F
Overall Diff          4    517   1.45   0.2161
```

Tests of differences between the groups at specific times (t) can be constructed using the ESTIMATE statement:

$$H_0: \sum_0^4 \beta_{1k} t^{[k]} = \sum_0^4 \beta_{2k} t^{[k]}. \tag{3.19}$$

```
*** Test Differences at Specific Times ***;
ESTIMATE 'Baseline Diff'  TREAT 1 -1;
ESTIMATE '2 weeks Diff'   TREAT 1 -1
                          TREAT*WEEKS 2 -2;
ESTIMATE '2 month Diff'   TREAT 1 -1
                          TREAT*WEEKS 8.67 -8.67
                          TREAT*WEEKS2 6.67 -6.67
                          TREAT*WEEKS8 0.67 -0.87;
```

Tests for differences in the change from baseline can also be constructed by dropping the intercept term TREAT from the ESTIMATE statement:

$$H_0: \sum_0^4 \beta_{1k} t^{[k]} - \beta_{10} = \sum_0^4 \beta_{2k} t^{[k]} - \beta_{20}. \tag{3.20}$$

```
ESTIMATE '2-week  change Diff' TREAT*WEEKS    2    -2 ;
ESTIMATE '2-month change Diff' TREAT*WEEKS  8.67 -8.67
                               TREAT*WEEKS2 6.67 -6.67
                               TREAT*WEEKS8 0.67 -0.67;
ESTIMATE '6-month change Diff' TREAT*WEEKS   26   -26
                               TREAT*WEEKS2  24   -24
                               TREAT*WEEKS8  18   -18;
```

3.5 Summary

- Event-driven designs are generally associated with repeated measures models.
- Time-driven designs are associated with growth curve models.
- The recommended model building process starts by defining a fully parameterized model for the means $(X_i\beta)$, then identifying the structure of Σ_i, and finally simplifying the mean structure.

CHAPTER 4

Missing Data

4.1 Introduction

Missing self-assessments of HRQoL occur in most longitudinal studies. Because the patients participating in these trials are free-living individuals and often experience disease- and treatment-related morbidity and mortality, missing assessments are inevitable. Missing HRQoL data may occur for reasons totally unrelated to the subjects' current quality of life (a missed appointment due to a snowstorm) or may be intimately related (severe episodes of nausea or vomiting). The term *missing* is sometimes used to include only assessments expected according to the guideline of the protocol; another term used for this narrow definition is *noncompliance*. The term *missing* often has a broader meaning to include missing for any reason, including unavoidable *attrition* due to death or termination of follow-up as specified in the protocol.

Terminology

This book uses the term *missing* to include both *attrition* and *noncompliance*. The term *dropout* will refer to the discontinuation of the outcome measures, Y_i. The term *censoring* will refer to incomplete follow-up of the time to an event associated with dropout, T_i^D; see Table 4.1.

Why are missing data a problem?

The first potential problem associated with missing data is loss of power to detect clinically meaningful differences as a result of a reduced number of observations. However, in many large (Phase III/IV) clinical studies, the sample size is often based on differences in a binary outcome such as survival. These sample sizes are generally more than sufficient to detect clinically meaningful differences in the HRQoL endpoints. The loss of power may be an issue in small studies, but the problem can be addressed by increasing the planned sample size of the trial. If the objectives associated with the HRQoL assessment are not of sufficient importance to warrant this increase in sample size, then the investigators should consider omitting the HRQoL assessments altogether rather than burdening patients when the design is inadequate in terms of sample size.

Why are missing data a problem?

Fewer Observations → Loss of Power
Nonrandomly Missing Data → Bias

Table 4.1. Summary of terms.

Attrition	No assessment due to termination of HRQoL assessment as specified in protocol
Noncompliance	No assessment but expected per protocol
Missing	No assessment when information at time of the scheduled assessment was not obtained, regardless of whether the assessment was required per protocol
Dropout	Discontinuation of the observation of the outcome
Censoring	Discontinuation of observation of the time to an event associated with dropout

The second problem is the potential bias of estimates due to missing data. For example, patients who are experiencing poorer HRQoL because of increased morbidity or mortality may be less likely to complete HRQoL assessments as a result of treatment-related toxicity, progressing disease, or death. If we ignore the presence of missing data and the analyses are based only on the observed data of patients who are doing well, HRQoL is overestimated. Alternatively, it is possible that individuals will drop out of a study when they are no longer experiencing the signs or symptoms of their diseases, in which case HRQoL is underestimated.

Why subjects fail to complete HRQoL assessments

Patient misses a specified appointment
Staff forgets to administer questionnaire
Translation not available in patient's language
Patient drops out from study because no longer ill
Patient refuses to complete questionnaire
Patient states he or she is too ill to complete questionnaire
Staff does not approach patient because of health status
Patient dies

How much data can be missing?

There are no magic rules about how much missing data is acceptable in a clinical trial. When the proportion of missing assessments is very small ($<5\%$), the potential impact on power or bias may be very minor. In some cases, 10 to 20% missing data will have little or no effect on the results of the study. In other studies, 10 to 20% may matter. As the proportion of missing data increases to 50%, the conclusions one is willing to draw will be restricted. The seriousness of the problem depends on the reasons for the missing data, the objectives of the study, and the intended use of the results. For example,

PATTERNS OF MISSING DATA								71

results from trials influencing regulatory issues of drug approval or health policy decisions may require more stringent criteria than those used to design future studies. The challenge for the analyst is to provide either a convincing argument that conclusions drawn from the analysis are insensitive to the missing data or clear limits for interpretation of the results. The concepts and tools to do that are the focus of this and the following chapters.

Similar patterns of dropout among intervention arms

A common question is whether missing data can be ignored if there are similar proportions of missing data across all study arms. Although experience indicates that comparisons between treatment arms are often less sensitive than the estimates of change over time to missing data, there is always the possibility that this is not a safe assumption.

Prevention

Although analytic strategies exist for missing data, their use is much less satisfactory than initial prevention. Some missing data, such as that due to death, is not preventable. However, both primary and secondary prevention are desirable. In terms of primary prevention, missing data should be minimized at both the design and implementation stages of a clinical trial [37, 171]. Strategies are discussed in Chapter 2. Secondary prevention consists of gathering information that is useful in the analysis and interpretation of the results. This includes collection of data on factors that may contribute to missing assessments and data that are likely to predict the missing HRQoL measures. Thus, one should prospectively document reasons for missing data. The classifications that are used should be specified in a manner that helps the analyst decide whether the reason is related to the individual's HRQoL. For example, "Patient refusal" does not clarify this, but reasons such as "Patient refusal due to poor health" and "Patient refusal unrelated to health" will be useful. Other strategies for secondary prevention may include gathering concurrent data on toxicity, evaluations of health status by the clinical staff, or HRQoL assessments from a caretaker. Use of this type of data is discussed in later chapters.

4.2 Patterns of missing data

Patterns of missing data can be considered either terminal dropout (monotone) or intermittent (nonmonotone). Examples of both patterns are shown in Table 4.2. In the second case, an observation on a patient may be missing, but a subsequent observation is observed. In the first case, no observations are made on a patient after a certain point in time. Within these two patterns of missing data, the causes of missing data are either related or unrelated to the patient's HRQoL. Similarly, the causes are planned (by design) or unplanned.

In patients with chronic diseases, terminal dropout may occur because a treatment works or the patient is no longer experiencing the signs and

Table 4.2. Terminal dropout and intermittent missing data.

Terminal dropout (Monotone)					Intermittent (Nonmonotone)				
X	X	X	X	X	X	X	X	X	X
X	X	X	X	—	X	X	X	—	X
X	X	X	—	—	X	—	X	X	X
X	X	—	—	—	⋮				
X	—	—	—	—	X	—	X	—	X

symptoms that prompted him or her to obtain treatment. In patients with progressive or fatal diseases, such as advanced cancer and AIDS, there are considerable missing HRQoL data or dropout due to death. Intermittent missing data might include missed clinical visits because of weather or episodes of severe acute toxicity. Causes such as the weather are unrelated to the subject's HRQoL, whereas causes such as toxicity are related to the subject's QoL.

Example: NSCLC study

In most studies both patterns exist, possibly within the same patient. In the NSCLC study (Table 4.3), the majority of missing data fits the terminal dropout pattern (76% of patients, including complete cases and those with no data). A smaller proportion of subjects (14%) have an intermittent or mixed pattern (intermittent followed by dropout).

4.3 Mechanisms of missing data

Understanding the missing data mechanism is critical to the analysis and interpretation of HRQoL studies. All possible analytic methods for longitudinal data depend on assumptions about the missing data. The robustness of analytic methods to violations of the assumptions varies. If the assumptions are incorrect, then the resulting estimates will be biased. Thus, examination of available evidence for or against these assumptions is the first major task in the analysis of HRQoL studies.

Notation

Consider a longitudinal study where n_i assessments of HRQoL are planned for each subject over the course of the study. As defined in Chapter 3, Y_{ij} indicates the jth observation of HRQoL on the ith individual.

Y_i = the *complete data* vector of n_i *planned* observations of the outcome for the ith individual, which includes both the *observed* data (Y_i^{obs}) and *missing* observations (Y_i^{mis}) of HRQoL.

MECHANISMS OF MISSING DATA

Table 4.3. Patterns of observations in the NSCLC study.

Pattern	Assessment No.				N	%
	1	2	3	4		
Complete case	X	X	X	X	146	25.4
Monotone dropout	X	X	X	—	98	17.0
	X	X	—	—	94	16.4
	X	—	—	—	133	23.1
No data	—	—	—	—	26	4.5
Intermittent	X	X	—	X	15	2.6
	X	—	X	X	11	1.9
	X	—	—	X	11	1.9
	—	X	X	X	5	0.9
	—	X	—	X	2	0.4
	—	—	—	X	1	0.2
Mixed	X	—	X	—	18	3.1
	—	X	X	—	3	0.5
	—	X	—	—	11	1.9
	—	—	X	—	1	0.2

X indicates the HRQoL assessment completed.

R_i = a vector of indicators of the missing data pattern for the ith individual, where $R_{ij} = 1$ if Y_{ij} is observed and $R_{ij} = 0$ if Y_{ij} is missing.

Note that the term *complete data* is defined as the set of responses that one would have observed if all subjects completed all possible assessments. This is in contrast to the term *complete cases*, which is defined as the set of responses on only those subjects who completed all possible assessments ($R_{ij} = 1$ for all possible Y_{ij} from the ith subject). In some of the following chapters, we will differentiate data from these complete cases (Y_i^C) and data from incomplete cases (Y_i^I). Table 4.4 is a summary of terms.

Example

If a study were planned to have four HRQoL assessments at 0, 4, 13, and 26 weeks and the HRQoLs of the ith subject were missing at 4 and 26 weeks, then that subject's data might look like

$$Y_i = \begin{bmatrix} 78 \\ \text{NA} \\ 58 \\ \text{NA} \end{bmatrix} \quad \text{and} \quad R_i = \begin{bmatrix} 1 \\ 0 \\ 1 \\ 0 \end{bmatrix} \quad \text{or} \quad \begin{aligned} Y_i^{\text{obs}} &= \begin{bmatrix} 78 \\ 58 \end{bmatrix} \\ Y_i^{\text{mis}} &= \begin{bmatrix} \text{NA} \\ \text{NA} \end{bmatrix} \end{aligned},$$

Table 4.4. Summary of terms.

Complete data	Y	All responses that one would have observed if all subjects had completed all possible assessments
Observed data	Y^{obs}	All responses that were observed
Missing data	Y^{mis}	All responses that were not observed
Complete cases	Y^C	Responses from cases (or subjects) where all possible responses were observed
Incomplete cases	Y^I	Responses from cases (or subjects) where one or more possible responses are missing

where NA indicates a missing observation. Notice that the vector of the observed data (Y_i^{obs}) contains the first (78) and third (58) observations and the vector of the missing data (Y_i^{mis}) contains the second and fourth observations.

The corresponding design matrix for this subject in a model estimating an intercept and a linear trend over time would appear as

$$X_i = \begin{bmatrix} 1 & 0 \\ 1 & 4 \\ 1 & 13 \\ 1 & 26 \end{bmatrix} \quad \text{and} \quad \begin{aligned} X_i^{\text{obs}} &= \begin{bmatrix} 1 & 0 \\ 1 & 13 \end{bmatrix} \\ X_i^{\text{mis}} &= \begin{bmatrix} 1 & 4 \\ 1 & 26 \end{bmatrix} \end{aligned}.$$

Even though the dependent variable Y_i is missing at some time points, X_i is fully observed if one assumes that the time of the observation is the planned time of the second and fourth HRQoL assessments.

The concept

There are three major classes of missing data, differing by whether the reasons for missingness are related to the subject's quality of life. For example, if HRQoL data are missing because the patient moved out of town or the staff forgot to administer the assessment, the data are *Missing Completely at Random* (MCAR). At the other extreme, if data are missing because of increased toxicity, progressive disease, and death, they are nonignorable or *Missing Not at Random* (MNAR). Intermediate cases are referred to as *Missing at Random* (MAR). In this case, missingness depends on the subject's observed HRQoL, generally the most recently observed HRQoL. Table 4.5 is an overview.

The remainder of this chapter presents the general concepts of these three mechanisms in more detail and suggests methods for distinguishing among them. Formal statistical definitions are presented in Appendix III. The subsequent chapters describe methods of analysis that can be used under the various assumptions.

Table 4.5. Simple overview of missing data mechanisms.

	Dependent on...	Independent of...
MCAR[a]	Covariates	Observed HRQoL
		Missing HRQoL
MAR	Covariates	Missing HRQoL
	Observed HRQoL	
MNAR	Missing HRQoL	

[a]And covariate-dependent dropout.

MCAR: Missing completely at random

The concept

The strongest assumption about the missing data mechanism is that the data are missing completely at random (MCAR). The basic assumption is that the reason for a missing HRQoL assessment is entirely unrelated to HRQoL. Examples might include a patient moving or staff forgetting to provide the assessment. (Note that this accounted for about 2% of the missing data in Example 1 and 8.5% in Example 2.) Assessments might be changed as a result of appointments delayed because of scheduling problems. Finally, some patients may not be able to participate because translations of the questionnaire are not available in their languages.

Covariate-dependent dropout

Dropout solely dependent on treatment, but constant within each treatment group irrespective of the outcome (Y_i), is also MCAR [64] conditional on treatment. If this assumption is true, then the patients with missing data are a random sample of all patients in each treatment group. Thus, there is no bias attributable to missing data. In the context of HRQoL studies, it is difficult to imagine scenarios where this is true. Dropout related to side effects or lack of effectiveness is likely to affect HRQoL and would not fit this condition. The missingness may also be associated with covariates (X_i) measured prior to randomization or treatment assignment. An example of covariate-dependent dropout is the cultural influences on follow-up observed in an international trial of breast cancer patients [116], where the proportion of missing assessments differed among the cultural groups. When these covariates are included in the analysis, the resulting estimates are adjusted for the covariate-dependent dropout.

In summary, while some missingness of HRQoL assessments is completely random in clinical trials, it is rare that this assumption holds for the majority of the missing data.

Identifying covariate-dependent missingness

The first step in the process of exploring the missing data process is to identify covariates that predict missing observations. One method is to examine the correlation between an indicator of missing observations (r_{ijk}) and possible covariates. Kendal's τ_b is useful when one variable is dichotomous, such as the missing data indicator, and the other variables are a mixture of dichotomous, ordered categorical, and continuous variables. A second approach is to perform a series of logistic regression analyses to model the probability of a missing assessment. From a practical standpoint, patient characteristics (covariates) that are likely to be also related to the subject's HRQoL should be given priority. The reasons for this will become more obvious in the later sections of this chapter and later chapters.

Example: NSCLC study

In the NSCLC study, missing assessments were weakly associated with physical characteristics such as older age, male gender, performance status, and disease symptoms at the time of randomization. Similar results were obtained using either bivariate correlation (Table 4.6) or multivariate logistic regression (Table 4.7).

In most studies, because prerandomization covariates are not directly related to the reasons for dropout, they are likely to be only weakly predictive of missing data. We see this in the NSCLC study. Although statistically significant, none of these covariates individually explains more than 2% of the variation in the likelihood of a missing assessment as indicated by the squared value of the correlation coefficients displayed in Table 4.6. It should be noted that this procedure is an exploratory first step in understanding the missing data mechanism. Because of the number of comparisons, there is

Table 4.6. Correlation (Kendall τ_b) of missing assessments with baseline covariates. Positive correlations indicate increased likelihood of missing assessment.

	Correlation coefficients			
	Assessment no.			
	1	2	3	4
Older age at randomization	−0.00	0.09**	0.04	0.07*
Poorer performance status	0.01	0.12**	0.13**	0.09*
Metastatic disease symptoms	0.01	0.00	0.06	0.10*
Systemic disease symptoms	0.01	0.09*	0.08*	0.04
Randomized to Taxol regimen	−0.01	−0.13**	−0.07	−0.06

Nonsignificant correlations: gender, weight loss in last 6 months, primary disease symptoms, associated chronic diseases, prior radiation therapy, assigned to G-CSF arm.

* $p < 0.05$, ** $p < 0.01$, *** $p < 0.001$.

Table 4.7. Prerandomization patient characteristics associated with missing HRQoL assessments.

Assessment	Characteristic	OR	(95% CI)
Baseline	≥5% weight loss prior 6 months	0.72	(0.52, 1.00)
6 weeks	Older age	1.24[a]	(1.02, 1.50)
	Poorer performance status	1.72	(1.16, 2.53)
	Taxol therapy	0.55	(0.38, 0.79)
12 weeks	Poorer performance status	1.71	(1.20, 2.44)
26 weeks	Older age (decades)	1.25	(1.04, 1.50)
	Systemic symptoms	1.53	(1.08, 2.19)

Notes: Odds ratios (OR) and 95% confidence intervals (CI) from logistic regression models of the probability of a missing observation at each of the four planned assessments. Associations identified using stepwise logistic regression with a selection criteria of 0.05.

Potential covariates include age, gender, ≥5% weight loss in 6 months prior to randomization, primary disease symptoms, metastatic disease symptoms, systemic disease symptoms, associated chronic diseases at the time of randomization, and prior radiation therapy.

[a] Age in years at randomization with OR estimated for 10-year difference.

the possibility of spurious correlations. This may be the explanation for the counterintuitive association of less missing data at baseline with prior weight loss.

Analytic methods

In general, analytic methods that assume the data are MCAR either exclude data for some individuals, such as methods that require complete cases for analysis (MANOVA), or ignore data obtained at other points in time, such as repeated univariate tests [105]. Detailed examples of these are presented in the following chapter.

MAR: Missing at random

The concept

The assumptions about the missing data mechanism are relaxed slightly when we assume the data are missing at random (MAR). Specifically, the missingness depends on observed HRQoL after conditioning on covariates. In most cases this is the initial (baseline) or previous HRQoL assessment, but it could possibly include subsequent HRQoL assessments. It is not uncommon for missing HRQoL data to depend on covariates and observed HRQoL scores. In most settings, individuals who are experiencing better health and HRQoL will generally be more likely to be available for follow-up and more likely to complete the self-assessments required for the evaluation of HRQoL. However, there are exceptions, such as individuals with an acute condition who drop out once they become well.

It is possible that data are MAR by design. Murray and Findlay [105] describe this in hypertension trials, where a subject is withdrawn from a trial by design because of inadequate blood pressure control. In this example, dropout is a function of a previously observed value of the outcome.

Identification of dependence on observed data (Y_i^{obs})

Differences between MCAR and MAR can be tested by examining the association of missing data with observed HRQoL scores. Various methods include graphical presentations, formal tests, correlational analyses, and logistic regression.

A graphical approach is displayed in Figure 4.1 for the NSCLC study. This plot displays the average observed FACT-Lung TOI in groups of patients defined by their pattern of missing data. Because the total number of patterns is large and the number of subjects with intermittent or mixed patterns is small (see Table 4.3), this plot was simplified by grouping subjects by the time of their last HRQoL assessment. The resulting figure suggests two things. First, subjects who dropped out earlier had poorer FACT-Lung TOI scores at baseline. Second, FACT-Lung TOI scores were lower at the time of the assessment just prior to dropout (the last observation). Since missingness depends on previously observed FACT-Lung TOI scores, the data are not MCAR. Fayers and Machin [45] describe an alternative graphical approach where the origin of the horizontal axis is the date of the last assessment. The HRQoL is then plotted backward in time.

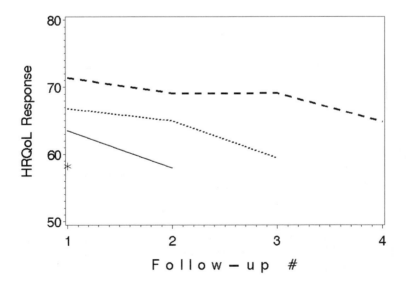

Figure 4.1. Average FACT-Lung TOI scores stratified by time of dropout.

Little [89] proposed a single test statistic for testing the assumption of MCAR vs. MAR. The basic idea is that if the data are MCAR, the means of the observed data should be the same for each pattern. If the data are not MCAR, then the means will vary across the patterns (as is observed in Figure 4.1). This test statistic is particularly useful when there is a large number of comparisons, either as a result of a large number of patterns or differences in missing data patterns across multiple outcome variables. The computational details of the statistic are shown in Section 4.3. In the NSCLC study, there is considerable evidence for rejecting the hypothesis of MCAR ($\chi^2 = 108.8$, df $= 26$, $p < 0.001$).

The next approach examines the association (correlation) between an indicator of missingness or dropout and the observed data. In the NSCLC study, we observe a moderate association between dropout and both the baseline and the most recent HRQoL scores (Table 4.8). The association is strongest for the scales measuring the physical or functional aspects of HRQoL such as functional well-being, physical well-being, and lung cancer symptoms, all of which are part of the FACT-Lung TOI.

We also wish to confirm that the missingness depends on the observed data after adjusting for the dependence on covariates. This can be tested by first forcing the baseline covariates identified in the previous step into a logistic model and then testing the baseline or previous measures of HRQoL. In the first set of models (Table 4.9), all subjects with baseline data are included in the logistic regression model. Age, performance status, and the presence of

Table 4.8. Correlation of missing assessments with baseline or previous HRQoL.

	Kendall τ_b correlation coefficients			
	Assessment no.			
	1	2	3	4
HRQoL at baseline assessment				
Physical well-being	NA	−0.18***	−0.21***	−0.20***
Functional well-being		−0.12**	−0.15***	−0.18***
Lung cancer subscale		−0.14***	−0.12***	−0.14***
Emotional well-being		−0.03	−0.10**	−0.03
Social/family well-being		0.03	−0.03	−0.05
HRQoL at previous assessment				
Physical well-being		−0.18***	−0.19***	−0.17***
Functional well-being		−0.12**	−0.18***	−0.21***
Lung cancer subscale		−0.14***	−0.17***	−0.23***
Emotional well-being		−0.04	−0.16***	−0.10
Social/family well-being		0.03	−0.06	−0.03

Note: Negative correlations indicate increased likelihood of missing assessment with poorer HRQoL scores.

* $p < 0.05$, ** $p < 0.01$, *** $p < 0.001$.

Table 4.9. Association (odds ratios) between baseline characteristics and either baseline or previous FCT-TOI assessment.

	Time of assessment		
	6 weeks	12 weeks	6 months
Age[a]	1.48***	1.17	1.40**
Performance status	1.18	1.22	1.02
Systemic symptoms	1.13	1.06	0.82
Baseline FACT-L TOI[b]	**0.76**^{***}	**0.74**^{***}	**0.66**^{***}
Age[a]	1.48***	1.03	1.46*
Performance status	1.18	1.18	0.72
Systemic symptoms	1.13	0.91	0.75
Previous FACT-L TOI[b]	**0.76**^{***}	**0.69**^{***}	**0.64**^{***}

Note: First set of OR is estimated from a logistic regression model for a missing observation regardless of patient status or missing data pattern. Second set of OR is estimated from a logistic regression model for dropout, given subject has completed previous assessment.

[a] Age in years at randomization with OR estimated for 10-year difference.

[b] OR estimated for 10-point difference in FACT-Lung TOI.

* $p < 0.05$, ** $p < 0.01$, *** $p < 0.001$.

systemic symptoms are forced into the model. For all follow-up assessments, poorer baseline HRQoL, as measured by the FACT-Lung TOI score, is highly predictive of missing data. Age is sometimes predictive, but baseline performance status and symptoms are no longer predictive in this multivariate model. In the second set of models, only those subjects who have completed the previous assessment are included. This is a model of the probability of missing observations given that an assessment occurred at the previous follow-up. Again, for all follow-up assessments, poorer HRQoL, as measured by the FACT-Lung TOI score, is highly predictive of missing data. These analyses reinforce the evidence that the missingness is dependent on observed HRQoL scores (Y_i^{obs}) and that in this NCSLC study we cannot assume that the observations are MCAR.

Analytic methods

In general, analytic methods that assume the missingness is MAR utilize all available HRQoL assessments. When the missing data are *ignorable*,* unbiased estimates can be obtained from likelihood based methods using all observed data (Y_i^{obs}) and covariates X_i that explain the missing data mechanism. Note that exclusion of part of the observed data or omission of information on covariates in the analysis may result in biased estimates. For example, if missingness is dependent on baseline scores and some individuals are excluded

* Formal definition of *ignorable* is presented in Appendix III.

MECHANISMS OF MISSING DATA   81

from an analysis of change from baseline differences because they do not have follow-up assessments, the estimates may not be unbiased. Similarly, if missingness is strongly dependent on a covariate and that covariate is ignored, the estimates are biased. Examples of methods assuming *ignorable* missing data are presented in Chapter 5 in more detail.

A test of MCAR vs. MAR for multivariate normal data

Notation

Consider a study designed to obtain J measurements. Let P be the number of distinct missing data patterns (R_i), where $J^{\{p\}}$ is the number of observed variables. $n^{\{p\}}$ is the number of cases with the pth pattern, and $\sum n^{\{p\}} = N$. Let $M^{\{p\}}$ be a $J^{\{p\}} \times J$ matrix of indicators of the observed variables in pattern P. The matrix has one row for each measure present consisting of $(J-1)$ 0s and one 1 identifying the observed measure. For example, in the NSCLC example, if the first and third observation were obtained in the 6th pattern, then

$$M^{\{6\}} = \begin{bmatrix} 1 & 0 & 0 & 0 \\ 0 & 0 & 1 & 0 \end{bmatrix}.$$

$\bar{Y}^{\{p\}}$ is the $J^{\{p\}} \times 1$ vector of means of the observed variables for pattern p. $\hat{\mu}$ and $\hat{\Sigma}$ are the ML estimates of the mean and covariance of Y_i, assuming that the missing data mechanism is ignorable. $\hat{\mu}^{\{p\}} = M^{\{p\}}\hat{\mu}$ is the $J^{\{p\}} \times 1$ vector of ML estimates corresponding to the pth pattern, and $\tilde{\Sigma}^{\{p\}} = [N/(N-1)] M^{\{p\}}\hat{\Sigma}M^{\{p\}\prime}$ is the corresponding $J^{\{p\}} \times J^{\{p\}}$ covariance matrix with a correction for degrees of freedom.

Test statistic

Little's [89] proposed test statistic, when Σ is unknown, takes the form

$$\chi^2 = \sum_{p=1}^{P} n^{\{p\}} (\bar{Y}^{\{p\}} - \hat{\mu}^{\{p\}})' \tilde{\Sigma}^{\{p\}-1} (\bar{Y}^{\{p\}} - \hat{\mu}^{\{p\}}). \quad (4.1)$$

Little shows that this test statistic is asymptotically χ^2 distributed with $\sum J^{\{p\}} - J$ degrees of freedom.

NSCLC example

The first step is to obtain the maximum likelihood estimates of the mean and covariance of the available data:

$$\hat{\mu} = \begin{bmatrix} 65.63 \\ 63.60 \\ 62.37 \\ 60.81 \end{bmatrix}, \quad \hat{\Sigma} = \begin{bmatrix} 258.6 & 144.2 & 121.8 & 113.4 \\ 144.2 & 262.3 & 178.1 & 142.2 \\ 121.8 & 178.1 & 280.0 & 142.2 \\ 113.4 & 142.2 & 142.2 & 261.1 \end{bmatrix}.$$

The second step is to split the data into the P patterns and obtain $J^{\{p\}}$ and $\bar{Y}^{\{p\}}$. $\hat{\mu}^{\{p\}} = M^{\{p\}}\hat{\mu}$ and $\tilde{\Sigma}^{\{p\}} = [N/(N-1)] M^{\{p\}}\hat{\Sigma}M^{\{p\}\prime}$ are then calculated

Table 4.10. Summary of $J^{\{p\}}$ and $\bar{\mathbf{Y}}^{\{p\}}$ by pattern.

p	$J^{\{p\}}$	$\bar{y}_1^{\{p\}}$	$\bar{y}_2^{\{p\}}$	$\bar{y}_3^{\{p\}}$	$\bar{y}_4^{\{p\}}$	$n^{\{p\}}$
1	4	71.83	69.63	68.99	65.39	146
2	3	66.63	65.24	60.02	.	98
3	3	69.25	66.06	.	59.88	15
4	2	63.27	57.50	.	.	94
5	3	67.47	.	72.61	63.10	11
6	2	66.63	.	53.21	.	18
7	2	73.03	.	.	69.85	11
8	1	58.26	.	.	.	133
9	3	.	70.21	78.68	69.85	5
10	2	.	71.48	75.49	.	3
11	2	.	51.12	.	62.54	2
12	1	.	61.86	.	.	11
13	1	.	.	73.81	.	1
14	1	.	.	.	47.32	1

for each of the patterns (Table 4.10). For example, in pattern 6:

$$\hat{\mu}^{\{6\}} = M^{\{6\}}\hat{\mu} = \begin{bmatrix} 1 & 0 & 0 & 0 \\ 0 & 0 & 1 & 0 \end{bmatrix} \begin{bmatrix} 65.63 \\ 63.60 \\ 62.37 \\ 60.81 \end{bmatrix} = \begin{bmatrix} 65.63 \\ 62.37 \end{bmatrix},$$

$$\tilde{\Sigma}^{\{6\}} = \frac{N}{N-1} M^{\{6\}} \hat{\Sigma} M^{\{6\}\prime} = \frac{549}{548} \begin{bmatrix} 258.6 & 121.8 \\ 121.8 & 280.0 \end{bmatrix}.$$

Combining all terms in Equation 4.1 yields $\chi_{26}^2 = 107.8$, $p < 0.001$.

Implementing in SAS

By combining output options from Proc MI* with the PROC IML capacity for matrix manipulation, we can save ourselves some tedious hand calculations. The first step is to create one record per subject, with the four repeated measures appearing as separate variables (TOI1 TOI2 TOI3 TOI4).

```
*** Create one record per subject ***;
PROC TRANSPOSE DATA=SASDATA.FACTL2(KEEP=CASEID FUNO FACT_T2)
   OUT=WORK.TRANS PREFIX=TOI;
BY CASEID;
VAR FACT_T2;
ID FUNO;
RUN;
```

The second step is to obtain the pattern-specific means $\bar{\mathbf{Y}}^{\{p\}}$ and the pooled estimates $\hat{\mu}^{\text{obs}}$ and $\hat{\Sigma}^{\text{obs}}$. Proc MI calculates all of these quantities when the

---

* Experimental procedure available in SAS 8.1 for Multiple Imputation.

MECHANISMS OF MISSING DATA

default (MCMC) technique is used. The ODS statement creates temporary data sets containing the desired information.

```
*** Obtain means for each pattern ***;
ODS OUTPUT MISSINGPATN=PATTERN INITPARM=ESTIMATE;
PROC MI DATA=WORK.TRANS IMPUTE=1;
 VAR TOI1 TOI2 TOI3 TOI4;
RUN;
```

Next, the information from the two data sets is read in Proc IML to create the matrices containing the pattern-specific means (PATMEAN) and the pooled estimates $\hat{\mu}^{\text{obs}}$ (MEAN) and $\hat{\Sigma}^{\text{obs}}$ (SIGMA).

```
*** Calculate Statistic ***;
PROC IML;
 *** Read data into PROC IML ***;
 USE WORK.ESTIMATE;
 READ ALL VAR{TOI1 TOI2 TOI3 TOI4}
         WHERE((TYPE='MEAN')&(IMPUTATION=1))
         INTO MEAN[COLNAME=COLNAME];
 READ ALL VAR{TOI1 TOI2 TOI3 TOI4}
         WHERE((TYPE='COV')&(IMPUTATION=1))
         INTO COVAR[ROWNAME=NAME COLNAME=COLNAME];
 PRINT 'Pooled Mean', MEAN [FORMAT=5.2];
 PRINT 'Pooled Covariance', COVAR [FORMAT=5.2];

 USE WORK.PATTERN;
 READ ALL VAR{TOI12 TOI22 TOI32 TOI42} INTO PATMEAN;
 READ ALL VAR{GROUP} INTO M;
 READ ALL VAR{FREQ} INTO N;
 PRINT 'Observed Means for Pattern', M PATMEAN [FORMAT=5.2] ;
```

Finally, the test statistic is calculated.

```
 *** Calculate statistic for test ***;
 STAT=0; DF=0;                       * Initializes STAT and DF *;
 DO P=1 TO NROW(PATMEAN);
  PATP=((PATMEAN[P,])>0);   * Indicator of non-missing value *;
  LOCP=LOC(PATP>0);         * Location of non-missing value  *;
  JP=SUM(PATP);             * # of non-missing values        *;
  IF JP^=0 THEN DO;
   DP=DIAG(PATP)[LOCP,];
   VP=DP*COVAR*DP';                  * Covariance for pattern *;
   RP=MEAN[,LOCP]-PATMEAN[P,LOCP];   * Difference in means    *;
   STAT=STAT+N[P]*(RP*INV(VP)*RP');  * Sums statistic         *;
   DF=DF+JP;                         * Sums degrees of freedom*;
  END;
 END;
 DF=DF-NCOL(MEAN);                   * Adjusts  df  *;
 PVALUE=1-PROBCHI(STAT,DF);          * Calculates p-value *;
 PRINT STAT DF PVALUE;
QUIT;
```

MNAR: Missing not at random

The concept

The final classification for missing data mechanisms, MNAR, has the least-restrictive assumptions. In this classification, the missingness is dependent on the HRQoL at the time the assessment is missing as well as on covariates and observed data. This might occur because assessments are more likely to be missing when an individual is experiencing side effects of therapy, such as nausea/vomiting or mental confusion. Alternatively, subjects might be less willing to return for follow-up (and be more likely to have missing assessments) if their HRQoL has improved as a result of the disappearance of their symptoms.

Analytic methods

In the past few years, there has been an increase in the amount of theoretical research on the analysis of nonrandom missing data [21, 23, 26, 30, 57, 66, 92, 103, 129, 133, 166–168, 170]. Little [92] has published a comprehensive review of most of the methods published prior to 1995. More recent reviews include Hogan and Laird [67]. There are three widely studied approaches to the analysis of longitudinal studies with nonrandom missing data: selection models, mixture models, and joint shared-parameter models. In all, the joint distribution of the longitudinally measured outcome Y_i and either the dropout time T_i^D or the missing data indicators R_i are modeled.

Selection models factor the joint distribution into the product of the complete data, $f(\mathbf{Y})$, and the missing data mechanism, $f(T^D|\mathbf{Y})$ or $f(\mathbf{R}|\mathbf{Y})$. Because the complete data are not fully observed, the analyst must make untestable assumptions about the form of $f(T^D|\mathbf{Y})$.

Mixture models factor the joint distribution into the product of $f(\mathbf{Y}|\mathbf{M})$ and $f(\mathbf{M})$, where $\mathbf{M}$ is either dropout time T_i^D, the pattern of missing data R_i, or a random coefficient β_i. The complete data, $f(Y)$, is characterized as a mixture (weighted average) of the conditional distribution $f(Y|\mathbf{M})$ over the distribution of dropout times, the patterns of missing data, or the random coefficients. Pattern mixture models are a special case of the mixture models, where the complete data are a mixture over the missing data patterns ($\mathbf{R}$). In mixture models, because the complete data are not fully observed, some of the parameters characterizing $f(\mathbf{Y}|\mathbf{M})$ cannot be estimated without imposing untestable restrictions.

An important feature of these models is that all of the proposed methods are based on assumptions that, while reasonable, cannot be tested or proved. Because we do not observe the missing outcome, all of these models are *underidentified*. This means it is impossible to estimate all parameters in the response and dropout models without making assumptions that are not testable with the available data. However, even though these models rely on assumptions that often cannot be verified, they can be useful. Examples of their usefulness are presented in more detail in Chapters 8 and 9.

Identification of dependence on unobserved data, Y_i^{mis}

Because we have not observed the missing HRQoL score, it is not possible to test formally a hypothesis that missingness does not depend on HRQoL at the time the assessment is missing. The data that we need to test the hypothesis are missing. However, it is possible to gather evidence that suggests the data are MNAR. Specifically, when there are other available measures of the disease or outcomes of treatment that are strongly associated with HRQoL, it may be possible to test for an association between missing observations and these measures. For example, if missingness is associated with more severe side effects and/or disease progression, then there is a reasonable likelihood that the data are MNAR.

Example: NSCLC study

In the NSCLC study, we have already shown that the missingness depends on both the initial and the most recent HRQoL scores. The question that remains is whether, given the observed HRQoL scores (and possibly the baseline covariates), there is additional evidence that missing assessments are more frequent in individuals who are experiencing events likely to impact HRQoL. The first step is to identify these events on a theoretical, a clinical, or an observational basis. Ideally, we want to identify variables associated with the missing HRQoL scores, but we only have access to observed data. Thus, we have to assume that the relationship between the observed HRQoL measures and these events is similar to the relationship between the missing HRQoL measures and these events.

In the NSCLC study, we might expect toxicity, disease progression, and nearness to death to impact both HRQoL and missingness. A plot of the FACT-Lung TOI during the months prior to death (Figure 4.2) illustrates the strong relationship between this measure and the proximity to death. Because one would expect that increased toxicity is associated with poorer HRQoL, indicators of toxicity were included in this exploratory analysis. We did not observe as strong a relationship between toxicity and observed HRQoL scores. However, this may have occurred because toxicity was recorded as the maximum toxicity score any time the patient was on treatment and not as the grade of toxicity experienced during the same time frame as the HRQoL assessment.

The final step is to determine if these events or outcomes are associated with missingness after adjusting for the covariates and observed HRQoL identified as associated with missingness. Obviously, death is a perfect predictor of missingness. After forcing age and prior FACT-Lung TOI score into a logistic regression model for missing assessments among survivors, progressive disease during the first six cycles of therapy and death within 2 months of the planned assessment are strong predictors of missing assessments (Table 4.11). This suggests that the data are MNAR. Unexpectedly, missing assessments were less likely among individuals with more toxicity. One possible explanation is that

Table 4.11. Patient outcomes associated with missing HRQoL.

Assessment	Characteristic	Odds ratio	(95% CI)
6 weeks	Age[a]	1.44	(1.13, 1.84)
	Prior FACT-L TOI[b]	0.86	(0.75, 0.99)
	Neurotoxicity[c]	0.74	(0.61, 0.91)
	PD[d] within 6 cycles	1.23	(1.23, 3.07)
	Death within 2 months	4.40	(2.45, 7.93)
12 weeks	Age[a]	1.19	(0.90, 1.57)
	Prior FACT-L TOI[b]	0.80	(0.68, 0.95)
	PD[d] within 6 cycles	2.84	(1.66, 4.87)
	Death within 2 months	5.34	(2.20, 12.9)
6 months	Age[a]	1.31	(0.96, 1.77)
	Prior FACT-L TOI[b]	0.76	(0.63, 0.92)
	Other Toxicity[c]	0.74	(0.61, 0.91)
	Death within 2 months	2.70	(1.25, 5.84)

Note: Logistic regression model of missing assessment among survivors with age and prior FACT-Lung TOI were forced into the model; potential covariates included maximum grade of hematological, neurological, and other toxicity; best response of complete or partial remission; progression of disease within the first six cycles of therapy and death within 2 months of planned HRQoL assessment.

[a] Age in years at randomization, with OR estimated for 10-year difference.

[b] OR estimated for 10-point difference in FACT-L TOI.

[c] Maximum NCI Common Toxicity Criteria (CTC) grade.

[d] Progressive disease.

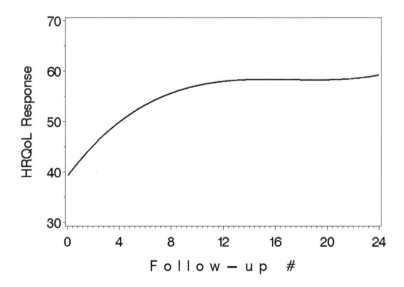

Figure 4.2. Change in FACT-Lung TOI prior to death in NSCLC study.

these patients are more likely to have follow-up visits and thus more likely to be available for HRQoL assessments.

A caveat is necessary. The lack of an identified relation between these additional variables and missingness is *not* proof that the data are not MNAR. Although it may increase the analyst's comfort with that assumption, there is always the possibility that important indicators of the dropout process were not measured in the trial or the analyst failed to identify them. Often, evidence for the potential for nonrandom missing data will come from sources outside the data. Clinicians may provide the most useful anecdotal information that suggests the presence of nonrandom missing data. A knowledge of the disease and its treatment is critical. Some of the analytic models for MNAR data [30, 133] will also provide evidence that dropout is MAR. But the absence of evidence from one particular model does not prove the null hypothesis of randomness. There is an infinite number of possible models for the nonrandom mechanism. Just because one model has been tested and there is no evidence of a nonrandom mechanism under that set of assumptions, we cannot rule out other mechanisms.

4.4 Renal cell carcinoma study

Examining the missing data mechanism in the renal cell carcinoma study is a bit more difficult than in the NSCLC study because of the greater variation in timing of the observations. Even when defining windows of time for each assessment, we see a complicated pattern with a large number of nonmonotone patterns (Table 4.12). Although the majority (65%) of patients have a monotone pattern of dropout, a substantial number have intermittent missing data prior to dropout.

The test MCAR vs. MAR proposed by Little [89] and described in Section 4.3 yields strong evidence against the MCAR assumption ($\chi^2_{118} = 1320$, $p < 0.001$). This is confirmed by examining a plot of estimates as a function of the time of dropout (Figure 4.3). The three dropout groups were defined so that approximately a third of the patients were in each group. There is a general trend for subjects who remain on the study longer to both start with higher FACT-BRM TOI scores and maintain higher FACT-BRM TOI scores over time.

Simplifying the remaining exploratory analysis, dropout during the early and middle periods was examined using logistic regression. In both periods, the predictors of dropout are the baseline FACT-BRM TOI scores and the duration of the patient's survival (Table 4.13). The odds of dropout are reduced by about a third in both periods, with a 10-point increase in the baseline FACT-BRM TOI scores. The odds are reduced by about half in the early period for every doubling of the survival time.*

---

* Solely for the purposes of this exploratory analysis, censoring of the survival times was ignored. Note that the majority had died (75%) and the minimum follow-up was 2 years; thus, the missing information would have only a moderate effect when the length of survival was expressed on a log scale.

Table 4.12. Summary of patterns of missing data in renal cell carcinoma trial.

Last measure	Monotone	1	2	3	4	5	6	Frequency	Percent
Complete 1 year	Yes	X	X	X	X	X	X	8	3.8
	No	.	X	X	X	X	X	1	0.5
	No	X	.	X	X	X	X	2	0.9
	No	X	X	.	X	X	X	2	0.9
	No	X	.	.	X	X	X	1	0.5
	No	.	.	.	X	X	X	1	0.5
	No	X	X	X	.	X	X	1	0.5
	No	.	X	X	.	X	X	1	0.5
	No	X	X	.	.	X	X	1	0.5
	No	X	X	X	X	.	X	3	1.4
	No	X	.	X	X	.	X	1	0.5
	No	X	X	.	X	.	X	1	0.5
	No	X	X	X	.	.	X	1	0.5
	No	.	X	X	.	.	X	1	0.5
	No	X	X	.	.	.	X	1	0.5
	No	.	X	.	.	.	X	1	0.5
8 months	Yes	X	X	X	X	X	.	12	5.7
	No	.	X	X	X	X	.	3	1.4
	No	X	.	X	X	X	.	3	1.4
	No	X	X	.	X	X	.	2	0.9
	No	X	X	X	.	X	.	6	2.8
	No	.	X	X	.	X	.	1	0.5
	No	X	X	.	.	X	.	6	2.8
	No	X	.	.	.	X	.	3	1.4
	No	.	.	.	.	X	.	1	0.5
4 months	Yes	X	X	X	X	.	.	19	9.0
	No	.	X	X	X	.	.	2	0.9
	No	X	.	X	X	.	.	5	2.4
	No	.	.	X	X	.	.	1	0.5
	No	X	X	.	X	.	.	4	1.9
	No	X	.	.	X	.	.	4	1.9
8 weeks	X	X	X	.	.	.	44	20.8	
	No	.	X	X	.	.	.	3	1.4
	No	X	.	X	.	.	.	5	2.4
2 weeks	Yes	X	X	.	.	.	.	33	15.6
	No	.	X	.	.	.	.	6	2.8
Baseline	Yes	X	.	.	.	.	.	22	10.4

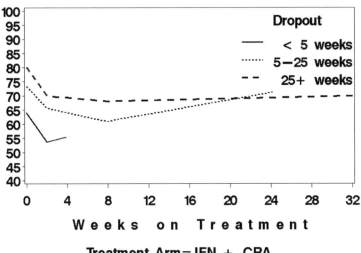
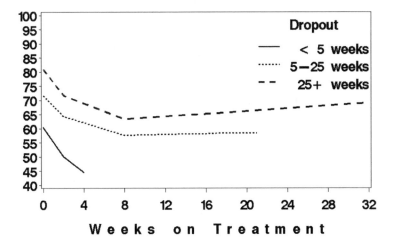

Figure 4.3. Change in FACT-BRM TOI displayed by time of last assessment.

Plotting outcome by dropout

The plots displayed in Figures 4.1 and 4.3 are easily generated. Using the model developed in Chapter 3, we add a variable defining groups in terms of their missing data patterns (DROP_GRP). In this example, we have chosen to define the groups by the time of their last HRQoL assessment. The first step is to generate a data set WORK.PLOTDATA containing the predicted values of the outcome. The variable defining the groups is included in the CLASS statement and as an interaction with every term in the MODEL statement.

```
PROC MIXED DATA=EXAMPLE3;
  CLASS TREAT DROP_GRP;
```

Table 4.13. Predictors of dropout in renal cell carcinoma trial. Results of exploratory multivariate logistic regression models.

Period	Characteristic	OR	(95% C.I.)
<5 weeks	Baseline FACT-BRM TOI[a]	0.66	(0.50, 0.87)
	ln survival[b]	0.46	(0.34, 0.62)
5 to <25 weeks	Baseline FACT-BRM TOI[a]	0.67	(0.47, 0.94)
	ln survival[b]	0.27	(0.16, 0.45)

[a]Odds ratio estimated for 10-point difference in FACT-BRM TOI.

[b]Odds ratio estimated for doubling of the length of survival (0.693 units on the natural log scale).

```
* Piecewise Regression Model *;
MODEL TOI=TREAT*DROP_GRP TREAT*WEEKS*DROP_GRP
        TREAT*WEEKS2*DROP_GRP TREAT*WEEKS8*DROP_GRP
  /NOINT SOLUTION OUTPM=WORK.PLOTDATA;
```

The data set is then sorted by treatment group, dropout group, and time. Two plots are then generated, one for each treatment group, by specifying treatment in the BY statement. Predicted values are plotted over time (PRED*WEEKS) within each dropout group (=DROP_GRP).

```
PROC SORT DATA=WORK.PLOTDATA;
  BY TREAT DROP_GRP WEEKS;
PROC GPLOT DATA=WORK.PLOTDATA;
  WHERE TOI NE .; * Excludes BLUPS *;
  BY TREAT;
  PLOT PRED*WEEKS=DROP_GRP;
  SYMBOL1 I=JOIN L=1  V=NONE C=BLACK;
  SYMBOL2 I=JOIN L=2  V=NONE C=BLACK;
  SYMBOL3 I=JOIN L=20 V=NONE C=BLACK;
```

If the first group is defined as having only a single (baseline) assessment, as in the NSCLC example, then a symbol (STAR) is substituted for the line.

```
SYMBOL1 V=STAR C=BLACK;
```

4.5 Summary

- It is important to understand the missing data patterns and mechanisms in HRQoL studies. This understanding comes from a knowledge of the disease or condition under study and its treatment as well as statistical information.
- MCAR vs. MAR can be tested when the data have a repeated measures structure using the test described by Little [89] (see Section 4.3).
- Graphical techniques are useful when examining the assumption of MCAR for studies with mistimed assessments (Figures 4.1 and 4.3).

SUMMARY

- It is not possible to test MAR vs. MNAR without assuming a specific model (see Chapter 9); however, it may be useful to examine the relationship between missing data and other observed outcomes, such as indicators of toxicity and response, that are expected to be related to HRQoL.
- The lack of statistical evidence of MNAR when there is clinical information (based on data or anecdote) that suggests that missing data are related to the subject's HRQoL should not be interpreted as sufficient to ignore the missing data.
- A general strategy for missing data is as follows:
  1. Plan the study in a manner that avoids missing data.
  2. Collect covariates that explain variability in the outcome and missing data patterns.
  3. Document the reasons for missing data.
  4. Perform sensitivity analyses.

CHAPTER 5

Analytic Methods for Ignorable Missing Data

5.1 Introduction

There are several methods that are often misused for the analysis of HRQoL studies when the data are not MCAR. The objective of this chapter is to convey the relationship between the assumptions of MCAR or MAR and commonly used analytic procedures. When missingness depends on observed data (Y_i^{obs}) and the analytic procedure does not include all available data, the results are biased. If dropout is dependent on a covariate (X_i) and the covariate is not included in the analytic model, then the results are biased. Popular analytic methods such as repeated univariate analyses and MANOVA of complete cases are examples of procedures that exclude observed data; results from these analyses are unbiased only if the missing data are MCAR [105].

The magnitude of the bias depends on the amount of missing data and the strength of the association between the missing data (Y_i^{mis}) and the observed data (Y_i^{obs}) or the covariates (X_i). The safest approach is to use methods that make the least restrictive assumptions about the missing data. These include multivariate likelihood methods with *all* the available data, such as mixed-effects models or repeated measures for incomplete data.

Hypothetical example

This example illustrates how the various methods presented in this chapter perform when we know the underlying missing data mechanism. Because all values are known and the example is simple, it is possible to show how the analytic results are affected by the missing data assumptions.

Assume there are 100 subjects with two assessments. The scores are generated from a standard normal distribution ($\mu = 0$, $\sigma = 1$). Three sets of data are generated such that the correlations between the assessments (ρ_{12}) are 0.0, 0.5, and 0.9. Correlations of HRQoL assessments over time in clinical trials are generally in the range of 0.4 to 0.7. The extremes of 0.0 and 0.9 are outside this range but will serve to illustrate the concepts.

All subjects have the first assessment (T1), but 50% are missing at the second assessment (T2). This is a larger proportion of missing data than one would desire in a clinical trial, but setting it this high magnifies the effect we are illustrating. Finally, missing values are generated in two ways. In the first, observations are deleted in a completely random manner.* Thus, the

---
* Uniform selection: $\Pr[r_{i2} = 1] = 0.5$.

Table 5.1. Expected means for hypothetical examples with 50% missing data at T2.

		$\rho = 0.0$		$\rho = 0.5$		$\rho = 0.9$	
		MCAR	MAR	MCAR	MAR	MCAR	MAR
Complete cases $N = 50$							
T1	$\bar{y}_1^C$	0.00	0.57	0.00	0.57	0.00	0.57
T2	$\bar{y}_2^C$	0.00	0.00	0.00	0.28	0.00	0.51
Incomplete cases $N = 50$							
T1	$\bar{y}_1^I$	0.00	-0.57	0.00	-0.57	0.00	-0.57
T2	$\bar{y}_2^I$	(0.00)	(0.00)	(0.00)	(-0.28)	(0.00)	(-0.51)

( ) indicates the mean of the deleted observations.

data are missing completely at random, or MCAR. In the second, the probability of a missing assessment at the second time point depends on the observed values at the first time point.* Thus, the data are missing at random (MAR), conditional on the observed baseline data. The means for these hypothetical data are summarized in Table 5.1. Data from the complete cases are noted as Y^C and data from the cases with any missing data are noted as Y^I. For subjects with both the T1 and T2 assessments, $\bar{y}_1^C$ and $\bar{y}_2^C$ are the averages of the T1 and T2 scores. For subjects with only the T1 assessment, $\bar{y}_1^I$ is the average of the observed T1 scores. $\bar{y}_2^I$ is the average of the deleted T2 scores, which is known only because this is a simulated example.

5.2 Repeated univariate analyses

One of the most commonly used analytic approaches for data from a study with a repeated measures design is repeated univariate analysis at each time point using test procedures such as the t-test, ANOVA, or Wilcoxon rank sum test. Although simple to implement, this approach has several disadvantages [31, 97, 117]. The first is the restrictive assumption of MCAR. If missingness is associated with previous or future observations of HRQoL, then estimates based on only the HRQoL assessments at one point in time will be biased. This is illustrated in the hypothetical example for repeated univariate analysis (Table 5.2, first row), where the estimates of $\hat{\mu}_2$ utilize only the data available at T2 from the complete cases ($\bar{y}_2^C$).

$$\begin{bmatrix} \hat{\mu}_1 \\ \hat{\mu}_2 \end{bmatrix} = \begin{bmatrix} \pi \bar{y}_1^C + (1-\pi)\bar{y}_1^I \\ \bar{y}_2^C \end{bmatrix} = \begin{bmatrix} \bar{y}_1 \\ \bar{y}_2^C \end{bmatrix}, \qquad (5.1)$$

where π is the proportion of subjects with complete data. Note that when dropout depends on the measure of HRQoL at T1 and responses are correlated

---

* Probit selection: $\Pr[r_{i2} = 1|Y] = \phi(y_{i1})$.

Table 5.2. Estimates of means at T2 ($\hat{\mu}_2$) in hypothetical example.

	$\rho = 0.0$		$\rho = 0.5$		$\rho = 0.9$	
	MCAR	MAR	MCAR	MAR	MCAR	MAR
Repeated univariate	0.01	0.00	0.01	**0.28**	0.01	**0.50**
Complete case	0.01	0.00	0.01	**0.28**	0.01	**0.50**
All available data	0.00	0.00	0.00	−0.02	−0.01	−0.02
Baseline (naive)[a]	0.01	0.00	0.01	**0.28**	0.01	**0.50**
Baseline (correct)[b]	0.00	0.00	0.00	−0.02	−0.01	−0.02

Note: Average of 100 simulations. The true mean at T2 is 0. Bold estimates indicate bias larger than the average standard error of the mean.

[a] Simple regression with baseline as a covariate; analysis limited to subjects with both assessments.

[b] Means estimated at average baseline for all subjects.

($\rho \neq 0$), there is significant bias in the estimated T2 mean. The bias increases as the correlation increases.

There are other disadvantages to the repeated univariate approach. First, the pool of subjects is changing over time. Thus, the inferences associated with each comparison are relevant to a different set of patients. Second, the analyses produce a large number of comparisons that often fail to answer the clinical question but rather present a confusing picture. Further, the probability of concluding that there are significant differences in HRQoL when none exists (the Type I error) increases as the number of comparisons increases. Finally, these univariate methods can be difficult to implement if measurements are mistimed as a result of delays in therapy or other factors.

Summary	Repeated univariate analyses
Examples	Two-sample *t*-tests ANOVA Wilcoxon rank sum test
Assumption	MCAR (R_i does not depend on Y_i^{obs}) because analysis ignores *information* in Y_i^{obs} from other time points
Advantages	Easy to run Easy to describe
Disadvantages	Biased if data are not MCAR Compares different groups of subjects at each time Large number of comparisons that are difficult to interpret Increasing Type I error rate with more repeated measures

Table 5.3. Results of a repeated univariate analysis of the NSCLC trial.

Follow-up no.	Taxol	N(%)	Mean	(S.E.)	t	df	p
1	No	177(91%)	64.7	(1.21)			
	Yes	349(91%)	66.0	(0.87)			
	Diff		−1.34	(1.49)	−0.90	524	0.37
2	No	109(56%)	63.7	(1.51)			
	Yes	265(70%)	65.5	(0.99)			
	Diff		−1.77	(1.82)	−0.98	372	0.33
3	No	85(44%)	64.6	(1.95)			
	Yes	197(52%)	65.6	(1.09)			
	Diff		−0.99	(2.10)	−0.47	280	0.64
4	No	57(29%)	65.0	(1.99)			
	Yes	134(35%)	64.8	(1.36)			
	Diff		0.22	(2.45)	0.09	189	0.93

NSCLC example

Consider the NSCLC study. Repeated univariate analyses can be generated as simply as this:

```
PROC SORT DATA=EXAMPLE2 OUT=WORK.SORTED;
  BY FUNO;
  RUN;
PROC TTEST DATA=WORK.SORTED;
  BY FUNO;
  CLASS TAXOL;
  VAR FACT_T2;
  RUN;
```

The results are summarized in Table 5.3. First, note that the means are almost constant over time, suggesting no change in the outcome. However, the pool of subjects that is being compared is changing across time, with a higher proportion of the original sample being retained in the arms randomized to the Taxol therapy. Basically, we are comparing smaller and smaller subgroups of patients over time. It is likely that we are not evaluating the impact of the treatment on the HRQoL of all patients, but rather on a select group of patients in each treatment group.

5.3 Multivariate methods

The term *multivariate* can be used to indicate both models that include more than one explanatory (independent) variable (e.g., multivariate logistic regression) and models that include more than one outcome (dependent) variable. In this chapter, the term refers to repeated multiple outcome measures, either the same HRQoL scale measured over time or different HRQoL scales. Multivariate methods include multivariate analysis of variance (MANOVA) and maximum likelihood estimation (MLE) for mixed-effects models or repeated measures models. In these models, the multiple observations on each subject are assumed to be correlated and all observations are used simultaneously in the estimation of the parameters. In contrast, univariate methods use only the observations occurring at one point in time. Univariate methods are usually repeated for each of the scheduled follow-ups.

Among multivariate methods, the major distinction that is relevant to the missing data problem is whether or not the analytic approach uses all available data. For example, traditional software for MANOVA restricts the analysis to those cases that are observed on all occasions. This is often referred to as complete case analysis. In contrast, modern methods, developed almost 20 years ago, are available for mixed-effects and repeated measures models for incomplete data. These methods, described in detail in Chapter 3, produce maximum likelihood or restricted maximum likelihood estimates (MLE/REML). They have the important advantage of allowing us to use all available outcome data (Y_i^{obs}) when the covariates (X_i) are fully observed. MANOVA is a special case of the repeated measures model, where the design matrix X_i is the same for all subjects and the analysis is restricted to subjects with no missing data.

Complete case analysis (MANOVA)

Limiting the analysis to only those subjects who have completed all assessments is another widely used method of analysis. This is also referred to as casewise or listwise deletion. Traditional software for MANOVA automatically limits the analysis to the complete cases. When data are MCAR, the only consequence of choosing this approach is a loss of power due to the reduced number of subjects. However, when the missingness depends on observed HRQoL, the results of these analyses are biased. This is illustrated in the hypothetical example (see Table 5.2, second row). Casewise deletion results in an estimate of μ_1 that is the average of only the T1 assessments from the complete cases ($\bar{y}_1^c$) and an estimate of μ_2 that is the average of the T2 assessments ($\bar{y}_2^c$) from the complete cases.

$$\begin{bmatrix} \hat{\mu}_1 \\ \hat{\mu}_2 \end{bmatrix} = \begin{bmatrix} \bar{y}_1^C \\ \bar{y}_2^C \end{bmatrix}. \tag{5.2}$$

When the data are MCAR, these estimates are unbiased. However, when the data are MAR, both $\hat{\mu}_1$ and $\hat{\mu}_2$ are likely to be biased. This is illustrated in the hypothetical example where $\hat{\mu}_2$ is biased when the observations are correlated (see Table 5.2). In addition, $\hat{\mu}_1$ is always biased and this will bias the estimated change from T1 to T2 (Table 5.4).

$$[\hat{\mu}_2 - \hat{\mu}_1] = [\bar{y}_2^C - \bar{y}_1^C]. \tag{5.3}$$

Table 5.4. Estimates of change ($\hat{\mu}_2 - \hat{\mu}_1$) in hypothetical example.

	$\rho = 0.0$		$\rho = 0.5$		$\rho = 0.9$	
	MCAR	MAR	MCAR	MAR	MCAR	MAR
Complete cases	−0.01	**−0.56**	−0.00	**−0.28**	−0.01	**−0.07**
All available data	0.01	0.01	0.01	−0.01	−0.01	−0.01
Change (naive)[a]	−0.01	**−0.56**	−0.00	**−0.28**	−0.01	**−0.07**
Change (correct)[b]	0.01	0.01	0.01	−0.01	−0.01	−0.01

Note: Average of 100 simulations. The expected change is 0. Bold estimates indicate bias larger than the average standard error of the mean.

[a] Change from baseline analysis limited to subjects with two assessments.

[b] Includes baseline as a covariate, means estimated at average baseline for all subjects.

Summary	Multivariate analysis of complete cases
Example	MANOVA
Assumptions	MCAR (R_i does not depend on Y_i^{obs}); complete case analysis ignores *information* in Y_i^{obs} and X_i for individuals with missing data
Advantage	Familiar method
Disadvantages	Biased unless data are MCAR Loss of information from subjects with partial data MANOVA does not accommodate mistimed observations or time-varying covariates

NSCLC example

In most settings, an analysis based on only the complete cases will overstate the benefit of treatment because only patients for whom treatment is successful are included. In the NSCLC study, the analysis is limited to survivors who complete the 6-month follow-up assessment.

The first step in the MANOVA analysis is to create a data set with one record per subject using the TRANSPOSE procedure of SAS. The new data set contains the case identifier (CASEID), an indicator variable for assignment to one of the Taxol arms (TAXOL), and the four possible FACT-Lung TOI scores (TOI1, TOI2, TOI3, TOI4).

```
*** Transform data to one record per subject ***;
PROC TRANSPOSE DATA=BOOK.EXAMPLE2 OUT=WORK.ONEREC PREFIX=TOI;
  BY CASEID TAXOL;
  ID FUNO;
  VAR FACT_T2;
RUN;
```

The MANOVA analysis can be generated as follows:

```
*** Complete Case MANOVA ***;
PROC GLM DATA=WORK.ONEREC;
MODEL TOI1 TOI2 TOI3 TOI4 = TAXOL;

*** Univariate Estimates ***;
ESTIMATE 'TAXOL - NO' INTERCEPT 1;
ESTIMATE 'TAXOL - YES' INTERCEPT 1 TAXOL 1;
ESTIMATE 'TAXOL - DIFF' TAXOL 1;

*** Multivariate Tests ***;
*** Differences at T2, T3 and T4 ***;
MANOVA H=TAXOL M=TOI2,TOI3,TOI4;
*** Differences in change from Baseline ***;
MANOVA H=TAXOL M=TOI2-TOI1,TOI3-TOI1,TOI4-TOI1;
RUN;
```

The GLM procedure first selects the *complete cases* and then runs both univariate and multivariate analyses. In this example, only 146 cases from the original 575 subjects are included, with 20 and 28% of the subjects randomized to the Taxol and No Taxol arms, respectively. This is noted in the output:

```
               The GLM Procedure

          Number of observations    575

NOTE: Observations with missing values will not be included in this
analysis. Thus, only 146 observations can be used in this analysis.
```

The results of the multivariate analyses are summarized in Table 5.5. The estimated means from the complete cases are generally higher than those

Table 5.5. Results of a multivariate analysis of only complete cases from the NSCLC trial.

Follow-up no.	Taxol	$N(\%)$	Mean	(S.E.)	t	df	p
1	No	39(20%)	72.7	(2.19)			
	Yes	107(28%)	71.5	(1.32)			
	Difference		−1.23	(2.55)	−0.48	144	0.63
2	No	39(20%)	69.3	(2.21)			
	Yes	107(28%)	69.8	(1.33)			
	Difference		0.49	(2.58)	0.19	144	0.85
3	No	39(20%)	69.1	(2.29)			
	Yes	107(28%)	69.0	(1.38)			
	Difference		−0.12	(2.67)	−0.04	144	0.97
4	No	39(20%)	63.6	(2.38)			
	Yes	107(28%)	66.0	(1.44)			
	Difference		2.40	(2.78)	0.86	144	0.39

estimated from the repeated univariate measures. The biggest differences occur prior to therapy (follow-up no. 1).

Finally, multivariate tests are generated. Note that TAXOL is an indicator variable (0 if no Taxol, 1 if Taxol), and it is included in the model without the CLASS statement. The group not assigned to Taxol becomes the reference group and the model parameter for the intercept (INTERCEPT) is the mean for that group. The model parameter TAXOL is an estimate of the difference between the two groups. The mean for the group receiving Taxol must be calculated using an ESTIMATE statement. The MANOVA statement is used to test the two multivariate hypotheses. The first MANOVA statement (see p. 99) is a test of treatment differences across all follow-up assessments. TAXOL estimates the difference between the two arms, and the M= option allows us to select the post-treatment observations.

Multivariate Analysis of Variance

M Matrix Describing Transformed Variables

	toi1	toi2	toi3	toi4
MVAR1	0	1	0	0
MVAR2	0	0	1	0
MVAR3	0	0	0	1

MANOVA Test Criteria and Exact F Statistics for the Hypothesis of
No Overall TAXOL Effect on the Variables
Defined by the M Matrix Transformation

Statistic	Value	F Value	Num DF	Den DF	Pr > F
Wilks' Lambda	0.99351043	0.31	3	142	0.8187
Pillai's Trace	0.00648957	0.31	3	142	0.8187
Hotelling-Lawley Trace	0.00653196	0.31	3	142	0.8187
Roy's Greatest Root	0.00653196	0.31	3	142	0.8187

The second MANOVA statement (see p. 99) is a test of treatment differences in the change from baseline. Again, TAXOL estimates the difference between the two arms and the M= option allows us to specify the change from baseline.

Multivariate Analysis of Variance

M Matrix Describing Transformed Variables

	toi1	toi2	toi3	toi4
MVAR1	-1	1	0	0
MVAR2	-1	0	1	0
MVAR3	-1	0	0	1

MANOVA Test Criteria and Exact F Statistics for the Hypothesis of
No Overall TAXOL Effect on the Variables

MULTIVARIATE METHODS

	Defined by the M Matrix Transformation				
Statistic	Value	F Value	Num DF	Den DF	Pr > F
Wilks' Lambda	0.98936428	0.51	3	142	0.6768
Pillai's Trace	0.01063572	0.51	3	142	0.6768
Hotelling-Lawley Trace	0.01075006	0.51	3	142	0.6768
Roy's Greatest Root	0.01075006	0.51	3	142	0.6768

The standard MANOVA statistics for main effects and interactions can be generated automatically with a REPEATED TIME statement. With the exception of the TAXOL*TIME interaction, the statement does not generate the tests of interest and was not used.

Maximum likelihood estimation with all available data

If the data are missing at random, conditional on the observed data Y_i^{obs}, then the method used for the analysis should include all the information from Y_i^{obs}. In the hypothetical example, this is accomplished by a repeated measures model for the two possible assessments,

$$\underbrace{\begin{bmatrix} y_{i1} \\ y_{i2} \end{bmatrix}}_{Y_i} = \underbrace{\begin{bmatrix} 1 & 0 \\ 0 & 1 \end{bmatrix}}_{X_i} \underbrace{\begin{bmatrix} \mu_1 \\ \mu_2 \end{bmatrix}}_{\beta} + \underbrace{\begin{bmatrix} e_{i1} \\ e_{i2} \end{bmatrix}}_{e_i},$$

where the observations on each subject are allowed to be correlated,

$$\text{Var}\begin{bmatrix} y_{i1} \\ y_{i2} \end{bmatrix} = \begin{bmatrix} \sigma_{11} & \sigma_{12} \\ \sigma_{12} & \sigma_{22} \end{bmatrix}.$$

The maximum likelihood estimates of the means (μ_1, μ_2) are

$$\begin{bmatrix} \hat{\mu}_1 \\ \hat{\mu}_2 \end{bmatrix} = \left(\sum X_i' \hat{\Sigma}_i^{-1} X_i \right)^{-1} \sum X_i' \hat{\Sigma}_i^{-1} Y_i.$$

It is difficult to see how the estimates are calculated when written in matrix notation. Consider a special case where all subjects have their first assessment but only a proportion, π, have their second assessment. The resulting estimates of the means are

$$\begin{bmatrix} \hat{\mu}_1 \\ \hat{\mu}_2 \end{bmatrix} = \begin{bmatrix} \pi \bar{y}_1^C + (1-\pi) \bar{y}_1^I \\ \bar{y}_2^C + (1-\pi) \dfrac{\hat{\sigma}_{12}}{\hat{\sigma}_{11}} \left(\bar{y}_1^I - \bar{y}_1^C \right) \end{bmatrix}$$

$$= \begin{bmatrix} \bar{y}_1 \\ \bar{y}_2^C + (1-\pi) \dfrac{\hat{\sigma}_{12}}{\hat{\sigma}_{11}} \left(\bar{y}_1^I - \bar{y}_1^C \right) \end{bmatrix}. \qquad (5.4)$$

If the variances of Y_1 and Y_2 are equal,

$$\begin{bmatrix} \hat{\mu}_1 \\ \hat{\mu}_2 \end{bmatrix} = \begin{bmatrix} \bar{y}_1 \\ \bar{y}_2^C + (1-\pi) \hat{\rho} (\bar{y}_1^I - \bar{y}_1^C) \end{bmatrix}. \qquad (5.5)$$

The estimate of the mean at T1 is the simple average of all T1 scores ($\bar{y}_1$), because there are no missing data for the first assessment. With missing data at the second time point (T2), $\hat{\mu}_2$ is not the simple mean of all observed T2 assessments ($\bar{y}_2^C$) but is a function of the T1 and T2 scores as well as the correlation between them. The second term in Equation 5.5 ($(1-\pi)\hat{\rho}(\bar{y}_1^I - \bar{y}_1^C)$) is the adjustment of the simple mean ($\bar{y}_2^C$). If we use the information in Table 5.1 for $\rho = 0.5$,

$$\hat{\mu}_2 = \bar{y}_2^C + .5\hat{\rho}(\bar{y}_1^I - \bar{y}_1^C) = 0.28 + (0.5)(0.5)(-0.57 - 0.57) = 0.0.$$

(The discrepancy is due to rounding of values in Table 5.1).

The estimates of the T2 means, using MLE for all available data, are displayed in the third row of Table 5.2. Estimates of change from T1 to T2 are displayed in Table 5.4. Note that the ML estimates are unbiased for both simulated data sets.

Summary	Multivariate analysis of all available data
Examples	Mixed-effects models Repeated measures models
Assumptions	MAR (R_i depends on Y_i^{obs} and X_i but not on Y_i^{mis}); thus, estimates unbiased if model includes Y_i^{obs} and X_i
Advantages	Uses all available data (all subjects with at least one observation) Huge class of models Allows mistimed observations (mixed-effects models) Allows time-varying covariates (X_i) Software: SAS Proc Mixed, BMDP 5V, S-plus Oswald

NSCLC example

Chapter 3 describes the implementation of repeated measures and growth curve models in detail. In that chapter we illustrate a *cell means model* for repeated measures for the adjuvant breast cancer study. In this chapter we show an alternative *reference cell* model. The test statistics generated from both models are identical, but the parameters have different interpretations. As in the MANOVA analysis, the group not assigned to receive Taxol therapy is the reference group. In combination with the NOINT option and the CLASS statement, the term FUNO in the model statement has four levels corresponding to the reference group mean at each of the four time points. The term TAXOL*FUNO also has four levels corresponding to the *difference* between the two treatment groups at each of the four time points.

```
PROC MIXED DATA=BOOK.EXAMPLE2;
  CLASS FUNO;
  *** Model for the Fixed Effects ***;
```

MULTIVARIATE METHODS

```
MODEL FACT_T2=FUNO TAXOL*FUNO /NOINT SOLUTION;
*** Covariance Structure ***;
REPEATED /SUBJECT=CASEID TYPE=UN;
```

The resulting parameter estimates for the fixed effects appear as:

The Mixed Procedure
Solution for Fixed Effects

Effect	FUNO	Estimate	Standard Error	t Value	Pr > |t|
FUNO	1	64.6443	1.2085	53.49	<.0001
FUNO	2	61.8049	1.4401	42.92	<.0001
FUNO	3	61.7782	1.6540	37.35	<.0001
FUNO	4	60.4076	1.9290	31.32	<.0001
TAXOL*FUNO	1	1.4781	1.4831	1.00	0.3194
TAXOL*FUNO	2	2.5843	1.7259	1.50	0.1349
TAXOL*FUNO	3	0.8862	1.9857	0.45	0.6556
TAXOL*FUNO	4	0.6083	2.3080	0.26	0.7922

To estimate the means for the group receiving Taxol, ESTIMATE statements are added:

```
*** Estimates of Means ***;
ESTIMATE 'BASELINE NOTX' FUNO 1 0 0 0;
ESTIMATE 'WEEK 6   NOTX' FUNO 0 1 0 0;
ESTIMATE 'WEEK 12  NOTX' FUNO 0 0 1 0;
ESTIMATE 'WEEK 26  NOTX' FUNO 0 0 0 1;
ESTIMATE 'BASELINE TX' FUNO 1 0 0 0 FUNO*TAXOL 1 0 0 0;
ESTIMATE 'WEEK 6   TX' FUNO 0 1 0 0 FUNO*TAXOL 0 1 0 0;
ESTIMATE 'WEEK 12  TX' FUNO 0 0 1 0 FUNO*TAXOL 0 0 1 0;
ESTIMATE 'WEEK 26  TX' FUNO 0 0 0 1 FUNO*TAXOL 0 0 0 1;
```

The estimates from the analysis of all available data are summarized in Table 5.6. Note that the estimated means are consistently lower than those obtained when the analysis was limited to the complete cases. This analysis is also statistically more efficient than either of the two previous approaches, as reflected by the smaller standard errors.

```
*** Change from Baseline ***;
   ESTIMATE 'WEEK 6-0  NOTX' FUNO -1 1 0 0 ;
   ESTIMATE 'WEEK 12-0 NOTX' FUNO -1 0 1 0 ;
   ESTIMATE 'WEEK 26-0 NOTX' FUNO -1 0 0 1 ;

   ESTIMATE 'WEEK 6-0  TX' FUNO -1 1 0 0 FUNO*TAXOL -1 1 0 0;
   ESTIMATE 'WEEK 12-0 TX' FUNO -1 0 1 0 FUNO*TAXOL -1 0 1 0;
   ESTIMATE 'WEEK 26-0 TX' FUNO -1 0 0 1 FUNO*TAXOL -1 0 0 1;
```

The same multivariate tests can also be constructed:

```
*** Multivariate Tests (Contrasts) ***;
CONTRAST 'FU DIFFERENCES' FUNO*TAXOL 0 1 0 0,
                         FUNO*TAXOL 0 0 1 0,
```

Table 5.6. Results of the multivariate analysis of all available data from the NSCLC study.

Follow-up no.	Taxol	Mean	(S.E.)	t	df	p
1	No	64.6	(1.21)			
	Yes	66.1	(0.86)			
	Difference	1.48	(1.48)	1.00	549	0.32
2	No	61.8	(1.44)			
	Yes	64.4	(0.95)			
	Difference	2.58	(1.73)	1.50	549	0.13
3	No	61.8	(1.65)			
	Yes	62.7	(1.10)			
	Difference	0.89	(1.99)	0.45	549	0.66
4	No	60.4	(1.93)			
	Yes	61.0	(1.27)			
	Difference	0.61	(2.31)	0.26	549	0.79

```
                                 FUNO*TAXOL  0 0 0 1;
       CONTRAST 'CHANGE FROM T1' FUNO*TAXOL -1 1 0 0,
                                 FUNO*TAXOL -1 0 1 0,
                                 FUNO*TAXOL -1 0 0 1;
```

In the NSCLC example there are no differences in the conclusions between the results of the analyses of the complete cases and all available data, but that will not always be true unless the data are missing completely at random.

```
               Contrasts

               Num    Den
Label          DF     DF    F Value   Pr > F
FU differences  3     549      0.82   0.4843
Change from T1  3     549      0.42   0.7358
```

Further comments

Exclusion of subjects

Exclusion of subjects, and thus observed data, from the analysis also occurs in subtler ways. It is not uncommon to include only those subjects with a baseline and at least one follow-up assessment in the analysis. This strategy automatically excludes some subjects with observed data because they have only one observation. The assumption is that the reason they do not have at least two assessments is completely random. In practice this is rarely true. Often these are the sickest patients with the poorest HRQoL scores at baseline. In the NSCLC study, only 5% of the subjects are missing all four FACT-Lung TOI scores (Table 5.7). However, another 27% of the subjects are excluded

Table 5.7. Potential for exclusion of subjects in NSCLC study.

	No Taxol		Taxol		Total	
	N	(%)	N	(%)	N	(%)
No FACT-L TOI data	10	(5)	16	(4)	26	(5)
No baseline FACT-L TOI	7	(4)	16	(4)	23	(4)
No follow-up FACT-L TOI	56	(29)	77	(20)	133	(23)
Baseline + follow-up	121	(62)	272	(71)	393	(68)
Total subjects	194	(100)	381	(100)	575	(100)

if a baseline and at least one follow-up assessment are required for inclusion; 4% because of the requirement for a baseline assessment; and 23% because of the requirement for a follow-up assessment.

Taking this idea a bit further, patients with no HRQoL scores should not be completely excluded from analyses. If there are covariates that are strongly associated with both missingness and observed HRQoL, the values of the covariates from all subjects can be used to improve the estimates; this is illustrated later in this chapter.

Exclusion of observations

Exclusion of observations from the analysis should be performed very cautiously. In some settings, there is a valid conceptual reason to do so. For example, in the adjuvant breast cancer study, four assessments were excluded from the pretherapy assessments because they occurred after therapy started and two assessments were excluded from the on-therapy assessments because they occurred after therapy had been stopped. In other settings, the artificial attempt to force observations into a repeated measures model may result in the exclusion of observations. If the exclusion is not random or missingness at other occasions depends on the the value of these observations, the resulting analyses are biased.

5.4 Baseline assessment as a covariate

Another popular strategy for the analysis of repeated measures is to include the baseline assessment in the model as a covariate (X_i) rather than using it as one of the repeated measures. In this model,

$$y_{ij} = X_{ij}\beta_j + y_{i1}\gamma_j + \epsilon_{ij}, \qquad (5.6)$$

where y_{i1} is the baseline measure for the ith subject. This strategy partially addresses the issue of ignoring the observed data by including the information in the baseline assessment. However, it should be used cautiously if there are missing data in either the baseline or early follow-up assessments. Most analytic procedures will, by default, exclude individuals with missing baseline

HRQoL or no follow-up assessments from all aspects of the analysis. The potential result of excluding these subjects from the analysis is to bias the estimates of HRQoL.

Consider the hypothetical example where the model is

$$y_{i2} = \beta + y_{i1}\gamma + \epsilon_{i2}. \tag{5.7}$$

If the mean of the T2 scores is estimated using only the baseline data from the subjects with follow-up assessments (y_{i1}^C), then the mean HRQoL scores at T2 will be overestimated because $\bar{y}_1^C$ overestimates the baseline mean, μ_1. This is illustrated in Table 5.2 in the row identified as "Baseline (naive)."

$$\hat{\mu}_2 = \hat{\beta} + \bar{y}_1^C \hat{\gamma}. \tag{5.8}$$

In this simple case, the estimates of μ_2 are identical to those obtained for the complete case and the univariate analyses. In contrast, if all observed T1 assessments are included in the estimation of μ_2, the estimates are no longer biased. This is illustrated in Table 5.2 in the row identified as "Baseline (correct)."

$$\hat{\mu}_2 = \hat{\beta} + \bar{y}_1 \hat{\gamma}, \quad \bar{y}_1 = \pi \bar{y}_1^C + (1-\pi) \bar{y}_1^I. \tag{5.9}$$

When there are multiple follow-up assessments, the same issues of multivariate vs. univariate analyses apply. If missingness is related to both the baseline and previously observed assessments of HRQoL, then the appropriate analysis is a multivariate analysis of the follow-up assessments. With extended follow-up this will become more important, as there is a stronger relationship between dropout and the more recent assessments of HRQoL than with the initial baseline measure. Repeated univariate analyses will ignore information from the previous assessments and will be biased if dropout depends on the previously observed HRQoL.

Summary	Baseline as a covariate
Assumption	MAR, if means of all baseline data are included MCAR, if limited to subjects with baseline and follow-up data (many programs ignore *information* in the covariates X_i for subjects with missing data; must force $E[Y_i]$ to be estimated at the mean of X_i for all subjects)
Advantages	Easy to use Easy to describe
Disadvantage	Cannot estimate change from baseline
SAS note	To obtain unbiased estimates, use `LSMEANS .../AT MEANS E;` and data set must include rows for missing observations

NSCLC example

As a first step, the baseline FACT-Lung TOI scores (TOI1) from WORK.ONEREC are merged with the follow-up scores from BOOK.EXAMPLE2. The SQL procedure allows us to do this in one step:

```
PROC SQL;
  *** Merges Baseline Score and change ***;
  CREATE TABLE WORK.FOLLOWUP
    AS SELECT *,
       (FACT_T2-TOI1) AS CHANGEBL   /* Change */
    FROM BOOK.EXAMPLE2 AS L
    LEFT JOIN WORK.ONEREC AS R
    ON L.CASEID=R.CASEID
    HAVING L.FUNO>1              /* Selects FU 2, 3, 4*/
    ORDER BY L.CASEID,L.FUNO;
```

The repeated follow-up assessments are estimated using the MIXED procedure:

```
PROC MIXED DATA=WORK.FOLLOWUP NOCLPRINT;
  TITLE 'Baseline FACT-Lung TOI as a covariate - With AT MEANS';
  CLASS FUNO TAXOL;
  MODEL FACT_T2 = TAXOL*FUNO TOI1/NOINT SOLUTION  DDFM=SATTERTH;
  REPEATED /SUBJECT=CASEID TYPE=UN;
  LSMEANS TAXOL*FUNO/AT MEANS;
  RUN;
```

A portion of the LSMEANS output appears as follows:

The Mixed Procedure

Least Squares Means

Effect	FUNO	TAXOL	TOI1	Estimate	Standard Error
FUNO*TAXOL	2	No	65.58	62.7618	1.3248
FUNO*TAXOL	2	Yes	65.58	64.0660	0.8600
FUNO*TAXOL	3	No	65.58	61.8029	1.5891
FUNO*TAXOL	3	Yes	65.58	61.8082	1.0564
FUNO*TAXOL	4	No	65.58	59.6353	1.9326
FUNO*TAXOL	4	Yes	65.58	60.2863	1.2579

In the NSCLC study, analysis of the follow-up observations with the baseline scores as covariates limits the analysis to the 383 subjects with both baseline and at least one follow-up observation, just over two thirds of the randomized subjects (see Table 5.7). When the AT MEANS option is omitted from the LSMEANS statement, the means are estimated at a value that is the mean of the covariate across all observations with a nonmissing value of the outcome (FACT_T2). In this example, the value was 69.3 (Table 5.8, naive estimates).

Table 5.8. Results of multivariate analyses of three repeated follow-up measures with the baseline scores as a covariate compared with four repeated measures with baseline as a dependent variable (Table 5.6).

		Covariate				Four repeated measures	
		Naive estimates		Correct estimates			
Follow-up no.	Taxol	Mean	(S.E.)	Mean	(S.E.)	Mean	(S.E.)
2	No	64.7	(1.32)	62.8	(1.32)	61.8	(1.44)
	Yes	66.0	(0.86)	64.1	(0.86)	64.4	(0.95)
3	No	63.7	(1.59)	61.8	(1.59)	61.8	(1.65)
	Yes	63.7	(1.05)	61.8	(1.05)	62.7	(1.10)
4	No	61.6	(1.92)	59.6	(1.92)	60.4	(1.93)
	Yes	62.2	(1.26)	60.3	(1.26)	61.0	(1.27)
Baseline[a]		69.3		65.6			

[a] Baseline scores used to estimate LSMEANS.

We can add back some information from the subjects who had only a baseline assessment by including their baseline values when estimating the LSMEANS. When the AT MEANS option is included and records exist for all subjects at all possible times, the LSMEANS are estimated at a value that is the mean of the covariate across all subjects with a nonmissing value of the covariate (TOI1). In this example, this value is 65.6 (Table 5.8, naive estimates). The parameter estimates obtained from the naive analysis (with the AT MEANS option omitted) are contrasted with the corrected analysis in Table 5.8. The estimates from the naive procedure are consistently higher than from the correct procedure, although the differences between the groups are not affected. Note also that the estimates from the correct procedure are very similar to those obtained with the multivariate analysis of all available data (Table 5.6). The differences occur because of the small difference of 64.6 vs. 66.1 in the baseline scores between the two groups.

5.5 Change from baseline

Another popular method is the analysis of change from baseline. The strategy is to subtract the baseline scores from the follow-up scores:

$$y_{ij} - y_{i1} = X_{ij}\beta_j + \varepsilon_{ij}. \qquad (5.10)$$

The analysis is then limited to subjects with both baseline and follow-up assessments. This is another example of how an analysis that is not carefully implemented will result in biased estimates. Because the outcome is now the change from baseline, the data are MAR only if the missingness depends on the *observed* change. In our hypothetical example, this is not a valid assumption, as the missingness also depends on the change in those subjects where we have

CHANGE FROM BASELINE

not observed the change. The biased estimates of change resulting from this analysis are summarized in the row labeled "Change (naive)" in Table 5.4. Note that the estimates of change in this setting are the same as those obtained from the complete case analysis.

In this simple example, we can fix the problem by adding baseline as a covariate. Now the data are MAR, conditional on the observed baseline response.

$$y_{ij} - y_{i1} = X_{ij}\beta_j + y_{i1}\gamma_j + \varepsilon_{ij}. \tag{5.11}$$

The unbiased estimates of change resulting from this analysis are summarized in the row labeled "Change (correct)" in Table 5.4. Again, it is important to use the mean of all observed data at T1 ($\bar{y}_1$), and not just the mean at T1 for those subjects who have both T1 and T2 assessments ($\bar{y}_1^C$), when estimating the change.

Again, when there are multiple follow-up assessments, the arguments in favor of multivariate over univariate analyses apply. With extended follow-up, the use of a multivariate analysis will become more important, as there is a stronger relationship between dropout and the more recent assessments of HRQoL. These multivariate models may also become very complex, as the relationship (γ) between the baseline assessment and change is moderated by either time or the intervention. Specifically, the relationship may be different for each of the J time points or H groups.

NSCLC example

Analysis of the change from baseline scores limits the analysis to the same 67% of the randomized subjects with both baseline and at least one follow-up observation (Table 5.7). When missingness depends on the baseline scores, these estimates are biased because the scores of subjects with no follow-up are ignored in the analysis (Table 5.9). By adding baseline as a covariate and estimating the change at the mean for all subjects, we minimize that bias.

```
PROC MIXED DATA=WORK.FOLLOWUP;
   TITLE 'Change from Baseline with Baseline as a Covariate';
   CLASS FUNO TAXOL;
   MODEL CHANGEBL = TAXOL*FUNO TOI1/NOINT SOLUTION  DDFM=SATTERTH;
   REPEATED FUNO/SUBJECT=CASEID TYPE=UN;
   LSMEANS TAXOL*FUNO/AT MEANS;
   RUN;
```

Least Squares Means

Effect	FUNO	TAXOL	TOI1	Estimate	Standard Error
FUNO*TAXOL	2	No	65.58	-2.8200	1.3248
FUNO*TAXOL	2	Yes	65.58	-1.5158	0.8600

Table 5.9. Results of a multivariate analysis of the three changes from baseline scores compared with estimates of change obtained from model with four repeated measures (Table 5.6).

		Change from baseline scores				Four repeated measures	
		Without covariate		With covariate			
Follow-up no.	Taxol	Mean	(S.E.)	Mean	(S.E.)	Mean	(S.E.)
2	No	−4.03	(1.45)	−2.82	(1.32)	−2.84	(1.40)
	Yes	−2.64	(0.94)	−1.52	(0.86)	−1.73	(0.92)
3	No	−5.17	(1.75)	−3.77	(1.59)	−2.87	(1.69)
	Yes	−5.38	(1.16)	−3.77	(1.06)	−3.46	(1.13)
4	No	−8.41	(2.09)	−5.95	(1.93)	−4.24	(1.99)
	Yes	−7.56	(1.36)	−5.30	(1.26)	−5.10	(1.31)

```
FUNO*TAXOL   3   No    65.58   -3.7788   1.5891
FUNO*TAXOL   3   Yes   65.58   -3.7736   1.0564
FUNO*TAXOL   4   No    65.58   -5.9464   1.9326
FUNO*TAXOL   4   Yes   65.58   -5.2955   1.2579
```

5.6 Adding other baseline covariates

If dropout depends on certain patient characteristics, the previous discussion would suggest that it will be important to include corresponding covariates in all analysis models. However, in practice, the inclusion or omission of these baseline covariates rarely makes a difference when the intent is to compare treatment arms in a randomized clinical trial. First, if the characteristic is not correlated with the HRQoL measure, then its inclusion/exclusion will not affect the results. Second, if the characteristic is correlated with the HRQoL measure, much of the covariance with postrandomization measures is explained by the prerandomization baseline measure. However, it is advisable to perform a sensitivity analysis by repeating the analysis with these covariates.

In theory, the treatment arms should be balanced with respect to these patient characteristics. When there are apparent differences detected in baseline characteristics, two possibilities exist: (1) the differences are real or (2) there is no difference between the groups and a Type I error has occurred. In the first case, it is appropriate to adjust the estimates by inclusion of a covariate in the analysis, but in the second case the differences are ignored. Unfortunately, it is not possible to distinguish the two cases. Again, a sensitivity analysis is advisable.

Summary	Change from baseline
Examples	Baseline subtracted from all FU observations
Assumptions	MCAR (R_i cannot depend on the difference, $Y_{ij} - Y_{i1}$)
	Possibly MAR with baseline as a covariate
Advantages	Familiar method
	Possible strategy when there are initial (baseline) differences in Y
Disadvantage	Cannot estimate means and some summary measures

NSCLC example

Based on the results presented in Chapter 4, a sensitivity analysis with age, performance status, and symptoms of systemic disease appears warranted. There were no identified differences between the two treatment groups, so no additional variables were selected for this sensitivity analysis. As an alternative to using the LSMEANS option to obtain the *adjusted* estimates, in this example each of the variables is centered at its mean. The SQL procedure can be used to create three new variables (CNT_AGE, CNT_PS and CNT_SXSYS) in a single step:

```
PROC SQL;
  CREATE TABLE WORK.CENTERED AS
    SELECT *,
           L.AGE_TX-MEAN(L.AGE_TX) AS CNT_AGE,
           L.ECOGPS-MEAN(L.ECOGPS) AS CNT_PS,
           L.SX_SYS-MEAN(L.SX_SYS) AS CNT_SXSYS
    FROM BOOK.PATIENT2 AS L
    LEFT JOIN BOOK.FACTL2 AS R
    ON L.CASEID=R.CASEID
    ORDER BY CASEID;
```

or in a simple two-step process:

```
PROC SQL;
  CREATE TABLE WORK.TEMP AS
    SELECT CASEID,
           AGE_TX-MEAN(AGE_TX) AS CNT_AGE,
           ECOGPS-MEAN(ECOGPS) AS CNT_PS,
           SX_SYS-MEAN(SX_SYS) AS CNT_SXSYS
    FROM BOOK.PATIENT2
    ORDER BY CASEID;
DATA WORK.CENTERED;
  MERGE BOOK.FACTL2 WORK.TEMP;
  BY CASEID;
RUN;
```

Table 5.10. Results of the multivariate analysis of all available data with and without baseline covariates associated with dropout (age, performance status, symptoms of systemic disease) from the NSCLC study.

Follow-up no.	Taxol	Without covariates		With covariates	
		Mean	(S.E.)	Mean	(S.E.)
1	No	64.6	(1.21)	64.8	(1.17)
	Yes	66.1	(0.86)	66.2	(1.83)
	Difference	1.48	(1.48)	1.39	(1.43)
2	No	61.8	(1.44)	61.7	(1.38)
	Yes	64.4	(0.95)	64.0	(0.91)
	Difference	2.58	(1.73)	2.23	(1.66)
3	No	61.8	(1.65)	61.8	(1.59)
	Yes	62.7	(1.10)	62.6	(1.05)
	Difference	0.89	(1.99)	0.85	(1.90)
4	No	60.4	(1.93)	59.9	(1.85)
	Yes	61.0	(1.27)	60.2	(1.22)
	Difference	0.61	(2.31)	0.33	(2.22)

The MIXED procedure statements are identical to those used for the multivariate maximum likelihood estimation with all available data except for the inclusion of the covariates in the MODEL statement.

```
PROC MIXED DATA=WORK.CENTERED;
  TITLE 'ML WITH COVARIATES';
  CLASS FUNO;
  MODEL FACT_T2=FUNO TAXOL*FUNO CNT_AGE CNT_SXSYS CNT_PS
      /NOINT SOLUTION ;
  REPEATED /SUBJECT=CASEID TYPE=UN;
```

Because we have used *centered covariates*, none of the other statements needs to be changed.

Coefficients for performance status (CNT_PS) and symptoms of systemic disease (CNT_SXSYS) were significant ($p < 0.001$), and age was marginally nonsignificant ($p = 0.09$). The resulting estimates of the parameters, with and without the covariates, are displayed in Table 5.10. The results from the two analyses were quite similar.

5.7 Empirical Bayes estimates

In the mixed-effects model, the expected value (unconditional expectation) of an observation is

$$E[Y_i] = E[X_i\beta + Z_i d_i + e_i] = X_i\beta. \tag{5.12}$$

EMPIRICAL BAYES ESTIMATES

Linear functions of the fixed effects are called *estimable functions*. $X_i\beta$ is an estimable function if β is estimable, and $X_i\hat{\beta}$ is called the *best linear unbiased estimate* (BLUE) of $X_i\beta$.

The conditional expectation of **Y** given the random effects is

$$E[Y_i|d_i] = E[X_i\beta + Z_i d_i + e_i] = X_i\beta + Z_i d_i. \quad (5.13)$$

Linear functions of the fixed and random effects are called *predictable functions*. The solutions for estimates of β and d_i provide the *best linear unbiased predictor* (BLUP) of $X_i\beta + Z_i d_i$.

Some insight into the estimates obtained from the mixed-effects model is provided by further examination of the BLUPs of the responses for a particular individual, $\hat{Y}_i$. The *empirical Bayes* estimates of the random effects, $\hat{d}_i$, are the expectation of the random effect, d_i, conditional on the observed data Y_i^{obs}, where

$$E\begin{bmatrix} Y_i \\ d_i \end{bmatrix} = \begin{bmatrix} X_i\beta \\ 0 \end{bmatrix}, \quad (5.14)$$

$$\text{Var}\begin{bmatrix} Y_i \\ d_i \end{bmatrix} = \begin{bmatrix} \Sigma_i & Z_i D \\ DZ_i & D \end{bmatrix}, \quad (5.15)$$

$$E[d_i|Y_i] = 0 + DZ_i\Sigma_i^{-1}(Y_i - X_i\beta). \quad (5.16)$$

With a bit of algebraic manipulation, we see that the predicted values are a weighted combination of average *population* estimates, $X_i\hat{\beta}$, and observed data, Y_i [154, p. 119].

$$\begin{aligned}
\hat{Y}_i &= X_i\hat{\beta} + Z_i\hat{d}_i \\
&= X_i\hat{\beta} + Z_i DZ_i'\Sigma_i^{-1}(Y_i^{\text{obs}} - X_i\hat{\beta}) \\
&= (I - Z_i DZ_i'\Sigma_i^{-1})X_i\hat{\beta} + Z_i DZ_i'\Sigma_i^{-1}Y_i^{\text{obs}} \\
&= (\Sigma_i\Sigma_i^{-1} - Z_i DZ_i'\Sigma_i^{-1})X_i\hat{\beta} + Z_i DZ_i'\Sigma_i^{-1}Y_i^{\text{obs}} \\
&= \underbrace{\sigma_w^2 I \ \Sigma_i^{-1} X_i\hat{\beta}}_{\text{Within}} + \underbrace{Z_i DZ_i' \Sigma_i^{-1} Y_i^{\text{obs}}}_{\text{Between}}. \quad (5.17)
\end{aligned}$$

Recall that $\Sigma_i = Z_i DZ_i' + \sigma^2 I$ and note that the numerator of the weight on $X_i\hat{\beta}$, $\sigma^2 I$, is the within-subject residual covariance and the denominator is the total variance, Σ_i. Likewise, the numerator of the weight on Y_i^{obs} is the between subject variance, $Z_i DZ_i'$. As the portion of the variance that is attributed to between subject differences (D) increases, the weight on the observed data increases. Although it is not so obvious, the number and timing of the observations affect the weights. When there are two random effects, the second term will increase both as the number of observations increase and as they spread over time. For a subject with two observations at the beginning and end of the study, this term is greater than for a subject with only two early observations.

Note that the sufficient statistics in the EM algorithm [32], which is often used to to estimate the mixed-effects parameters, are constructed from these conditional expectations.

5.8 Summary

- In the presence of missing or mistimed data, it is advisable to employ analytic methods that use all of the observed data such as repeated measures models for incomplete data or mixed-effects models (Chapter 3).
- Methods that exclude subjects or observations from the analysis should be avoided unless one is convinced that the data are missing completely at random (MCAR). These methods include repeated univariate analyses, which ignore observations that occur at different times, and MANOVA, which deletes cases with any missing assessments.

CHAPTER 6

Simple Imputation

6.1 Introduction

Traditional use of imputation was motivated by the desire to avoid bias due to missing data and the unavailability of analytic methods for incomplete data. Prior to the mid-1980s, statistical software for longitudinal studies or repeated measures, such as MANOVA or MANCOVA, required the exclusion of all individuals with any missing data. This disadvantage has disappeared with the accessibility of software for incomplete data such as maximum likelihood estimation (MLE) for longitudinal studies with ignorable missing data [109, 115, 132] described in Chapter 5. When it is reasonable to assume that the missing data in a HRQoL study are either MCAR or MAR, these MLE procedures are appropriate and the need to impute missing observations diminishes.

There remain two situations where imputation may be useful in studies involving HRQoL measurement. The first situation occurs when there are missing explanatory (independent) variables or covariates in the analysis [153]. Missing covariates will result in the deletion of individuals with missing data from any analysis. The second situation occurs when HRQoL is the outcome (dependent) measure and there is a concern that the missing data are not ignorable. Imputation methods are useful as part of sensitivity analyses to examine the dependence of the results on specific assumptions about the HRQoL of individuals with missing observations [153]. However, imputation should not be considered either an easy fix or a definitive solution to the problem of missing data; in all cases imputation requires the analyst to make untestable assumptions concerning the missing data.

This chapter covers simple imputation techniques. Simple imputation is the process of substituting a single reasonable value for a missing observation. This procedure, if thoughtfully performed, may have a limited usefulness in examining the sensitivity of estimates of the means to various assumptions. Common simple imputation methods (Table 6.1) include techniques such as last value carried forward (LVCF) and substitution of predicted values from regression-based techniques. The choice among methods should be made only after careful consideration of why the observations are missing, the general patterns of change in HRQoL over time, and the research questions being addressed. Without this careful consideration, imputation may increase the bias of the estimates. For example, if missing HRQoL observations are more likely in individuals who are experiencing toxicity as a result of the treatment, the average value from individuals with observations (who are less likely to be experiencing toxicity) will likely overestimate the HRQoL of individuals with missing data.

Table 6.1. Examples of simple imputation methods.

Means	Mean of observed data
Predicted values	Predicted values from univariate or multivariate linear regression models
Hot deck	Randomly sampled observation
LVCF (LOCF)	Last value (observation) carried forward
MVCF	Minimum value carried forward
Low/high value	A theoretically justified low or high value; possibly the minimum or maximum observed value

Table 6.2. Selected patients from the NSCLC study.

No.	Taxol	Baseline	6 weeks	12 weeks	26 weeks	CR/PR	Months survival
12	No	**60.9**	M	X	X	No	2.5
13	No	**82.1**	M	X	X	No	2.7
60	Yes	**57.2**	**40.6**	M	X	No	3.6
527	Yes	**63.5**	**52.4**	M	M	No	7.2
277	Yes	**67.5**	**71.6**	M	M	No	7.8

Observed data are displayed in bold, M indicates missing and alive, X indicates patient has expired. CR/PR = complete or partial response.

Limitations of simple imputation

The most common criticism of simple imputation methods is that most analyses treat imputed values as if they were observed values. This results in underestimation of the variance of the parameter estimates. Without proper adjustments, simple imputation is inappropriate when the goal is to construct test statistics and confidence intervals. Naive implementation of these techniques may produce a false sense of confidence that we have solved the missing data problem when, in fact, we have just obscured it.

NSCLC example

Some of the problems with simple imputation cited above are illustrated by examining the results of simple imputation in the NSCLC study. Consider five patients selected from this trial (Table 6.2). All failed to respond to therapy. The first two (subjects 12 and 13) have a similar short survival and could only be assessed prior to therapy and at 6 weeks. The major difference between these two subjects is that one had a higher initial score than the other. The third subject is missing an assessment at 12 weeks and died prior to the time of the final assessment. The fourth and fifth subjects have similar survival and are both missing two assessments. Subject 277 reported very little change in his HRQoL, whereas subjects 60 and 527 both report a significant decline over the first 6 weeks of therapy. As different methods of simple imputation are presented in the next section, the imputed values are illustrated for these five subjects.

6.2 Mean value substitution

A common simple imputation technique is the substitution of the average value from the individuals who completed the measure of HRQoL for the missing observations. This mean may be computed across all individuals or may be specific to treatment groups or to individuals with similar characteristics. The method assumes that the reasons some individuals did not complete their HRQoL assessments is completely unrelated to their HRQoL. This may be valid if the missing data are due to administrative problems, but it is hard to justify in most situations. For example, even in the case where a subject with a missing assessment was documented to be experiencing toxicity and the mean HRQoL score was computed from responses among other individuals experiencing toxicity, there is still the assumption that the impact of the toxicity on the subject's HRQoL is equivalent among those who completed the HRQoL assessment and those who did not.

Table 6.3 displays mean imputation for five cases in the NSCLC study. Means were imputed separately for each treatment group, ignoring all other information about the patient. Thus, the first two subjects have the same imputed value at 6 weeks, even though subject 12 had a much lower baseline score than subject 13. The last three subjects have the same value at 12 weeks, irrespective of the differences in their survival. However, in the NSCLC study, we have observed that subjects with lower baseline HRQoL and those who are closer to death are more likely to have missing assessments; simple mean imputation is likely to result in biased estimates of the overall mean.

Table 6.3. Simple imputation using mean of observed data illustrated for selected patients in the NSCLC study.

No.	Taxol	Baseline	6 weeks	12 weeks	26 weeks	Months survival
12	No	**60.9**	*63.7*	X	X	2.5
13	No	**82.1**	*63.7*	X	X	2.7
60	Yes	**57.2**	**40.6**	**65.6**	X	3.6
527	Yes	**63.5**	**52.4**	**65.6**	*64.8*	7.2
277	Yes	**67.5**	**71.6**	**65.6**	*64.8*	7.8

Observed data are displayed in bold and imputed data in italics. X indicates patient has expired.

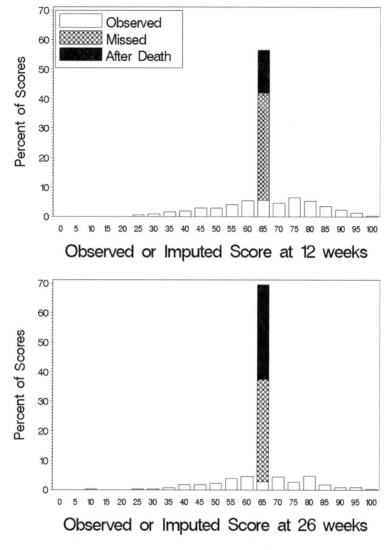

Figure 6.1. Distribution of observed and imputed values using group means.

The distributions of observed scores and imputed scores are displayed in Figure 6.1. The imputed values are centered relative to the observed scores, emphasizing the assumption that the missing values are MCAR.

6.3 Explicit regression models

In the explicit regression model approach, we identify a regression model to predict the missing observation. The explicit regression approach has the advantage that the regression model used to impute missing observations can readily use auxiliary information about the subject's HRQoL that could not be included in the model used for the ultimate analysis of the clinical trial. This additional information might include indicators of the side effects of treatment and the clinical course of the disease when the therapy succeeds or fails. Alternatively, it could include measures of HRQoL provided by a caregiver when the subject is no longer able to complete self-assessments.

Analytic model: $Y_i = X_i \beta + \epsilon_i$
Imputation model: $Y_i^* = X_i^* \mathcal{B}^* + \varepsilon_i^*$

Identification of the imputation model

Recall that one of the objectives of imputation is to obtain unbiased estimates of the missing observations. In the context of the explicit regression approach, we are looking for a model where the missingness in the imputation model depends only on the observed data (Y_i^*) and covariates in the imputation model (X_i^*). Basically, we are attempting to augment the analytic model with auxiliary outcome data (Y_i^*) or covariates (X_i^*), so that the MAR assumption in the imputation model seems reasonable. The primary candidates for covariates include measures that are strongly correlated with both the measure being imputed and the probability that it is missing. In the NSCLC example, this suggests adding covariates associated with toxicity, disease progression, and the proximity of the patient to death. Note that * is used to distinguish the covariates and corresponding parameters of the imputation model from those included in the analytic model.

Assuming that the objective of the analysis is the comparison of treatment groups, the following strategy is recommended for identification of the imputation model:

1. Identify patient characteristics, measures, and clinical outcomes that are strong predictors of the HRQoL outcome to be imputed.
2. Identify patient characteristics, measures, and clinical outcomes that predict missingness of the HRQoL outcome to be imputed.
3. Remove variables from the above lists if they are frequently missing. If $X_i^{*\mathrm{mis}}$ includes covariates that are missing, then we will be unable to impute values for Y_i^{mis}.
4. Select and test potential covariates in the imputation models, giving the highest priority to variables that are in both lists.
5. If the sample size is large, develop separate imputation models for each treatment group. Otherwise, force variables identifying treatment groups into the model. If models are not being developed separately for each treatment group, evaluate interactions between treatment and potential covariates. Failure to do this will bias the treatment comparisons toward the null hypothesis.

When the intent of the analysis extends beyond treatment comparisons, all important explanatory variables on which inference is planned should be included as explanatory variables in the imputation model to avoid biasing the evidence toward the null hypothesis.

Simple univariate regression

The parameters of the imputation model for the jth assessment, $\hat{\mathcal{B}}_j^*$, are estimated using the observed data with the model

$$Y_{ij}^{\text{obs}} = X_{ij}^{*\text{obs}}\mathcal{B}_j^* + \varepsilon_{ij}^*. \tag{6.1}$$

The predicted values are then computed for the missing values:

$$Y_{ij}^{*\text{mis}} = X_{ij}^{*\text{mis}}\hat{\mathcal{B}}_j^*. \tag{6.2}$$

This approach will result in unbiased estimates if the regression model satisfies the assumptions. Specifically, the missingness should depend only on covariates that were included in the imputation model. In practice, this approach will require the careful documentation of the reasons for missing data and the luck or foresight to measure the patient characteristics and outcomes (covariates) that explain the missing data mechanism.

Table 6.4 displays the imputed values for the same five cases from the NSCLC study for simple unconditional imputation. Imputed values are the predicted values from simple linear regression models. For the first two cases, the predicted value at 6 weeks for subjects on the Etoposide arm is

$$Y_{ij1}^{*\text{mis}} = X_{ij}^{*\text{mis}}\hat{\mathcal{B}}_j^* = 63.4 + 6.6 \times X_{ij1}^* - 12.4 \times X_{ij2}^*, \quad j = 2, \tag{6.3}$$

where $X_{1j}^* = 1$ if the best response is a complete or partial response or 0 otherwise and $X_{ij2}^* = 1$ if the patient will expire within 2 months of the jth assessment or 0 otherwise. For both cases, $X_{i21} = 0$ and $X_{i22} = 1$; therefore, the predicted value is 51.0. At 12 weeks, the predicted value for subjects on the Taxol arm is

$$Y_{ij}^{*\text{mis}} = X_{ij}^{*\text{mis}}\hat{\mathcal{B}}_j^* = 63.8 + 6.7 \times X_{ij1}^* - 20.2 \times X_{ij2}^*, \quad j = 3. \tag{6.4}$$

Because subject 60 is within 2 months of death ($X_{i32}^* = 1$), the imputed value is much lower than for subjects 277 and 527. These values are much more intuitively appealing than the simple means, especially for subjects closer to death. The assumptions about the missing data have been relaxed slightly.

Table 6.4. Simple imputation using linear regression models with covariates.

| No. | Taxol | Weeks postrandomization | | | | Months survival | CR/PR |
		0	6	12	26		
12	No	**60.9**	*51.0*	X	X	2.5	No
13	No	**82.1**	*51.0*	X	X	2.7	No
60	Yes	**57.2**	**40.6**	*43.6*	X	3.6	No
527	Yes	**63.5**	**52.4**	*63.8*	*50.9*	7.2	No
277	Yes	**67.5**	**71.6**	*63.8*	*50.9*	7.8	No

Observed data are displayed in bold and imputed data in italics. NSCLC example. CR/PR = complete or partial response.

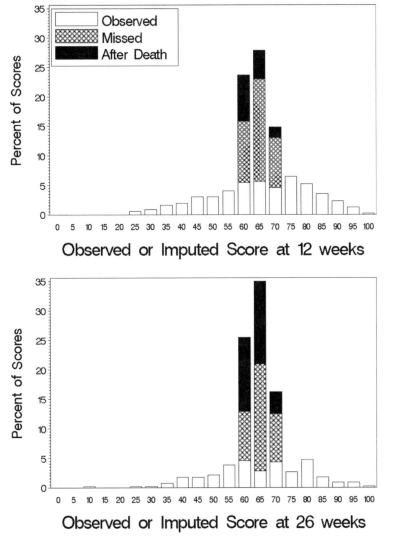

Figure 6.2. Distribution of observed and imputed values using simple regression with baseline characteristics (treatment group, performance status, prior weight loss, symptoms of primary and systemic disease).

We are still assuming that relationships between HRQoL and clinical outcomes such as response and survival are the same for subjects with missing data as for those with observed HRQoL.

The distributions of observed scores and imputed scores, predicted by simple linear regression, are displayed in Figures 6.2 and 6.3. In the first set of plots (Figure 6.2), the explanatory variables in the regression models are limited to baseline characteristics. The imputed values remain centered relative to the

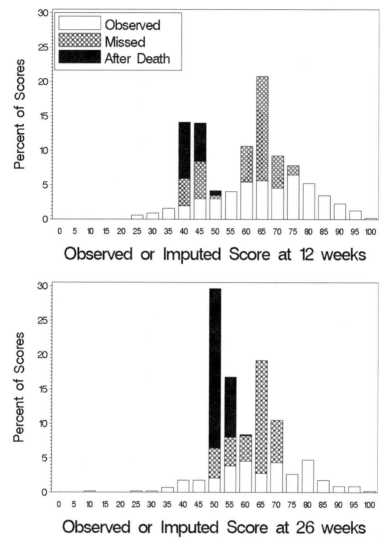

Figure 6.3. Distribution of observed and imputed values using simple regression with baseline characteristics (treatment group, performance status, prior weight loss, symptoms of primary and systemic disease) and outcome (best response and death within 2 months).

observed scores. In the second set of plots, two covariates are added: complete or partial response and death within 2 months. The distribution of imputed values is shifting down slightly, especially for those subjects who are within the last 2 months of their lives. Note that the range of imputed values is much smaller than the range of observed values. The implications of this are discussed later in this chapter.

Conditional predicted values

In the longitudinal setting, the likelihood of missing data often depends on such observed data (Y_i^{obs}) as previous HRQoL assessments. If we wish to obtain unbiased estimates, it is critical that we include the observed data in the imputation procedure. Specifically, we want to predict values of the missing HRQoL scores using the previously observed HRQoL scores from that individual. These conditional estimates are referred to as either empirical best linear unbiased predictors (EBLUP) or Buck's conditional means [11, 88]. (See Section 5.6 for more details on EBLUPs.) For both the repeated measures and random-effects models, the estimates take the form

$$E\big[Y_i^{\text{mis}}\big|Y_i^{\text{obs}},\hat{\mathcal{B}}^*\big] = X_i^{\text{mis}}\hat{\mathcal{B}}^* + \hat{\Sigma}_{mo}\hat{\Sigma}_{oo}^{-1}\big(Y_i^{\text{obs}} - X_i^{\text{obs}}\hat{\mathcal{B}}^*\big), \qquad (6.5)$$

$$\text{Var}\begin{bmatrix}Y_i^{\text{obs}}\\Y_i^{\text{mis}}\end{bmatrix} = \begin{bmatrix}\Sigma_{oo} & \Sigma_{om}\\ \Sigma_{mo} & \Sigma_{mm}\end{bmatrix}. \qquad (6.6)$$

For a mixed-effects model (Equation 3.9), the estimates are a special case:

$$\begin{aligned}E\big[Y_i^{\text{mis}}\big|Y_i^{\text{obs}},\hat{\mathcal{B}}^*,\hat{d}_i^*\big] &= X_i^{*\text{mis}}\hat{\mathcal{B}}^* + Z_i^{*\text{mis}}\hat{d}_i^*\\&= X_i^{*\text{mis}}\hat{\mathcal{B}}^* + Z_i^{*\text{mis}}\hat{D}Z_i^{*\text{obs}\prime}\hat{\Sigma}_{oo}^{-1}\big(Y_i^{\text{obs}} - X_i^{*\text{obs}}\hat{\mathcal{B}}^*\big). \end{aligned}\qquad (6.7)$$

Note that the observed data (Y_i^{obs}) are now included in the equation used to predict the missing values for each individual. When the observed HRQoL scores for the ith subject are higher (or lower) than the average scores for similar subjects, the difference ($Y_i^{\text{obs}} - X_i^{*\text{obs}}\hat{\mathcal{B}}^*$) is positive (or negative). As a result, the imputed conditional predicted value is larger (or smaller) than the imputed unconditional value ($X_i^{*\text{mis}}\hat{\beta}$). Further, when HRQoL scores within the same individual are more strongly correlated, the second term in these equations, $\hat{\Sigma}_{mo}\hat{\Sigma}_{oo}^{-1}(Y_i^{\text{obs}} - X_i^{*\text{obs}}\hat{\mathcal{B}}^*)$ or $Z_i^{*\text{mis}}\hat{d}_i^*$, is larger in magnitude and the difference between the conditional and unconditional imputed values will increase.

Table 6.5 displays the imputed values for the same five cases from the NSCLC study for conditional predicted. Imputed values are computed using the results of a repeated measures model of all available data. For the subjects

Table 6.5. Simple imputation using (EBLUPs) conditional predicted values.

No.	Taxol	Baseline	6 weeks	12 weeks	26 weeks	Months survival
12	No	**60.9**	*51.0*	X	X	2.5
13	No	**82.1**	*61.8*	X	X	2.7
60	Yes	**57.2**	**40.6**	*34.4*	X	3.6
527	Yes	**63.5**	**52.4**	**54.9**	*43.0*	7.2
277	Yes	**67.5**	**71.6**	**65.9**	*51.2*	7.8

Observed data are displayed in bold and imputed data in italics. NSCLC example.

on the Etoposide arm who will survive less than 2 months after the scheduled 6-week assessment, the unconditional predicted values at baseline and 6 weeks are

$$Y_{ij}^{*\text{mis}} = X_{ij1}^{*\text{mis}} \hat{\beta}_1^* = 65.1 + 5.4 X_{ij1}^{*\text{mis}} - 10.4 X_{ij2}^{*\text{mis}} = 65.1, \quad j = 1, \quad (6.8)$$

$$Y_{ij}^{*\text{mis}} = X_{ij2}^{*\text{mis}} \hat{\beta}_2^* = 62.1 + 6.7 X_{ij1}^{*\text{mis}} - 9.0 X_{ij2}^{*\text{mis}} = 53.1, \quad j = 2. \quad (6.9)$$

The conditional predicted value for the 6-week assessment given the baseline assessment is

$$Y_{i2}^{*\text{mis}} | Y_{i1}^{\text{obs}} = X_{i2}^{*\text{mis}} \hat{\beta}_2^* + \hat{\sigma}_{21} \hat{\sigma}_{11}^{-1} \left(Y_{i1}^{\text{obs}} - X_{i1}^{*\text{obs}} \hat{\beta}_1^* \right). \quad (6.10)$$

Specifically, for subjects 12 and 13,

$$Y_{i2}^{*\text{mis}} | Y_{i1}^{\text{obs}} = 53.1 + \frac{123.9}{243.4} \left(Y_{i1}^{\text{obs}} - 65.1 \right)$$
$$= 53.1 + 0.51(60.9 - 65.1) = 51.0 \text{ for subject 12}$$
$$= 53.1 + 0.51(82.1 - 65.1) = 61.8 \text{ for subject 13}.$$

Note that because subject 13 had a much higher than average baseline value, the imputed value at 6 weeks is also higher. The equations for the remaining three subjects are messy and involve the inversion and multiplication of matrices. For subject 60:

$$\left[Y_{i3}^{*\text{mis}} \middle| \begin{array}{c} Y_{i1}^{*\text{obs}} \\ Y_{i2}^{*\text{obs}} \end{array} \right]$$

$$= X_{i3}^* \hat{\mathcal{B}}_3^* + [\hat{\sigma}_{31} \quad \hat{\sigma}_{32}] \begin{bmatrix} \hat{\sigma}_{11} & \hat{\sigma}_{12} \\ \hat{\sigma}_{21} & \hat{\sigma}_{22} \end{bmatrix}^{-1} \left(\begin{bmatrix} Y_{i1}^{*\text{obs}} \\ Y_{i2}^{*\text{obs}} \end{bmatrix} - \begin{bmatrix} X_{i1}^{*\text{obs}} \\ X_{i2}^{*\text{obs}} \end{bmatrix} \begin{bmatrix} \hat{\mathcal{B}}_1^* \\ \hat{\mathcal{B}}_2^* \end{bmatrix}' \right)$$

and for subjects 277 and 527:

$$\begin{bmatrix} Y_{i3}^{*\text{mis}} \\ Y_{i4}^{*\text{mis}} \end{bmatrix} \middle| \begin{bmatrix} Y_{i1}^{*\text{obs}} \\ Y_{i2}^{*\text{obs}} \end{bmatrix} = \begin{bmatrix} X_{i3}^{*\text{obs}} \\ X_{i4}^{*\text{obs}} \end{bmatrix} \begin{bmatrix} \hat{\mathcal{B}}_3^* \\ \hat{\mathcal{B}}_4^* \end{bmatrix}' + \begin{bmatrix} \hat{\sigma}_{31} & \hat{\sigma}_{32} \\ \hat{\sigma}_{41} & \hat{\sigma}_{42} \end{bmatrix} \begin{bmatrix} \hat{\sigma}_{11} & \hat{\sigma}_{12} \\ \hat{\sigma}_{21} & \hat{\sigma}_{22} \end{bmatrix}^{-1}$$
$$\times \left(\begin{bmatrix} Y_{i1}^{*\text{obs}} \\ Y_{i2}^{*\text{obs}} \end{bmatrix} - \begin{bmatrix} X_{i1}^{*\text{obs}} \\ X_{i2}^{*\text{obs}} \end{bmatrix} \begin{bmatrix} \hat{\mathcal{B}}_1^* \\ \hat{\mathcal{B}}_2^* \end{bmatrix}' \right).$$

The imputed values are easily obtained using existing software (e.g., SAS Proc Mixed). Note that in Table 6.5 the imputed values at 12 and 26 weeks reflect both the earlier death of subject 60 and the previously observed scores for all three subjects.

The entire distribution of observed scores and imputed scores, predicted by multivariate linear regression, is displayed in Figure 6.4. The same set of explanatory variables used to generate the data in Figure 6.3 was used to generate these values. However, the imputed values now include information about the patient's previous HRQoL. As a result, the distribution of the imputed values appears to be shifted down and the range of values has greatly expanded, but is still smaller than for the observed scores.

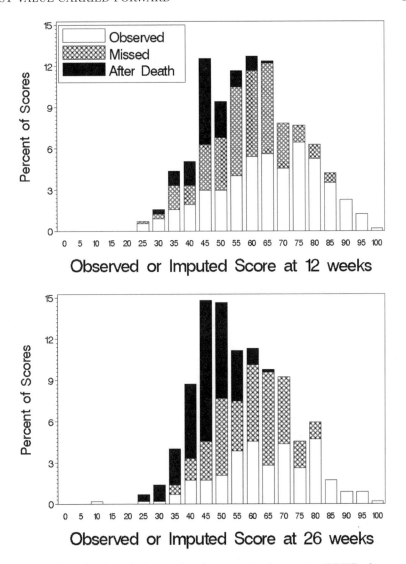

Figure 6.4. Distribution of observed and imputed values using BLUPs from a repeated measures model with baseline characteristics (treatment group, performance status, prior weight loss, symptoms of primary and systemic disease) and outcome (best response and death within 2 months).

6.4 Last value carried forward

Another popular approach is to use the last value (or observation) carried forward (LVCF or LOCF), where the patient's last available assessment is substituted for each of the subsequent missing assessments. Although analyses using LVCF are often reported, the authors rarely justify the use of LVCF or examine the pattern of change in HRQoL as a function of dropout [120].

Table 6.6. Simple imputation—LVCF.

No.	Taxol	Baseline	6 weeks	12 weeks	26 weeks	Months survival
12	No	**60.9**	*60.9*	X	X	2.5
13	No	**82.1**	*82.1*	X	X	2.7
60	Yes	**57.2**	**40.6**	*40.6*	X	3.6
527	Yes	**63.5**	**52.4**	*52.4*	*52.4*	7.2
277	Yes	**67.5**	**71.6**	*71.6*	*71.6*	7.8

Observed data are displayed in bold and imputed data in italics. NSCLC example.

This approach assumes that the last available response of a patient withdrawing from a study is the response that the patient would have if the patient had remained in the trial. The assumption that HRQoL does not change after dropout seems inappropriate in most studies. Thus, this approach has limited utility [60, 64, 94] and should be employed with great caution.

Consider a situation where treatment may be associated with toxicity, such as the study of adjuvant therapy for breast cancer previously described. In this study, most women reported poorer HRQoL during therapy than they were experiencing prior to therapy. Thus, carrying forward their previous baseline assessment would create an overly optimistic picture of the HRQoL of subjects on that treatment arm, giving a possible benefit to the therapy with more dropout. As a second example of possible misuse, consider a study where HRQoL is decreasing over time. In this situation, LVCF would make a treatment with early dropout appear better than a treatment where tolerance to the therapy was higher.

Table 6.6 displays the imputed values for the same five cases from the NSCLC study with the last value carried forward. In each of these cases, this value is greater than that imputed using information about response, survival, and prior HRQoL. The entire distribution of observed scores and imputed scores, using the LVCF, is displayed in Figure 6.5. Imputed scores cover the entire range of possible scores, with the distribution of imputed scores much closer to the observed scores than observed in Figure 6.4. In this trial, we are assuming that a patient's HRQoL is the same after dropout as when the patient completed the last assessment. In this particular setting, that does not seem to be a reasonable assumption.

δ-Adjustments

Diehr et al. [34] describe a variation on LVCF to address the problem of differences in HRQoL between individuals who were able to complete HRQoL assessments and those who were not. In the proposed procedure, a value k is subtracted from (or added to) the last observed value. If this value can be justified, then this approach is a useful option in a sensitivity analysis. In Diehr's example, a value of 15 points on the SF-36 physical function scale was proposed, where 15 points is justified as the difference in scores between

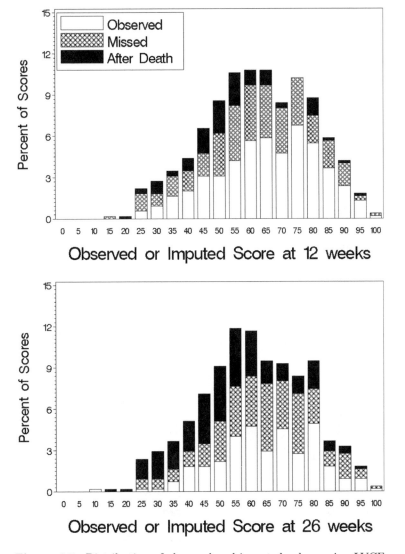

Figure 6.5. Distribution of observed and imputed values using LVCF.

individuals reporting their health as unchanged vs. those reporting worsening [157].

Arbitrary high or low value

Another example of simple imputation is the substitution of an arbitrary high or low value for the missing assessments. This is most commonly used when the missing HRQoL data are the result of an adverse event such as death [43, 120]. In some cases a value of 0 is used; in others a value just below the minimum of all observed scores is substituted for the missing data. Both approaches can be partially justified, but neither can be completely defended.

Table 6.7. Strategy for simple imputation of ranks. Assumes that all subjects who completed the study have an observed response (Y_i^{obs}) and all others are missing data.

	Outcome	N	Assumed value	Rank value
1	Died	n_1	$Y_i^{\text{mis}} = 0$	Lowest tied rank
2	Withdrawal due to lack of efficacy or toxicity	n_2	$0 < Y_i^{\text{mis}} < \min(Y_i^{\text{obs}})$	Next lowest tied rank
3	Completed study	n_3	Y_i^{obs}	R_i^{obs}
4	Withdrawal with cure	n_4	$\max(Y_i^{\text{obs}}) < Y_i^{\text{mis}}$	Highest tied rank
5	Withdrawal not related to toxicity or efficacy	n_5	Omitted	

Lowest tied rank = $\text{avg}(1,\ldots,n_1)$. Next lowest tied rank = $\text{avg}(n_1+1,\ldots,n_1+n_2)$. $R_i^{\text{obs}} = n_1 + n_2 + $ Rank of Y_i^{obs} among those who completed the study. Highest tied rank = $\text{avg}(n_1+n_2+n_3+1,\ldots,n_1+n_2+n_3+n_4)$.

One approach that avoids some of the controversy is an analysis based on the ranked HRQoL scores [43, 60, 120], for example, the Wilcoxon Rank Sum test. Gould [60] suggests classifying the subjects into four groups. The idea is extended to five groups in Table 6.7.

The strategy for imputing missing data has the advantage that one only has to assume a relative ordering of the HRQoL. For example, we are assuming that the HRQoL of subjects who died is poorer than of those that remain alive. However, even with this seemingly straightforward procedure, it is important to consider the assumptions very carefully. In practice it will not be easy to classify all dropouts into one of the three groups (2, 4, and 5) defined in Table 6.7. Heyting [64] and Pledger and Hall [114] describe situations where this strategy may not be appropriate. Also note that when a large proportion of the subjects expire, this approach becomes an approximation to the analysis of survival rather than an analysis of HRQoL.

6.5 Underestimation of variance

The major disadvantage of simple imputation techniques is the underestimation of the variance of the observations. There are several reasons for the underestimation. First, when we use means or predicted values, we are assuming that there is no variability among the missing observations (i.e., $\text{Var}[\epsilon_{hij}] = 0$). Second, we assume that we know the true mean or predicted value (i.e., $\text{Var}[\hat{\mu}] = 0$ or $\text{Var}[X\hat{\beta}] = 0$), when, in fact, we have estimated these values. Finally, we assume that we have observed the HRQoL of all subjects rather

Table 6.8. Naive estimation of standard deviation (S.D.) and standard error (S.E.) in the NSCLC study; 26-week estimates for survivors.

Imputation	Taxol	Observed (n)	Mean	S.D. $(\hat{\sigma})$	S.E. $\left(\frac{\hat{\sigma}}{\sqrt{n-1}}\right)$	Ratio[a] of S.E.
None	No	57	65.0	15.0	1.99	1.00
	Yes	134	64.8	15.7	1.36	1.00
Simple mean	No	125	65.0	10.1	0.90	0.45
	Yes	265	64.8	11.1	0.68	0.63
Covariates	No	125	62.8	11.3	1.01	0.51
	Yes	265	63.6	11.9	0.73	0.54
Conditional	No	125	61.1	13.1	1.18	0.59
	Yes	265	62.4	13.5	0.83	0.61
LVCF	No	121	63.9	15.9	1.45	0.73
	Yes	259	64.3	15.6	0.97	0.73

[a]Reference (denominator) is the standard error with no imputation.

than just a subset of the subjects. As a result, test statistics and confidence intervals based on a naive analysis of the observed and imputed data will not be valid.

This is illustrated in the NCSLC study. Consider the scores at 6 months (26 weeks); the estimated standard deviation of the observed data is roughly 15 to 16 points.

$$\hat{\sigma} = \sqrt{\sum_{i=1}^{n}(Y_{hij} - \bar{Y}_{hj})^2/(n-1)}. \qquad (6.11)$$

When we impute values for the missing data using the mean value of the observed data and use a naive estimate of the variance, we add nothing to the squared terms because $Y_{hij}^{\text{mis}} - \bar{Y}_{hj} = 0$, but we do increase the apparent number of observations. The effect of this is illustrated in Table 6.8, where the naive estimate of the standard deviation decreases by almost one third as we increase the apparent number of observations by about twofold. In the simple univariate case, the underestimation of the variance is roughly proportional to the amount of missing data. The naive estimate of the variance of y_i is

$$\hat{\sigma}^2 = \frac{\sum^{n^{\text{obs}}}(y_i^{\text{obs}} - \bar{y}_i^{\text{obs}})^2 + n^{\text{mis}}(\bar{y}_i^{\text{obs}} - \bar{y}_i^{\text{obs}})^2}{n^{\text{obs}} + n^{\text{mis}} - 1}$$

$$= \frac{(n^{\text{obs}} - 1)\hat{\sigma}_{\text{obs}}^2 + 0}{(n-1)} = \frac{n^{\text{obs}} - 1}{n-1}\hat{\sigma}_{\text{obs}}^2.$$

When $\hat{\sigma}_{\text{obs}}^2 \approx \sigma^2$, then $E[\hat{\sigma}^2] \approx n^{\text{obs}}/n\sigma^2$. The standard deviation is underestimated by a factor proportional to the square root of the amount of missing data. While it is straightforward to adjust the estimate of the variance using mean imputation, it becomes a much more difficult task for other imputation procedures.

The problem with the underestimation of the variance of the observations is compounded when we attempt to estimate the standard errors of means or regression parameters. This in turn affects test statistics and confidence intervals. For example, the naive estimate of the standard error of the mean (S.E.$(\hat{\mu}) = \sqrt{\hat{\sigma}^2/n}$) assumes that we have information on all n individuals rather than the n^{obs} individuals who completed the HRQoL assessments. In the 6-month estimates for survivors of the NSCLC study, we analyze a data set with 389 observations when only 191 subjects were observed. The effect is illustrated in Table 6.8, where the naive standard errors are roughly half the true standard errors. This makes a substantial difference in the test statistics. Consider a small difference of 3 points ($\frac{1}{5}$ S.D.) in the means of the two groups. With no imputation, the t-statistic for a test of differences is 1.24 ($p = 0.22$). With mean imputation, the t-statistic is 2.65 ($p = 0.008$), a highly significant difference. For the other simple imputation methods displayed in Table 6.8, the estimates of the standard deviations are biased for all approaches but LVCF, and the standard errors are biased toward zero for all approaches.

6.6 Sensitivity analysis

Despite the limitations of simple imputation, these methods are useful as part of a *limited* analysis of the sensitivity of results. Visual comparison of the means or medians is helpful, but comparisons of test statistics are inappropriate. Several authors have used simple imputation combined with nonparametric analysis to examine the sensitivity of their results to the assumptions made about the missing data. Raboud et al. [120] used this approach in a study of antimicrobial therapy in patients with HIV to demonstrate the sensitivity of estimates of treatment effects to different rates of dropout and survival. Fairclough et al. [43] demonstrated the consistency of their conclusions, in a clinical trial of adjuvant therapy for breast cancer, to the assumptions made about the missing data. The means displayed in Table 6.8 illustrate an example of such an analysis. The sensitivity of the results to these different methods of simple imputation should not be unexpected for a study with extensive dropout. Estimates of the means vary from 61.1 to 65.0 for patients not receiving Taxol and from 62.4 to 64.8 for those receiving Taxol. These differences are approximately $\frac{1}{4}$ of the standard deviation.

6.7 Summary

- The primary limitation of simple imputation is the underestimation of the variance of any estimate and the corresponding effect on any test statistic.
- Last value carried forward (LVCF), if used, should be well justified and any underlying assumptions verified. This approach will not be conservative in all cases and may, in some settings, bias the results in favor of a treatment that results in more dropout associated with morbidity.

CHAPTER 7

Multiple Imputation

7.1 Introduction

The major criticism of simple imputation methods is the underestimation of the variance (see previous chapter). Multiple imputation [125, 126] retains many of the advantages of single imputation but rectifies this problem. Multiple imputation of missing values will be worth the effort only if there is a substantial benefit that cannot be obtained using maximum likelihood methods for the analysis of incomplete data (Chapter 5). Two quotes summarize the issues:

> Multiple imputation is not a panacea. Although it is a powerful and useful tool applicable to many missing data settings, if not used carefully it is potentially dangerous. The existence of software that facilitates its use requires the analyst to be careful about the verification of assumptions, the robustness of imputation models, and the appropriateness of inferences. For more complicated models (e.g., longitudinal or clustered data) this is even more important. (Norton and Lipsitz [107])

> It is clear that if the imputation model is seriously flawed in terms of capturing the missing data mechanism, then so is any analysis based on such imputation. This problem can be avoided by carefully investigating each specific application, by making the best use of knowledge and data about the missing-data mechanism. (Barnard and Meng [4])

7.2 Overview of multiple imputation

The basic strategy of multiple imputation is to impute 3 to 20 sets of values for the missing data that incorporate both the variability of the HRQoL measure and the uncertainty about the missing observations. Each set of data is then analyzed using complete data methods and the results of the analyses are then combined. The general strategy is summarized in four steps:

Step 1: Selection of the imputation procedure

Although the least technical, selection of an appropriate imputation procedure is the most difficult step. There is a variety of implicit and explicit methods that can be used for multiple imputation [125]. Explicit methods generally utilize regression models, whereas implicit methods utilize sampling techniques. Four specific examples of these strategies are described in the subsequent sections.

There are three desirable properties of an imputation procedure. The first objective is that it produce unbiased estimates. This is particularly difficult when there is a suspicion that the missingness depends on the HRQoL of the individual at the time the observation was to be made (MNAR). Second, the procedure should incorporate the appropriate variation to reflect the randomness of the observations, the loss of information due to the missing observations, and the uncertainty about the reason for nonresponse. Finally, the procedure should not distort the covariance structure of the repeated measurements in longitudinal studies, especially when the analyses involve estimation of changes in HRQoL over time. The challenge is to select an appropriate model and fully understand the assumptions that are being made when that model is implemented. This is the focus of the subsequent sections.

Step 2: Generation of M imputed data sets

Once the model and procedure for imputing the missing observations are selected, the details for implementing the procedure are generally well worked out (see Sections 7.3 through 7.5). One of the questions often asked is, "How many datasets should be imputed?" There is no straightforward answer. The recommendations generally range from 3 to 10. As the proportion of missing data increases, the between imputation variance will increase (see Section 7.7) and will become more important in the calculation of the overall variance. Increasing the number of imputed data sets (M) will improve the precision of this estimate. Imputing more rather than fewer (10 or 20) data sets is recommended, as the additional time required is a trivial part of the entire analytic effort with modern computing power.

Step 3: Analysis of M data sets

Each of the M data sets is then analyzed using either complete data or maximum likelihood methods such as MANOVA or mixed-effects models. In this step, estimates of the primary parameters ($\hat{\beta}^{(m)}$) and their variance (Var[$\hat{\beta}^{(m)}$]) are obtained for each of the M complete data sets. Step 3 is often expanded to include hypothesis testing (H_0: $\theta = C\beta = 0$) with the estimation of secondary parameters ($\hat{\theta}^{(m)} = C\hat{\beta}^{(m)}$) and their variance (Var[$\hat{\theta}^{(m)}$]).

Step 4: Combining results of M analyses

The results of the M analyses are then combined by averaging the parameter estimates from each of the M data sets. Finally, the variance of these estimates is computed by combining within and between components of the variance of the estimates from the M data sets. As is shown later, it is the combination of the imputation procedures and the computation of the variance estimates that results in the appropriate estimates of variance. Full details for this procedure are presented in Section 7.7.

7.3 Explicit univariate regression

In the explicit regression model approach to multiple imputation, we identify a regression model to predict the missing observation. This is basically the same model that is used for the simple imputation procedure described in the previous chapter. However, the multiple imputation procedure differs in two ways. First, because the true parameters of the imputation model are unknown, random error is added to the estimated parameters ($\hat{\mathcal{B}}^*$).* These new values of the parameters ($\beta^{(m)}$) are then used to predict the average HRQoL for a subject with specific characteristics defined by the covariates ($X^{*(\text{mis})}$). Then, additional random error is added to these values to reflect the natural variability of the individual outcome measures ($\text{Var}[Y_i]$).

Analytic model: $\quad Y_i = X_i \beta + \epsilon_i$

Imputation model: $\quad Y_i^{*\text{obs}} = X_i^{*\text{obs}} \mathcal{B}^* + \varepsilon_i^*$

Identification of the imputation model

The explicit regression approach has the advantage that the regression model used to impute missing observations can readily use auxiliary information about the subject's HRQoL that could not be included in the model used for the ultimate analysis of the clinical trial. This additional information might include indicators of the side effects of treatment and the clinical course of the disease when the therapy succeeds or fails. Alternatively, it could include measures of HRQoL provided by a caregiver when the subject is no longer able to complete self-assessments.

Recall that one of the objectives of imputation is to obtain unbiased estimates of the missing observations. In the context of the explicit regression approach, we are looking for a model where the missingness in the imputation model depends only on the observed data included in the imputation model (Y_i^*) and the covariates in the imputation model (X_i^*). Basically, we are attempting to augment the analytic model with auxiliary outcome data (Y_i^*) or covariates (X_i^*), so that the MAR assumption in the imputation model seems reasonable. The primary candidates for covariates include measures that are strongly correlated with both the measure being imputed and the probability that it is missing. In the NSCLC example, this suggests adding covariates associated with toxicity, disease progression, and the proximity of the patient to death. Assuming that the objective of the analysis is the comparison of treatment groups, the same strategy outlined in Section 6.2 is recommended for identification of the imputation model. To avoid biasing the comparison of treatment groups toward the null hypothesis, it is critical that imputation of

---

* We use the superscript asterisk to differentiate the imputation model from the analytic model.

postrandomization data either be done separately for each treatment group or include treatment as a covariate.

Computation of imputed values

The general procedure for imputing M sets of missing values for univariate data is as follows [21, 94, 126]:

1. Estimate the parameters of the regression model ($Y_i^{*\text{obs}} = X_i^{*\text{obs}} \mathcal{B}^* + \epsilon_i^*$) using the observed data.

$$\hat{\mathcal{B}}^* = \left(\sum X_i'^{*\text{obs}} X_i^{*\text{obs}}\right)^{-1} \sum X_i'^{*\text{obs}} Y_i^{*\text{obs}}, \qquad (7.1)$$

$$\hat{\sigma}^{*2} = \sum (Y_i^{*\text{obs}} - \hat{\mathcal{B}}^* X_i^{*\text{obs}})^2 / (n^{\text{obs}} - p^*), \qquad (7.2)$$

where p^* is the number of unknown parameters in $\mathcal{B}^*$.

2. Generate M sets of model parameters ($\beta^{(m)}$ and $\sigma^{2(m)}$) by adding random error to the estimates reflecting the uncertainty of the estimates.

$$\sigma^{2(m)} = \hat{\sigma}^{2*} \times (n^{obs} - p^*) / \mathcal{K}^{(m)}, \qquad (7.3)$$

$$U_\beta' U_\beta = \text{Var}[\hat{\mathcal{B}}^*] = \sigma^{2(m)} \left(\sum X_i'^{*\text{obs}} X_i^{*\text{obs}}\right)^{-1}, \qquad (7.4)$$

$$\beta^{(m)} = \hat{\beta}^* + U_\beta \mathcal{Z}_\beta^m, \qquad (7.5)$$

where
$\mathcal{K}^{(m)}$ = a randomly drawn number from a χ-square distribution with $n^{\text{obs}} - p^*$ degrees of freedom
U_β = the upper triangular matrix of the Cholesky decomposition of the variance of $\hat{\mathcal{B}}^*$
$\mathcal{Z}_\beta^{(m)}$ = a vector of p^* random numbers drawn from a standard normal distribution

The Cholesky decomposition is also referred to as the square root method. In this procedure, we have assumed that the parameters have a normal distribution with variance approximately equal to $\sigma^2 (\sum X_i'^{*\text{obs}} X_i^{*\text{obs}})^{-1}$. This is a reasonable assumption for large studies but may not be valid for smaller studies. When there is concern about these assumptions, more complex methods of generating these parameters are required [129].

3. Generate the imputed values of Y_i^{mis}, for the mth imputation, by adding random error corresponding to the between- and within-subject variability of the outcome ($\text{Var}[Y_i] = \hat{\sigma}^{*2}$).

$$Y_i^{\text{mis}(m)} = X_i^{\text{mis}} \beta^{(m)} + \sigma^{(m)} \mathcal{Z}_Y^{(m)}, \qquad (7.6)$$

where $\mathcal{Z}_Y^{(m)}$ is a random number drawn from a standard normal distribution.

4. The second and third steps are repeated for each of the M data sets.

Practical considerations

There are two major barriers to implementing this procedure. The first is a small sample size. The second is the lack of strong predictors of the HRQoL measure. When the sample size is small, the analyst is unable to obtain precise estimates of the imputation model parameters ($\hat{\mathcal{B}}^*$). This will result in a wide range of values of $\beta^{(m)}$. Thus, the imputed values may only add noise to the observed data. The lack of strong predictors will have similar consequences. If the variation in the outcome explained by the imputation model is small (the R^2 is small), the values of $\sigma^{2(m)}$ will be large and, again, the imputed values may only add noise to the observed data. An additional nuisance associated with both problems is that some of the predicted values may lie outside the possible range of values of the HRQoL scale.

The above description of the procedure for identifying the imputation model does not specify a cutoff for the significance of potential covariates. This aspect of the model-fitting procedure is as much art as it is science. Adding more covariates to the imputation model will improve the procedure by increasing the R^2 and reducing $\sigma^{2(m)}$, thus decreasing the statistical noise added in Equation 7.6. However, this is balanced by adding parameters with large variance and increasing the statistical noise added in Equation 7.5. Thus, adding covariates that result in small increases in the R^2 is unlikely to improve the imputation procedure, even when the statistical significance of a particular parameter is large.

Extensions to longitudinal studies

The above procedure was developed for cross-sectional studies. However, in most clinical trials HRQoL is measured longitudinally. Little and Yau [94] suggest a sequential procedure for a monotone missing data pattern. The procedure is first to fill in the missing values of the first observation (Y_{i1}), generating M sets of data for the first observation (Equation 7.7). The second step is to fill in the missing values of the second observation (Y_{i2}), given the observed (Y_{i1}) or imputed values ($Y_{i1}^{(m)}$) of the first observation (Y_{i1}). Note that in this step, only one set of new values is generated for each of the M data sets. Subsequent missing values are imputed using all previously observed and imputed data (Equations 7.8 and 7.9). The imputation models at each step are

$$Y_{i1}^{*\text{obs}} = X_{i1}^{*\text{obs}} \beta_1^* + \varepsilon_{i1}^*, \tag{7.7}$$

$$Y_{i2}^{*\text{obs}} = X_{i2}^{*\text{obs}} \beta_2^{*(m)} + Y_{i1}^{(m)} \beta_{2|1}^{*(m)} + \varepsilon_{i2}^*, \tag{7.8}$$

$$Y_{i3}^{*\text{obs}} = X_{i3}^{*\text{obs}} \beta_3^{*(m)} + Y_{i1}^{(m)} \beta_{3|1}^{*(m)} + Y_{i2}^{(m)} \beta_{3|2}^{*(m)} + \varepsilon_{i3}^*. \tag{7.9}$$

Assumptions

When we impute the missing observations using this model, we are making at least two assumptions that are not testable. First, we are assuming that the relationship between the explanatory variables and HRQoL is the same when individuals complete the HRQoL assessments and when they do not complete the assessments. Basically, we are assuming that $Y_i^{*\text{obs}} = X_i^{*\text{obs}} \mathcal{B}^* + \varepsilon_i$ and $Y_i^{*\text{mis}} = X_i^{*\text{mis}} \mathcal{B}^* + \varepsilon_i$ are both true. Second, we are assuming that we have identified *all* the important relevant covariates such that the missingness no longer depends on the missing HRQoL value (Y_i^{mis}). As previously mentioned, we have no way formally to test the assumption that the missing data are MAR, given the observed data ($Y_i^{*\text{obs}}$) and covariates in the imputation model ($X_i^{*\text{obs}}$).

Less critical assumptions in this procedure are that the residual errors (ε_i^*) and the parameter estimates ($\hat{\mathcal{B}}^*$) of the imputation model are normally distributed. The first assumption can be assessed by examining the residual errors (ε_i^*), and the second is true for studies with moderate sample sizes.

NSCLC example

Although the procedure described above sounds straightforward, one quickly realizes that there are many choices to be made. One issue is how to handle the small proportion of subjects with nonmonotone missing data patterns. In the following example, we have ignored later observations rather than excluded these individuals from the analysis. A second choice is whether to run the imputation procedures separately for each treatment group or to include treatment as a covariate in all imputation models. By taking the second option, we run the risk of missing a potential interaction between one of the covariates and treatment but gain precision in the estimation of the parameters when the relationships are the same in each treatment group. This later advantage is more important when the sample size is small. Another decision is how to handle imputed values that are out of the range of the scale. As will be demonstrated later, this is a very minor issue and does not affect the results.

The covariate (X_{ij}^*) selection process had three steps. The first was to identify potential variables. This selection was made on a conceptual basis and summarized in Table 7.1. For example, treatment assignment should not have any impact on the baseline scores if patients did not know their treatment assignment prior to completing the FACT-Lung questionnaire. Similarly, treatment outcomes were not considered as predictors of the baseline scores but were considered for all follow-up assessments. Potential covariates with more than 5% missing data were not considered. The second step was to eliminate variables where the correlation with the TOI scores was weaker ($p > 0.001$). Finally, a backward elimination procedure was used with multivariate regression where the selection criterion was set at $\alpha = 0.01$. Because the intent of the final analysis is to compare the treatment groups, the treatment indicator (TAXOL) was forced into all imputation models even though it was nonsignificant. Previously imputed values from the first set of imputed values ($m = 1$) were included in these regression analyses. The variables excluded in this third step would have explained only 1 to 2% more variation. The resulting

Table 7.1. Covariate selection for multiple imputation with sequential univariate regression models.

Potential	Assessment no.			
covariate	1	2	3	4
Taxol		X	X	X
Age	−	−	−	−
Gender	−	−	−	−
Performance status	+	−	−	−
Weight loss	+	−	−	−
Prior radiotherapy	−	−	−	−
Primary disease symptoms	+	−	−	−
Metastatic disease symptoms	−	−	−	−
Systemic symptoms	+	−	−	−
Associated chronic diseases	−	−	−	−
Baseline TOI score		+	−	+
6-week TOI score			+	−
12-week TOI score				+
Cycles of therapy		−	−	−
Complete or partial response		−	+	−
Hemotological toxicity		−	−	−
Neurological toxicity		−	−	−
Withdrawal due to progressive disease		−	−	−
Survival (log transformation)		+	+	+
R^2	0.19	0.32	0.35	0.34

X indicates forced into model; − indicates tested but not included; + indicates included.

R^2 values, summarized in Table 7.1, explain a moderate amount of the variation in FACT-Lung TOI scores.

SAS Versions 8.1 and 8.2 have an experimental procedure (`Proc MI`) that can be used to implement this series of imputations. Because the dropout pattern is not strictly monotone and the covariates differ over time, a series of imputations will be necessary. The first step is to create a data set (`WORK.ONEREC`) with one record per subject containing the four possible FACT-Lung TOI scores (`TOI1, TOI2, TOI3, TOI4`) and the covariates to be used in the MI procedure. Next, the missing values for the baseline assessment (`TOI`) are imputed with the selected baseline covariates (`WT_LOSS ECOGPS SX_SYS SX_PRI`). The MI procedure with a `MONOTONE METHOD=REGRESSION;` statement sequentially imputes missing data using

$$Y_j = \beta_0 + \beta_1 Y_1 + \cdots + \beta_{j-1} Y_{j-1}$$

for the $Y_1, \ldots, Y_j$ identified in the `VAR` statement, with the restriction that the missing data pattern is monotone among the variables for the order specified.

```
PROC MI DATA=WORK.ONEREC OUT=WORK.MIDATA1 NIMPUTE=20;
  MONOTONE METHOD=REGRESSION;
  VAR WT_LOSS ECOGPS SX_SYS SX_PRI TOI1;
  RUN;
```

This creates a new data set with 20 sets of imputed values for missing baseline assessments. In the following steps we are going to use separate models for each of the two treatment groups. We will use imputed missing baseline values (TOI1) in the imputation model for the 6-week values (TOI2), imputed 6-week values (TOI2) in the imputation model for the 12-week data (TOI3), etc. To do this we are going to rename the variable that identifies these 20 sets from _IMPUTATION_ to _M_ and sort the data by imputation number and treatment group.

```
PROC SORT DATA=WORK.MIDATA1
          OUT=WORK.MIDATA2(RENAME=(_IMPUTATION_=_M_);
  BY _IMPUTATION_ TAXOL;
  RUN;
```

From this point on, we are going to impute only one set of values for each of the 20 sets generated in the first step using the log of the survival times (LN_SURV), best response (CRPR), and previous FACT-Lung TOI scores as explanatory variables.

```
PROC MI DATA=WORK.MIDATA2 OUT=WORK.MIDATA3 NIMPUTE=1;
  BY _M_ TAXOL;
  MONOTONE METHOD=REGRESSION;
  VAR LN_SURV TOI1 TOI2;
  RUN;
PROC MI DATA=WORK.MIDATA3 OUT=WORK.MIDATA4 NIMPUTE=1;
  BY _M_ TAXOL;
  MONOTONE METHOD=REGRESSION;
  VAR LN_SURV CRPR TOI1 TOI2 TOI3;
  RUN;
PROC MI DATA=WORK.MIDATA4 OUT=WORK.MIDATA5 NIMPUTE=1;
  BY _M_ TAXOL;
  MONOTONE METHOD=REGRESSION;
  VAR LN_SURV TOI1 TOI2 TOI3 TOI4;
  RUN;
```

Figure 7.1 displays the observed and imputed scores at the third and fourth assessment. As expected in this study, the distribution of the imputed scores is lower than the observed scores. A very small proportion, less than 0.1%, of the scores lie outside of the possible range of 0 to 100. Low values (<0) represent 0.01, 0.03, 0.16, and 1.84% of the scores at each of the four assessments. High values (>100) represent 0.14, 0.22, 0.19, and 0.26% of the scores, respectively. Even when these out-of-range scores are replaced with 0 and 100, there is little impact on the overall distribution of scores (Figure 7.1) or on the results of the analysis of the imputed data sets (Table 7.2).

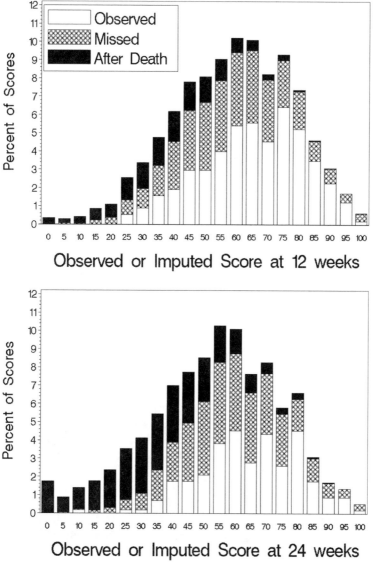

Figure 7.1. Distribution of observed and multiply imputed values generated with sequential univariate regression.

A more difficult decision is how to handle the observations that would have occurred after the death of the patients. There is considerable controversy about imputing HRQoL scores after the patient has died. I am not going to attempt to resolve the existential question about rating the quality of life after death. I would like to point out the statistical implications of not using imputed values after death in the analyses. When observations occurring after death are missing, we assume that the data are MAR and that HRQoL in the

Table 7.2. Results of the sequential univariate MI procedures ($M = 20$).

Estimate	Taxol	Out-of-range not replaced		Out-of-range replaced		After death excluded	
		Mean	(S.E.)	Mean	(S.E.)	Mean	(S.E.)
Baseline	No	64.8	(1.2)	64.8	(1.2)	64.8	(1.2)
	Yes	66.1	(0.9)	66.1	(0.9)	66.1	(0.9)
6 weeks	No	59.7	(1.6)	59.7	(1.6)	60.7	(1.6)
	Yes	62.8	(1.1)	62.8	(1.1)	63.7	(1.0)
12 weeks	No	58.0	(1.6)	58.0	(1.7)	60.1	(1.6)
	Yes	59.9	(1.5)	59.9	(1.4)	61.8	(1.2)
26 weeks	No	50.9	(2.9)	51.0	(2.8)	57.2	(2.0)
	Yes	54.0	(2.3)	54.2	(2.0)	59.8	(1.3)
6-week change	No	−5.1	(1.6)	−5.1	(1.6)	−4.1	(1.6)
	Yes	−3.3	(1.1)	−3.3	(1.0)	−2.3	(1.0)
	Diff	1.8	(1.7)	1.8	(1.7)	1.8	(1.7)
12-week change	No	−6.8	(1.8)	−6.8	(1.8)	−4.7	(1.6)
	Yes	−6.2	(1.6)	−6.1	(1.5)	−4.2	(1.3)
	Diff	0.7	(2.1)	0.7	(2.1)	0.5	(2.0)
26-week change	No	−13.9	(3.0)	−13.8	(2.9)	−7.6	(2.1)
	Yes	−12.0	(2.3)	−11.8	(2.1)	−6.3	(1.3)
	Diff	1.8	(2.7)	1.9	(2.6)	1.3	(2.5)

patient who has died is similar to HRQoL in the survivors (conditional on the observed scores). As discussed in Chapter 5, values used in the E-step of the EM algorithm are imputed using the BLUPs. In Figure 7.2A, the average estimates of the observed and imputed data are displayed by the time of death (<6 weeks, 6 to 12 weeks, 12 to 24 weeks, >24 weeks). The averages decline over time, more quickly in patients who die earlier. Figure 7.2B displays the corresponding estimates where observations after death are replaced by the BLUPs generated by the MIXED procedure, with FACT-Lung TOI scores after death set to missing. Regardless of whether the decision is to include or exclude the imputed values after death, plots similar to Figures 7.2A and B are essential to the interpretation of the results.

7.4 Closest neighbor and predictive mean matching

There are many variations on the explicit regression model approach to multiple imputation. Both closest neighbor [126, 153] and predictive mean matching [63, 125] have the advantage that it is not possible to impute a value that is out of range for the HRQoL scale. They are also more likely to be robust to deviations from the normality assumptions. But the more critical assumption is that of equivalent models for subjects with observed data and subjects with missing data.

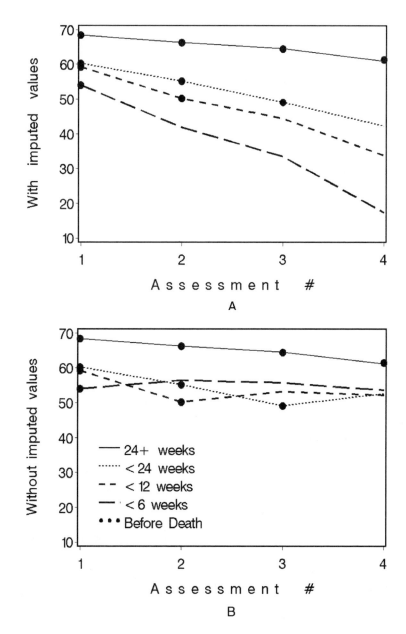

Figure 7.2. Average FACT TOI scores by time of death. (A) Estimates include imputed values after death; (B) estimates include BLUP for values after death.

Closest neighbor

The initial steps for the closest neighbor procedure are the same as those for the explicit regression procedure. M sets of parameter estimates for the imputation model are generated as previously described (Equations 7.1 through 7.5). The difference is in the third step.

3. Predicted values are generated for subjects with both observed and missing data:

$$E\bigl[Y_i^{\mathrm{obs}(m)}\bigr] = X_i^{\mathrm{obs}} \beta^{(m)}, \qquad (7.10)$$

$$E\bigl[Y_{i'}^{\mathrm{mis}(m)}\bigr] = X_{i'}^{\mathrm{mis}} \beta^{(m)}. \qquad (7.11)$$

4. For each subject (i') with a missing observation, the subject with the closest predicted value, $E[Y_i^{\mathrm{obs}(m)}]$, is selected and that subject's actual observed value, Y_i^{obs}, is the imputed value for subject i'.

5. Repeat steps 2 to 4 for M data sets.

Predictive mean matching

1. In the initial step of predictive mean matching [63, 125], M bootstrap samples are generated from the subjects with observed data. This consists of sampling N^{obs} subjects at random with replacement.

2. The parameters of the imputation model ($\hat{\beta}^{(m)}$) are then estimated within each of the M samples.

3. Predicted values are generated for both the cases with observed data and the cases with missing data (Equations 7.10 and 7.11).

4. The five nearest matches among the subjects with observed data are identified for each subject with missing data and one of the five is selected at random. The observed value of the HRQoL measure from that subject is the imputed value.

7.5 Approximate Bayesian bootstrap

An alternative to explicit model-based imputation is implicit or sampling-based imputation. One commonly used method is approximate Bayesian bootstrap (ABB). This was proposed initially for ignorable missing data from simple random samples [125–127]. The basic concept is first to draw a set of *potential* responses, at random with replacement, from a subset of subjects with the same characteristics (X^*). In the second step, the imputed values are drawn from the set of potential responses. This double sampling ensures proper variation of the responses [127], assuming large enough sets of subjects with the same set of covariates.*

---

* The alternative procedure, simple hot-deck imputation, of simply drawing the imputed values from the set of observed values does not properly reflect sampling variability [125].

Table 7.3. ABB imputation for a bivariate response (Y) with a dichotomous covariate (X) with a monotone missing data pattern.

Subject(i)	X_i	Y_{i1}	Y_{i2}
1	A	1	1
2	A	1	0
3	A	0	0
4	B	1	1
5	B	1	(1, 1)
6	B	2	1
7	B	2	2
8	B	(1, 2)	(1, 2)

The two sets ($M = 2$) of imputed values are indicated as (*,*).

The basic procedure

To illustrate the procedure, consider the following simple example with a bivariate response (Y_1, Y_2), a dichotomous covariate and monotone missing data pattern (Table 7.3). Two subjects have missing observations. Both outcomes are missing for subject 8 and the second is missing for subject 5. For purposes of illustration, we will let $M = 2$.

1. Impute M values of the first response variable for all subjects with missing values (Y_{81} in our example) matching on the covariate X.

   a. Draw n_{obs} values from the n_{obs} subjects with observed data for the first response and matching covariates. There is a pool of four potential subjects (4, 5, 6, and 7) with matching values of the covariate for subject 8. For the first imputation, draw four values of Y_1 at random with replacement from the responses for those four subjects (e.g., 1, 1, 1, 2).
   b. Draw a single value (e.g., 1) randomly from that set of potential values.
   c. Repeat the same procedure M times. In our example, the second potential set of values may consist of 1, 2, 2, 1 and the value 2 is drawn from that set.

2. Impute values for subjects who are missing the second response variable (y_{52} and y_{82}), using the original data set with $y_{81} = 1$ for the first imputation and then with $y_{81} = 2$ for the second imputation. In the first imputation, subject 4 is the only possible subject with $X = B, Y_1 = 1$ to impute the values of y_{52} and y_{82}. In the second imputation, subject 4 is still the only possible subject with $X = B, Y_1 = 1$ to impute y_{52}, whereas subjects 6 and 7 are possible donors for y_{82}.

More formally, the procedure is as follows. Consider a set of n subjects with the same values of X, where a univariate outcome was observed for n_{obs} and missing for n_{mis} subjects ($n = n_{obs} + n_{mis}$). For $m = 1, \ldots, M$, first randomly select a set of n_{obs} possible values with replacement from the n_{obs} values.

Then choose n_{mis} observations at random with replacement from each of the M potential samples.

Extensions to longitudinal studies

This procedure can be extended to situations where there are multiple measurements $(Y_1, \ldots, Y_J)$ with a monotone missing data pattern. The assumption is that the values of Y_j are missing at random conditional on X and $Y_1, \ldots, Y_{j-1}$. After imputing M sets of values for the first measurement (Y_1), subjects are grouped by both X and Y_1. Within these groups, a possible sample of n_{obs} observations of Y_2 is randomly selected from which the n_{mis} imputed values are randomly selected. This procedure is repeated for each subsequent measure for each of the M sets of imputations. Although this extension is theoretically possible, the practical limitations quickly become apparent. With each step to impute missing values of Y_k, the possible combinations of X and $Y_1, \ldots, Y_{j-1}$ increase so that ultimately there are insufficient subjects with a particular combination to provide an adequate sample. When Y_1 is continuous, the possible combinations of X and Y_1 can be extremely large, and it will not be possible to impute values of Y_2 using this procedure without some modifications.

Propensity scores

In the previously described procedure, the first step was to identify patient strata with increasing likelihood for missing observations. These strata could be defined by one or two patient characteristics as well as the previously observed HRQoL measures. In the NSCLC study, tumor responses, length of survival, cycles completed, and progressive disease during therapy are possible candidates. As noted above, the number of strata becomes unmanageable when the number of characteristics used to define the strata increases or if the characteristics are continuous.

To solve this problem, Lavori et al. [84] propose a strategy based on a *propensity score* for the probability of dropout. The idea is to find a univariate score that summarizes the multiple variables defining the history of each patient, stratify patients based on that score, and then use ABB to impute the missing values within each stratum. In this approach, a logistic model is used to estimate the probability of a missing assessment, which can be a function of multiple covariates and previously observed and imputed HRQoL scores. Strata are then formed on the basis of quintiles or quartiles of the predicted probability of a missing observation.

Practical issues

Although the procedure sounds straightforward, there are a number of challenges in the implementation of this procedure for HRQoL in longitudinal studies. Again, the sample size needs to be large enough to implement the procedure. To guard against biasing the results toward the null hypothesis, the imputation procedures must be done within treatment groups when the objective of the subsequent analysis is to compare treatment groups. Within the treatment groups, it may become necessary to reduce the number of strata when the stratum with the highest propensity for missing data has too few observed values.

In many studies, the missing data pattern will not be strictly monotone as was the case for the study described by Lavori et al. [84]. In the NSCLC example, approximately 15% of the cases have a missing assessment followed by an observed assessment. One option is not to impute values for these missing data. If documentation of the reasons for missing observations indicates that this is a random event, such as an administrative error, then this is a reasonable strategy. Because we now have readily available software for longitudinal analyses that will not exclude these subjects, it is not necessary to impute every value. The other option is to ignore the subsequent observations when imputing the missing data. This is a preferable strategy if these intermittent missing values tend to be associated with episodes of acute toxicity or other conditions likely to impact HRQoL.

The assumptions

The critical assumption of the ABB procedure is that the data are *missing at random* conditional on a set of covariates (X) and previously observed values of the outcome. However, when the propensity scores are used to define strata, the missing data are assumed to occur *completely at random* within the strata defined by the propensity score. This is a strong assumption that is difficult to justify for HRQoL studies where there is a strong association between missing data and clinical outcomes. Increasing the number of strata defined by the propensity scores would improve the likelihood that this assumption is correct. But this may also result in strata with too few subjects available for drawing the imputed values.

Another limitation occurs when estimates of longitudinal change are of interest. The ABB procedure with propensity scores uses only the information about the association of patient characteristics and previous HRQoL with whether the HRQoL values are missing. It does not use any information about the correlation among the variables. Thus, it is useful when the intent of the analysis is to make cross-sectional comparisons among groups, but it is not appropriate for the estimation of change over time. Similarly, if missing values of covariates are imputed with this approach, then the relationship between the covariate and the outcome may be underestimated.

Nonignorable missing data

To deal with nonignorable missing data, Rubin and Schenker [127] suggest independent draws of the n_{obs} possible values, where the probability of sampling an observation is proportional to some function of Y (e.g., Y^2 or $\sqrt{Y}$) to increase the proportion of large or small values of Y. Another approach that would increase the probability of drawing a smaller (or larger) value to replace the missing observation is to randomly draw k (usually 2 or 3) observations and take the minimum (or maximum) of the k draws. VanBuuren et al. [153] suggest a *delta-adjustment* where a predetermined constant is subtracted from the imputed value. Unfortunately, the difficult choice among these possible approaches cannot be made on the basis of the observed data or any statistical tests. In practice, testing a range of choices as part of a sensitivity analysis is appropriate.

7.6 Multivariate procedures for nonmonotone missing data

To this point, we have discussed methods for monotone missing data patterns. The Markov Chain Monte Carlo (MCMC) method was adapted to handle the more complex problem of nonmonotone patterns. Extending the univariate regression methods described in Section 7.3 to the multivariate setting requires the generation of random numbers for multidimensional and often intractable probability distributions. The MCMC method simulates the joint posterior distribution, assuming the data are from a multivariate normal distribution. A detailed description of this method is beyond the scope of this book, and the interested reader is referred to Schafer [129].

NSCLC example

Following the same logic as in Section 7.3, we will use separate imputation models for the missing baseline and follow-up data. The imputation of the missing baseline data is exactly the same as before. In contrast to the previous procedure, where the follow-up assessments were imputed in three steps, one single step is used to impute missing scores for TOI2, TOI3, TOI4 with the MCMC procedure, including the log transform of the survival time (LN_SURV), an indicator of a complete or partial response (CRPR), and the baseline scores (TOI1). One of the variables in this application is dichotomous and thus does not have a normal distribution. However, in moderately large data sets when dichotomous (and other non-normal) variables are included as an explanatory variable rather than one of the variables to be imputed, the consequences of violating the multivariate normal assumptions will be minimal. When transformations are possible (such as for the survival times), they should be utilized.

```
PROC MI DATA=WORK.MIDATA2 OUT=WORK.MIDATA5 NIMPUTE=1;
  BY _M_ TAXOL;
  MCMC;
  VAR LN_SURV CRPR TOI1 TOI2 TOI3 TOI4;
  RUN;
```

The distribution of the resulting data and the estimates are almost identical to those displayed in Figures 7.1 and 7.2.

7.7 Combining the M analyses

For each of the imputed data sets, the parameter estimates and their variance are computed using an appropriate analytic method (Table 7.4). In addition, linear combinations of the parameters ($\hat{\theta}^{(m)} = C\hat{\beta}^{(m)}$), which will be used to test specific hypotheses (for example, $H_0\colon \hat{\theta}^{(m)} = 0$) and the corresponding variance ($U_\theta^{(m)} = \text{Var}(\hat{\theta}^{(m)})$), may be estimated using each of the M data sets. The combined parameter estimates ($\bar{\beta}$ and $\bar{\theta}$) are obtained by averaging the M within-imputation estimates ($\hat{\beta}^{(m)}$ and $\hat{\theta}^{(m)}$). The total variance of the parameter estimates incorporates both the average within imputation variance of the estimates ($\bar{U}_\beta$ and $\bar{U}_\theta$) and the between imputation variability of the M estimates (B_β and B_θ). The total variance is computed by the sum of the within-imputation component ($\bar{U}$) and the between-imputation component (B) weighted by a correction for a finite number of imputations $(1 + M^{-1})$.

The fraction of information about the parameters that is missing due to nonresponse (γ) for each parameter can be estimated from the ratio of the between-imputation variance to the total variance. As the amount of missing data increases, γ increases. In contrast, as the amount of information about the missing data in the covariates of the imputation model increases, γ decreases.

Table 7.4. Computations for combining the analyses of the M data sets.

Within imputation	
Estimates	$\hat{\beta}^{(m)}$
Variance of estimates	$U_\beta^{(m)} = \text{Var}(\hat{\beta}^{(m)})$
Between imputation	
Variance between estimates	$B_\beta = \frac{1}{M-1}\sum_{m=1}^{M}(\hat{\beta}^{(m)} - \bar{\beta})^2$
Pooled analyses	
Pooled estimates	$\bar{\beta} = \sum_{m=1}^{M}\hat{\beta}^{(m)}/M$
Pooled within imputation variance	$\bar{U}_\beta = \sum_{m=1}^{M}U_\beta^{(m)})/M$
Total variance	$V_\beta = \bar{U}_\beta + (1+\frac{1}{M})B_\beta$
Miscellaneous	
Between to within variance ratio	$r_\beta = (1+M^{-1})B_\beta/\bar{U}_\beta$
Fraction of missing information[a]	$\gamma_\beta = (1+M^{-1})B_\beta/V_\beta$
Univariate test statistics and confidence intervals	
Degrees of freedom[b]	$\nu_\beta = (M-1)(1+r_\beta^{-1})^2$
t-statistic	$t_\beta = \bar{\beta}/V_\beta^{1/2} \sim t_{\nu_\beta}$
$100(1-\alpha)\%$ interval	$\bar{\beta} \pm t_{\nu_\beta,(1-\alpha/2)}V_\beta^{1/2}$

[a]Fraction of information about β (or θ) that is missing due to nonresponse ($\gamma = r/(1+r)$).

For tests with a single degree of freedom (θ is scalar), confidence interval estimates and significance levels can be obtained using a t-distribution with ν degrees of freedom [125, 126]. For tests with multiple degrees of freedom (θ is a $k \times 1$ vector of linear contrasts), significance levels can be obtained using the multivariate analogue [127]. The statistic

$$F = (\theta_0 - \bar{\theta})' U_\theta^{-1} (\theta_0 - \bar{\theta}) / [(1+r)k] \tag{7.12}$$

has an approximate F distribution with ν_1 and ν_2 degrees of freedom. $\nu_1 = k$ and

$$r_\theta = \left(1 + \frac{1}{M}\right) \text{trace}(B_\theta U_\theta^{-1})/k.$$
$$\nu_2 = 4 + [k(M-1) - 4](1 + a/r)^2,$$
$$a = 1 - 2/[k(M-1)] \quad \text{if} \quad k(M-1) > 4, \text{ or}$$
$$\nu_2 = (k+1)(M-1)(1+r)^2/2 \quad \text{if} \quad k(M-1) \le 4.$$

Both procedures assume the data set is large enough that if there were no missing values, the degrees of freedom for standard errors and denominators of F statistics would be effectively infinity. Barnard and Rubin [5] suggest an adjustment for the degrees of freedom for small sample cases. However, in most cases, if the data set is large enough to use multiple imputation techniques, this adjustment will not be necessary.

SAS example

In the following example, `PROC MIXED` is used to generate estimates of the primary and secondary parameters. Now that the data are *complete*, other estimation procedures could also be used. In this example, the M imputations are identified by the variable `_IMPUTATION_`. For the model, `FACT_T2=FUNO`, the primary parameters are the means at each time point. These are stored in a table labeled `SOLUTIONF` and exported to a SAS data set using the `ODS` statement below. Secondary parameters are generated by the `ESTIMATE` statement and also exported to a SAS data set. In this example, these are the estimates of change from baseline. The resulting `WORK.MIXPARMS` and `WORK.MIXESTS` data sets will each contain M sets of parameter estimates. They are merged and the results are combined using a macro labeled `MI_SUM`.

```
ODS LISTING CLOSE; * Suppresses listing of Proc Mixed output *;

*** Run analysis of multiply imputed data ***;
PROC MIXED DATA=WORK.TOI3;
  BY _IMPUTATION_;
  CLASS FUNO;
  MODEL FACT_T2=FUNO/NOINT SOLUTION COVB;
  REPEATED FUNO/SUBJECT=CASEID TYPE=UN;
  ESTIMATE '6 WK CHANGE'  FUNO -1 1 0 0;
  ESTIMATE '12 WK CHANGE' FUNO -1 0 1 0;
```

COMBINING THE M ANALYSES

```
   ESTIMATE '6 MO CHANGE'   FUN0 -1 0 0 1;
   ODS OUTPUT SOLUTIONF=WORK.MIXPARMS
              ESTIMATES=WORK.MIXESTS;
   RUN;


ODS LISTING; * Turns listing back on *;

*** Runs macro that combines the results ***;
%MI_SUM(_IMPUTATION_,WORK.MIXPARMS,WORK.MIXESTS,WORK.SUMDATA2,FUN0);
```

Details of the SAS Macro MI_SUM are as follows. The code assumes that primary and secondary parameter estimates are exported from Proc MIXED (V8.1) using SOLUTIONF and ESTIMATES options.

```
%MACRO MI_SUM(M_VAR,BDATA,TDATA,SUMDATA,FIXED);
*******************************************************************;
*** Macro designed to be used when data are analyzed       ***;
***    using PROC MIXED                                    ***;
*** USER SUPPLIED ARGUMENTS:                               ***:
***   M_Var - Variable that identifies imputation #        ***;
***   BDATA - SAS dataset created by ODS SOLUTIONF statement ***;
***   TDATA - SAS dataset created by ODS ESTIMATES statement ***;
***   SUMDATA - Output dataset                             ***;
***   FIXED - List of covariates in the MODEL statement    ***;
*******************************************************************;

*** Combines primary and secondary parameter estimates ***;
DATA WORK.POOLED;
  SET &BDATA &TDATA;
  BY &M_VAR;
  *** Creates Identifier of Parameter ***;
  IF FIRST.&M_VAR THEN ESTNO=0;
  ESTNO=ESTNO+1;
  RETAIN ESTNO;
  *** Compute Variance ***;
  VAR=STDERR*STDERR;
RUN;

*** Between and Within Imputation Calculations ***;
PROC SUMMARY DATA=WORK.POOLED NWAY MISSING;
   CLASS ESTNO EFFECT &FIXED LABEL;
   VAR ESTIMATE VAR;
   OUTPUT OUT=WORK.SUMSTATS MEAN=THETA WITHIN VAR=BETWEEN DUMMY;
RUN;

*** Compute pooled estimates and statistics ***;
DATA &SUMDATA;
   SET WORK.SUMSTATS(DROP=_TYPE_ DUMMY RENAME=(_FREQ_=M));
   TOTAL=WITHIN+(1+(1/M))*BETWEEN;
   TOT_SE=SQRT(TOTAL);
```

```
        RATIO=((1+(1/M))*BETWEEN)/WITHIN;
        GAMMA=((1+(1/M))*BETWEEN)/TOTAL;
        T_STAT=THETA/TOT_SE;
        DF=(M-1)*(1+(1/RATIO))**2;
        P_VALUE=(1-PROBT(ABS(T_STAT),DF))*2;
        LABEL M='# Imputations'
              THETA='Estimate'
              WITHIN='Within- Imputation Var'
              BETWEEN='Between- Imputation Var'
              TOTAL='Total Variance'
              TOT_SE='Total S.E.'
              RATIO='Between-to-within ratio'
              GAMMA='Fraction Missing Information'
              T_STAT='T Statistic (Ho: EST=0)'
              P_VALUE='P (2-sided)';
        FORMAT THETA WITHIN BETWEEN TOTAL TOT_SE RATIO
               GAMMA T_STAT P_VALUE 7.4 DF 6.;
     RUN;

   *** Print results ***;
   PROC PRINT DATA=&SUMDATA LABEL;
     TITLE5 'MULTIPLE-IMPUTATION PARAMETER SUMMARY';
     ID ESTNO;
     VAR EFFECT &FIXED LABEL M;
     RUN;
   PROC PRINT DATA=&SUMDATA LABEL;
     TITLE5 'MULTIPLE-IMPUTATION VARIANCE INFORMATION';
     ID ESTNO;
     VAR BETWEEN WITHIN TOTAL RATIO GAMMA;
     RUN;
   PROC PRINT DATA=&SUMDATA LABEL;
     TITLE5 'MULTIPLE-IMPUTATION PARAMETER ESTIMATES';
     ID ESTNO;
     VAR THETA TOT_SE T_STAT P_VALUE;
     RUN;
     TITLE5 '    ';
   %MEND MI_SUM;
```

7.8 Sensitivity analyses

Many of the articles describing multiple imputation incorporate sensitivity analyses as part of the presentation. These sensitivity analyses include both comparisons of multiple imputation with simple methods [19, 21, 84] and explorations of the effects of assumptions that have been made in the process of imputing the missing observations [63, 94, 153]. There are several outcomes of these sensitivity analyses. The analyses may demonstrate that the estimates and inference are insensitive to the results. Or, if the results do depend on

7.9 Imputation vs. analytic models

If the multiple imputation models use only the same data that is used in the analytic models (the observed response data and baseline covariates), the resulting estimates are almost identical to those obtained using the maximum likelihood method with the same information. This is illustrated in Table 7.5, where the estimates obtained using a repeated measures analysis of incomplete data are almost identical to those obtained after multiple imputation using the four FACT-Lung TOI scores and treatment group (TAXOL). In contrast, when additional information about the patient, which is potentially related to his or her HRQoL when the observation is missing, is added to the imputation procedure, the resulting estimates may be dramatically different. This is illustrated in Table 7.5, where the length of survival and number of cycles of therapy started were included in the imputation procedure and the estimated rate of decline in the FACT-Lung TOI scores more than doubled. Reiterating the points: (1) multiple imputation is the hard way to analyze data where missingness is MAR and (2) it will only provide a benefit when the analyst has additional information (data) that is related to HRQoL both when the response is observed and when it is missing.

Table 7.5. Comparison of estimates obtained using maximum likelihood estimation of all available FACT-Lung TOI data (MLE), multiple imputation using all available data (MI Obs), and multiple imputation with additional outcome data (MI Plus).

Parameter	MLE Obs[a]		MI Obs[b]		MI Plus[c]	
	Est	(S.E.)	Est	(S.E.)	Est	(S.E.)
Mean 0 weeks	65.69	(0.70)	65.70	(0.70)	65.74	(0.69)
Mean 6 weeks	63.63	(0.79)	63.65	(0.78)	61.72	(0.85)
Mean 12 weeks	62.40	(0.91)	62.44	(0.94)	58.92	(1.16)
Mean 6 months	60.84	(1.06)	60.83	(1.11)	53.25	(1.29)
Change 6 weeks	−2.05	(0.77)	−2.05	(0.85)	−4.02	(0.78)
Change 12 weeks	−3.29	(0.94)	−3.26	(0.98)	−6.82	(1.16)
Change 6 months	−4.85	(1.09)	−4.87	(1.14)	−12.49	(1.23)

[a]MLE Obs: REML with repeated measures design of all available data (SAS Proc MIXED).

[b]MI Obs: Multiple imputation using MCMC method limited to the four repeated measures of the FACT-Lung TOI, $M = 20$ (SAS Proc MI).

[c]MI Plus: Multiple imputation using MCMC method including the four repeated measures of the FACT-Lung TOI plus log transformation of survival and number of cycles of therapy started, $M = 20$ (SAS Proc MI).

Includes 548 patients with at least one observation and no missing covariate data.

7.10 Implications for design

If multiple imputation is proposed as an analysis strategy for a clinical trial, a number of factors should be considered. As mentioned above, these procedures all require large data sets. Initially, multiple imputation was developed for large surveys. Application of multiple imputation to smaller clinical trials should be proposed cautiously. How large is necessary will depend on how much auxiliary information (strong covariates) is available and how much missing data is expected.

Anticipating the use of multiple imputation, it is wise to ensure the collection of auxiliary information that is required. When, as a result of careful planning of a study, there is adequate documentation of the reasons for missing data along with information that will link these reasons to changes in HRQoL, it is possible to develop a good imputation model. For example, a possible strategy is to use surrogate assessments of HRQoL or related measures obtained from the health-care providers or caregivers. These measures can be obtained both concurrently with the patients' assessments of HRQoL and also when the patients' assessments are missing. Although there has been considerable documentation of the discrepancies between the patients' self-evaluations of HRQoL and those of others, these assessments may be stronger predictors than other measures. This strategy is particularly useful in settings where subjects are expected to be unable to provide their own assessment of HRQoL over the course of the study, for example, patients with brain tumors or Alzheimer's disease.

7.11 Summary

- Multiple imputation provides a flexible way of handling missing data from multiple unrelated causes or when the mechanism changes over time. For example, separate models can be used for early and late dropout.
- Multiple imputation will provide a benefit only when the analyst has additional information (data) that is related to HRQoL both when the response is observed and missing.
- Multiple imputation will be difficult to implement in studies with mistimed observations and where the sample size is small.
- Sequential univariate regression will be useful when the missing data patterns are predominately monotone and the variables explaining dropout are very different over time.
- MCMC will be useful when the missing data pattern is not strictly monotone and the same set of variables explain dropout over time.
- ABB is not recommended for longitudinal studies, as it underrepresents the correlation of observations over time. It also makes stronger assumptions about the missing data mechanism than the explicit procedures (MCMC and regression).

CHAPTER 8

Pattern Mixture Models

8.1 Introduction

Non-ignorable missing data are the common type of missing data in HRQoL studies where there is dropout as a result of toxicity, disease progression, or even therapeutic effectiveness. Studies with this type of missing data are also the most difficult to analyze. The primary reasons are (1) there are a large number of possible models and (2) it is impossible to verify statistically the correctness of any model because the data required to distinguish between models are missing. In this chapter, we describe one group of models, *pattern mixture models*, that has been proposed for this problem. In pattern mixture models, the portion of the model specifying the missing data mechanism ($f[\mathbf{R}|\mathbf{X}, \Psi]$) does not depend on the missing values. Thus, for pattern mixture models, we only need to know the proportion of subjects with each pattern of missing data and we do not need to specify how missingness depends on Y_i^{mis}. This advantage is balanced by (1) the large number of potential patterns of missing data and (2) the difficulties of estimating all parameters in each pattern.

The basic concept [90–92] is that there are P different missing data patterns ($R_i \in M^{\{p\}}$). The distribution of the responses, Y_i, may differ across the P patterns with different parameters, $\beta^{\{p\}}$, and variance, $\Sigma^{\{p\}}$.

$$Y_i | M^{\{p\}} \sim N\big(X_i \beta^{\{p\}}, \Sigma_i^{\{p\}}\big), \qquad p = 1, \ldots, P.$$

For example, change in HRQoL among subjects in each pattern is described using a different intercept ($\beta_0^{\{p\}}$) and slope ($\beta_1^{\{p\}}$). This would allow patients who drop out earlier to have lower HRQoL scores initially and to decline more rapidly over time. The patients who drop out earlier also may have more or less variability in their scores (different variance) than patients who remain in the study.

The true distribution of the measures of HRQoL for the entire group of patients is a mixture of the distributions from each of the P groups of patients. The quantities of interest are the expected values of the parameters averaged over the missing data patterns:

$$E[\beta] = \sum^{P} \pi^{\{p\}} \beta^{\{p\}},$$

where $\pi^{\{p\}}$ is the proportion of subjects observed with the pth pattern.

The general method is to stratify the patients by the missing data pattern. Then, the parameters ($\beta^{\{p\}}, \Sigma^{\{p\}}$) are estimated within each of the strata.

Weights are determined by the number of subjects within each of the P missing data patterns ($\hat{\pi}^{\{p\}} = n^{\{p\}}/N$). The population estimates are the weighted average of the estimates from the P missing data patterns ($\hat{\beta} = \sum \hat{\pi}^{\{p\}} \hat{\beta}^{\{p\}}$).

The procedure sounds easy and straightforward, but there are some practical problems. The first difficulty is the large number of missing data patterns that occur where there may be only a few subjects with some patterns. In a study with J assessments over time, there are theoretically 2^J possible patterns. Thus, with only four assessments, there are 16 possible patterns.

The second difficulty is that, for most of the patterns, the model ($X_i \beta^{\{p\}}$) is *underidentified*. This means that all the parameters cannot be estimated in each pattern unless additional assumptions are made. Daniels and Hogan [26] cite three approaches to deal with the lack of information. Some options for solving these problems are presented in the following sections.

1. Impose explicit restrictions such as complete case restrictions (see Sections 8.2 and 8.3) or missing data assumptions (MAR).
2. Impose model restrictions such as selection model restrictions that assume a nonignorable mechanism (see Section 8.2).
3. Carry out a sensitivity analysis across a range of choices (see Section 8.2).

Option 1 is not viable when we believe the missing data are nonignorable. Other options apply only to a few limited situations. Further, the assumptions that allow us to estimate all of the parameters are often difficult to communicate and cannot be tested because they depend on the values of the missing data. This chapter focuses on the various restrictions and assumptions required to estimate parameters in these underidentified models. Sections 8.2 and 8.3 describe restrictions for bivariate data and monotone dropout, respectively. In Section 8.4, the use of parametric models to extrapolate growth curves is described.

NSCLC example

The existence of a large number of patterns is clearly illustrated in the NSCLC study. Of the 16 possible patterns, 15 were observed (see Table 4.2). Of the 15 patterns, 10 have less then 5% of the observations. If we simplify the problem by defining the patterns by the time of dropout, we still have five patterns. Average HRQoL scores are displayed for four of the patterns with any observations in Figure 8.1 (one pattern has no observations).

As mentioned before, the second difficulty is that, for most of the patterns, the unknown parameters of the model (β and Σ_i) are *underidentified*. If we were using a cell means model in the NSCLC example, we would need to estimate a mean at each time in each pattern ($\hat{\mu}_1^{\{p\}}, \hat{\mu}_2^{\{p\}}, \hat{\mu}_3^{\{p\}}, \hat{\mu}_4^{\{p\}}$) and the ten covariance parameters ($\hat{\sigma}_{11}^{\{p\}}, \hat{\sigma}_{12}^{\{p\}}, \ldots, \hat{\sigma}_{44}^{\{p\}}$). Without making additional assumptions, we could do that in only the one pattern with all four assessments. Even if we were considering a simple linear growth curve, we could only estimate both the intercept and slope in the patterns where there are at least two observations.

Table 8.1. All possible missing data patterns for two repeated measures.

Pattern	Y_1	Y_2	R
1	$Y_1^{\{1\}}$	$Y_2^{\{1\}}$	(1,1)
2	$Y_1^{\{2\}}$	?	(1,0)
3	?	$Y_2^{\{3\}}$	(0,1)
4	?	?	(0,0)

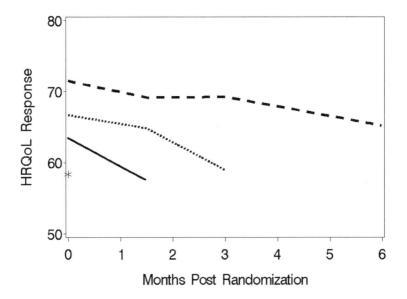

Figure 8.1. Patterns defined by timing of last assessment.

8.2 Bivariate data (two repeated measures)

The simplest case for longitudinal studies consists of two repeated measures. There are four possible patterns of missing data (Table 8.1). The first pattern, in which all responses are observed, contains the *complete cases*. The second and third patterns have one observation each. In the fourth pattern, none of the responses is observed.

In each of the four patterns, there are five possible parameters to be estimated: two means $(\hat{\mu}_1^{\{p\}}, \hat{\mu}_2^{\{p\}})$ and three parameters for the covariance $(\hat{\sigma}_{11}^{\{p\}}, \hat{\sigma}_{12}^{\{p\}}, \hat{\sigma}_{22}^{\{p\}})$. We can estimate 9 of the 20 total parameters from the data: all five parameters from pattern 1 $(\hat{\mu}_1^{\{1\}}, \hat{\mu}_2^{\{1\}}, \hat{\sigma}_{11}^{\{1\}}, \hat{\sigma}_{12}^{\{1\}}, \hat{\sigma}_{22}^{\{1\}})$ and two each from patterns 2 and 3 $(\hat{\mu}_1^{\{2\}}, \hat{\sigma}_{11}^{\{2\}}$ and $\hat{\mu}_2^{\{3\}}, \hat{\sigma}_{22}^{\{3\}})$. Thus, the model is under-identified and some type of restriction (assumption) is required to estimate the remaining parameters.

Table 8.2. Number of subjects with each missing data pattern for the initial and 12-week assessments in the NSCLC study.

Pattern	Y_1	Y_2	No Taxol	Taxol
1	$Y_1^{\{1\}}$	$Y_2^{\{1\}}$	83	190
2	$Y_1^{\{2\}}$	?	94	159
3	?	$Y_2^{\{3\}}$	2	7
4	?	?	15	25

Table 8.3. Identified parameters in each pattern. Covariance parameters were restricted to be equal across pattern but allowed to differ across treatment groups.

		Means		Covariance		
Pattern	$\hat{\pi}^{\{p\}}$	$\hat{\mu}_1^{\{p\}}$	$\hat{\mu}_2^{\{p\}}$	$\hat{\sigma}_{11}^{\{p\}}$	$\hat{\sigma}_{12}^{\{p\}}$	$\hat{\sigma}_{22}^{\{p\}}$
No Taxol						
1	0.43	68.4	64.1	249.5	118.3	320.7
2	0.48	61.4	?	249.5	?	?
3	0.01	?	84.2	?	?	320.7
4	0.08	?	?	?	?	?
Taxol						
1	0.50	69.9	65.2	245.7	101.2	242.0
2	0.42	61.4	?	245.7	?	?
3	0.02	?	75.0	?	?	242.0
4	0.07	?	?	?	?	?

NSCLC example

To illustrate the problem of identifying all parameters in the model, consider the initial and 12-week assessments in NSCLC study. The majority of subjects are in either the first or second pattern (Table 8.2). The estimable parameters for these first two patterns are summarized in Table 8.3.

Complete-case missing variable (CCMV) restriction

One possible set of restrictions is based on the complete cases [90]. The assumption is that the missing value distributions are equal to the complete case distributions. For the bivariate case shown in Table 8.1, the restrictions are

$$\theta_{[2\cdot 1]}^{\{2\}} = \theta_{[2\cdot 1]}^{\{1\}}, \quad \theta_{[1\cdot 2]}^{\{3\}} = \theta_{[1\cdot 2]}^{\{1\}}, \quad \text{and} \quad \theta^{\{4\}} = \theta^{\{1\}}, \tag{8.1}$$

where $\theta_{[2\cdot 1]}^{\{1\}}$ denotes the parameters from the regression of Y_2 on Y_1 (or the conditional distribution of Y_2 given Y_1) using the complete cases in pattern 1.

BIVARIATE DATA (TWO REPEATED MEASURES)

For a moment, consider an example where we have only the first two patterns. All subjects were observed initially, but some are missing at the second assessment. We estimate $\mu_1^{\{1\}}, \mu_2^{\{1\}}$, and $\mu_1^{\{2\}}$ directly from the data.

$$\hat{\mu}_1^{\{1\}} = \bar{Y}_1^{\{1\}} = \frac{1}{n^{\{1\}}} \sum Y_{i1}^{\{1\}}. \tag{8.2}$$

$$\hat{\mu}_2^{\{1\}} = \bar{Y}_2^{\{1\}} = \frac{1}{n^{\{1\}}} \sum Y_{i2}^{\{1\}}. \tag{8.3}$$

$$\hat{\mu}_1^{\{2\}} = \bar{Y}_1^{\{2\}} = \frac{1}{n^{\{2\}}} \sum Y_{i1}^{\{2\}}. \tag{8.4}$$

We then apply this complete-case missing variable restriction to estimate $\mu_2^{\{2\}}$. Consider the regression of Y_2 on Y_1:

$$Y_{i2}^{\{1\}} = \beta_{0[2\cdot1]}^{\{1\}} + \beta_{1[2\cdot1]}^{\{1\}} Y_{i1}^{\{1\}} + e_i, \tag{8.5}$$

$$Y_{i2}^{\{2\}} = \beta_{0[2\cdot1]}^{\{2\}} + \beta_{1[2\cdot1]}^{\{2\}} Y_{i1}^{\{2\}} + e_i. \tag{8.6}$$

Because we cannot estimate the parameters in the second equation due to missing data, we assume the same relationship holds in pattern 2 as in pattern 1.

$$\beta_{0[2\cdot1]}^{\{2\}} = \beta_{0[2\cdot1]}^{\{1\}}, \tag{8.7}$$

$$\beta_{1[2\cdot1]}^{\{2\}} = \beta_{1[2\cdot1]}^{\{1\}}. \tag{8.8}$$

The procedure is to estimate the intercept $\beta_{0[2\cdot1]}^{\{1\}}$ and slope $\beta_{1[2\cdot1]}^{\{1\}}$ using the complete cases in pattern 1; then, applying the restrictions, the estimated mean for the second assessment in pattern 2 is

$$\hat{\mu}_2^{\{2\}} = \hat{\beta}_{0[2\cdot1]}^{\{1\}} + \hat{\beta}_{1[2\cdot1]}^{\{1\}} \bar{Y}_1^{\{2\}}$$

$$= \bar{Y}_2^{\{1\}} - \frac{\hat{\sigma}_{12}^{\{1\}}}{\hat{\sigma}_{11}^{\{1\}}} \left(\bar{Y}_1^{\{1\}} - \bar{Y}_1^{\{2\}} \right). \tag{8.9}$$

The algebraic details for Equation 8.9 are at the end of this chapter. Combining the estimates for the two patterns, the overall estimates of the two means are

$$\hat{\mu}_1 = \hat{\pi}^{\{1\}} \hat{\mu}_1^{\{1\}} + \hat{\pi}^{\{2\}} \hat{\mu}_1^{\{2\}} = \hat{\pi}^{\{1\}} \bar{Y}_1^{\{1\}} + \hat{\pi}^{\{2\}} \bar{Y}_1^{\{2\}} = \bar{Y}_1, \tag{8.10}$$

$$\hat{\mu}_2 = \hat{\pi}^{\{1\}} \hat{\mu}_2^{\{1\}} + \hat{\pi}^{\{2\}} \hat{\mu}_2^{\{2\}} = \bar{Y}_2^{\{1\}} + \frac{\hat{\sigma}_{12}^{\{1\}}}{\hat{\sigma}_{11}^{\{1\}}} \left(\hat{\mu}_1 - \bar{Y}_1^{\{1\}} \right). \tag{8.11}$$

The algebraic details for Equation 8.11 are at the end of this chapter. Procedures for estimating the covariance parameters are outlined in detail by Little [90, 91].

Note that for this special case these estimates are the same as those obtained using MLE with all available data (see Chapter 5, Equation 5.4). In the example described above, the restrictions are equivalent to assuming that the missingness of Y_2 depends only on Y_1. Recall that this is exactly the definition

Table 8.4. Baseline and 12-week FACT-Lung TOI means estimated under the CCMV restrictions. Example limited to subjects with baseline assessments.

Pattern	No Taxol			Taxol		
	$\hat{\pi}^{\{p\}}$	$\hat{\mu}_1^{\{p\}}$	$\hat{\mu}_2^{\{p\}}$	$\hat{\pi}^{\{p\}}$	$\hat{\mu}_1^{\{p\}}$	$\hat{\mu}_2^{\{p\}}$
1	0.47	68.4	64.1	0.54	69.9	65.2
2	0.53	61.4	*60.8*	0.46	61.4	*61.6*
Pooled		64.7	62.3		66.0	63.6

of MAR. Thus, this restriction is helpful when trying to understand pattern mixture models, but it is not of much practical use when we believe that the data are MNAR.

NSCLC example

To illustrate the CCMV restriction, consider the baseline and 12-week assessments for subjects who had a baseline assessment. (This limitation is not required under the CCMV restriction, but it will simplify the illustration and allow comparison with the restriction presented in the next section.) The estimated means at 12 weeks for the subjects in pattern 2 follow from Equation 8.9 (Table 8.4). Notice that the 12-week estimates for pattern 2 are lower than those for pattern 1 (60.8 vs. 64.1 for patients not receiving Taxol, and 61.6 vs. 65.2 for patients receiving Taxol). This is because the baseline observations are lower in pattern 2 than in pattern 1 and the two measures are positively correlated.

Brown's protective restrictions

A second set of restrictions was proposed by Brown [10] for monotone dropout where patterns 1 and 2 are observed. The assumption is that the missingness of Y_2 depends on Y_2. This is the MNAR assumption. For the bivariate case, the restriction is $\theta_{[1 \cdot 2]}^{\{2\}} = \theta_{[1 \cdot 2]}^{\{1\}}$. (Note that this is the mirror image of the complete-case restriction.)

Again, consider the bivariate example where we have only the first two patterns. We need to estimate the second mean in the second pattern, $\mu_2^{\{2\}}$. This time, we will regress Y_1 on Y_2.

$$Y_{i1}^{\{1\}} = \beta_{0[1 \cdot 2]}^{\{1\}} + \beta_{1[1 \cdot 2]}^{\{1\}} Y_{i2}^{\{1\}} + e_i, \qquad (8.12)$$

$$Y_{i1}^{\{2\}} = \beta_{0[1 \cdot 2]}^{\{1\}} + \beta_{1[1 \cdot 2]}^{\{1\}} Y_{i2}^{\{2\}} + e_i. \qquad (8.13)$$

The assumption is that the same relationship holds in pattern 2 as in pattern 1:

$$\beta_{0[1 \cdot 2]}^{\{2\}} = \beta_{0[1 \cdot 2]}^{\{1\}}, \qquad (8.14)$$

BIVARIATE DATA (TWO REPEATED MEASURES)

$$\beta_{1[1\cdot 2]}^{\{2\}} = \beta_{1[1\cdot 2]}^{\{1\}}. \tag{8.15}$$

The procedure is to estimate the intercept $\beta_{0[1\cdot 2]}^{\{1\}}$ and slope $\beta_{1[1\cdot 2]}^{\{1\}}$ using the complete cases in pattern 1. To estimate $\mu_2^{\{2\}}$, we assume

$$\bar{Y}_1^{\{2\}} = \beta_{0[1\cdot 2]}^{\{1\}} + \beta_{1[1\cdot 2]}^{\{1\}} \hat{\mu}_2^{\{2\}} \tag{8.16}$$

and then solve for $\hat{\mu}_2^{\{2\}}$:

$$\hat{\mu}_2^{\{2\}} = (\bar{Y}_1^{\{2\}} - \hat{\beta}_{0[1\cdot 2]}^{\{1\}})/\hat{\beta}_{1[1\cdot 2]}^{\{1\}}$$

$$= \bar{Y}_2^{\{1\}} - \frac{\hat{\sigma}_{22}^{\{1\}}}{\hat{\sigma}_{12}^{\{1\}}} (\bar{Y}_1^{\{1\}} - \bar{Y}_1^{\{2\}}). \tag{8.17}$$

Combining the estimates for the two patterns, the overall estimates of the two means are

$$\hat{\mu}_1 = \hat{\pi}^{\{1\}} \hat{\mu}_1^{\{1\}} + \hat{\pi}^{\{2\}} \hat{\mu}_1^{\{2\}} = \hat{\pi}^{\{1\}} \bar{Y}_1^{\{1\}} + \hat{\pi}^{\{2\}} \bar{Y}_1^{\{2\}} = \bar{Y}_1, \tag{8.18}$$

$$\hat{\mu}_2 = \hat{\pi}^{\{1\}} \hat{\mu}_2^{\{1\}} + \hat{\pi}^{\{2\}} \hat{\mu}_2^{\{2\}} = \bar{Y}_2^{\{1\}} + \frac{\hat{\sigma}_{22}^{\{1\}}}{\hat{\sigma}_{12}^{\{1\}}} (\hat{\mu}_1 - \bar{Y}_1^{\{1\}}). \tag{8.19}$$

The algebraic details for Equations 8.17 and 8.19 are at the end of the chapter.

NSCLC example

To illustrate, again consider the subjects in patterns 1 and 2. Applying Equation 8.17, we compute the 12-week means in the second pattern ($\hat{\mu}_2^{\{2\}}$) to be 44.9 and 45.0 in the two treatment arms. Comparing these estimates of $\hat{\mu}_2^{\{2\}}$ with those made under the CCMV restrictions (see Table 8.4.), we see that they are approximately 20 points lower (Table 8.5). With roughly half of the cases in each pattern, the pooled estimates of the 12-week means are about 10 points lower under Brown's protective restrictions than those with the CCMV restrictions. The discrepancy between the estimates with the two different sets of restrictions is not surprising, as the first set of estimates was made under an assumption that the data were MAR and the later under an assumption that the data were MNAR. Three factors influence the magnitude of

Table 8.5. Baseline and 12-week FACT-Lung TOI means estimated under Brown's protective restrictions. Example limited to subjects with baseline assessments.

	No Taxol			Taxol		
Pattern	$\hat{\pi}^{\{p\}}$	$\hat{\mu}_1^{\{p\}}$	$\hat{\mu}_2^{\{p\}}$	$\hat{\pi}^{\{p\}}$	$\hat{\mu}_1^{\{p\}}$	$\hat{\mu}_2^{\{p\}}$
1	0.47	68.4	64.1	0.54	69.9	65.2
2	0.53	61.4	*44.9*	0.46	61.4	*45.0*
Pooled		64.7	53.9		66.0	56.0

the discrepancy. The differences between the estimates will increase as (1) the proportion of missing data increases, (2) the magnitude of the difference between the baseline means ($\bar{Y}^{\{1\}}$ and $\bar{Y}^{\{2\}}$) increases, and (3) the correlation between the baseline and 12-week scores decreases.* In this example, approximately 50% of the subjects are missing an assessment at 12 weeks, there is roughly a 7-point difference between the baseline means (≈ 0.5 S.D.), and the correlation between the baseline and 12-week score is 0.4.

Sensitivity analyses with intermediate restrictions

Although both approaches use the complete cases to define the restrictions, the first approach assumes that dropout is completely dependent on the initial measure of the outcome, Y_1, and the second approach assumes that dropout is completely dependent on the final measure of the outcome, Y_2. Reality is likely to be somewhere in between. Little [91] proposed a mixture of these two approaches in which missingness depends on $Y_1 + \lambda Y_2$.

$$\hat{\mu}_2 = \bar{Y}_2^{\{1\}} + b^{(\lambda)}(\hat{\mu}_1 - \bar{Y}_1^{\{1\}}), \qquad b^{(\lambda)} = \frac{\lambda \hat{\sigma}_{22}^{\{1\}} + \hat{\sigma}_{12}^{\{1\}}}{\lambda \hat{\sigma}_{12}^{\{1\}} + \hat{\sigma}_{11}^{\{1\}}}. \tag{8.20}$$

If $\lambda = 0$, this is equivalent to the CCMV restriction.

$$b^{(\lambda)} = \frac{\lambda \hat{\sigma}_{22}^{\{1\}} + \hat{\sigma}_{12}^{\{1\}}}{\lambda \hat{\sigma}_{12}^{\{1\}} + \hat{\sigma}_{11}^{\{1\}}} = \frac{\hat{\sigma}_{12}^{\{1\}}}{\hat{\sigma}_{11}^{\{1\}}}. \tag{8.21}$$

As $\lambda \to \infty$, by L'Hôpital's rule, we have

$$\lim_{\lambda \to \infty} b^{(\lambda)} = \lim_{\lambda \to \infty} \frac{\lambda \hat{\sigma}_{22}^{\{1\}} + \hat{\sigma}_{12}^{\{1\}}}{\lambda \hat{\sigma}_{12}^{\{1\}} + \hat{\sigma}_{11}^{\{1\}}} = \frac{\hat{\sigma}_{22}^{\{1\}}}{\hat{\sigma}_{21}^{\{1\}}}. \tag{8.22}$$

This is equivalent to Brown's protective restriction.

Unfortunately, we are unable to estimate λ. We can, however, use a range of values of λ to perform a sensitivity analysis. Sensitivity to λ will decrease as the correlation between Y_1 and Y_2 increases. For example, when the variance of Y is constant over time ($\sigma_{11}^{\{1\}} \approx \sigma_{22}^{\{1\}}$) and the correlation approaches 1, $b^{(\lambda)}$ will vary only slightly from a value of 1 regardless of the value of λ.

Large-sample inferences for μ_2

The large-sample variance of $\hat{\mu}_2$ is derived using Taylor series approximations [91]:

$$\begin{aligned}\text{var}(\hat{\mu}_2) = & \frac{\hat{\sigma}_{22}}{N} + (\mu_1 - \bar{Y}_1^{\{1\}})^2 V_b \\ & + \frac{n_2}{n_1 N}[\hat{\sigma}_{22}^{\{1\}} - 2b^{(\lambda)}\hat{\sigma}_{12}^{\{1\}} + b^{(\lambda)2}\hat{\sigma}_{11}^{\{1\}}],\end{aligned} \tag{8.23}$$

---

* Note that the quantity $\hat{\mu}_1 - \bar{Y}_1^{\{1\}}$ in Equation 8.19 is a function of both $\hat{\pi}^{\{2\}}$ and $\bar{Y}^{\{1\}} - \bar{Y}^{\{2\}}$ (see Section 8.6).

Table 8.6. Sensitivity analysis.

	No Taxol			Taxol			Difference	
λ	$\hat{\mu}_{11}$	$\hat{\mu}_{12}$	$\hat{\mu}_{1\Delta}$	$\hat{\mu}_{21}$	$\hat{\mu}_{22}$	$\hat{\mu}_{2\Delta}$	$\hat{\mu}_{22}-\hat{\mu}_{12}$	(S.E.)
0	64.7	62.3	−2.3	66.0	63.6	−2.4	1.31	(2.22)
1	64.7	59.6	−5.1	66.0	61.4	−4.6	1.79	(2.52)
2	64.7	58.2	−6.5	66.0	60.2	−5.8	1.96	(2.89)
4	64.7	56.8	−7.9	66.0	58.9	−7.1	2.07	(3.40)
∞	64.7	53.9	−10.8	66.0	56.0	−10.0	2.40	(4.82)

Example limited to NSCLC subjects with baseline assessments. μ_{hk} is the mean at the kth assessment for the hth treatment group. $\mu_{h\Delta}$ is the change between the initial and 12-week assessments for the hth treatment group.

where $\hat{\sigma}_{11}^{\{1\}}, \hat{\sigma}_{12}^{\{1\}}, \hat{\sigma}_{22}^{\{1\}}$ are the parameters of the covariance of Y_1 and Y_2 estimated from the complete cases in pattern 1,

$$\hat{\sigma}_{11} = \frac{1}{N}\sum(Y_{i1}-\hat{\mu}_1)^2,$$

$$\hat{\sigma}_{22} = \hat{\sigma}_{22}^{\{1\}} + b^{(\lambda)2}(\hat{\sigma}_{11}-\hat{\sigma}_{11}^{\{1\}}),$$

$$V_b = \mathrm{var}(b^{(\lambda)}) = \frac{\left(\hat{\sigma}_{11}^{\{1\}}\hat{\sigma}_{22}^{\{1\}}-\hat{\sigma}_{12}^{\{1\}2}\right)\left(\lambda^2\hat{\sigma}_{22}^{\{1\}}+2\lambda\hat{\sigma}_{12}^{\{1\}}+\hat{\sigma}_{11}^{\{1\}}\right)^2}{n_1\left(\lambda\hat{\sigma}_{12}^{\{1\}}+\hat{\sigma}_{11}^{\{1\}}\right)^4}.$$

NSCLC example

Application of this type of sensitivity analysis is illustrated in Table 8.6. Although the estimates of the 12-week means ($\hat{\mu}_{h2}$) and of the change over time ($\hat{\mu}_{h2}-\hat{\mu}_{h1}$) are very sensitive to the value of λ, the differences between the two treatments are very insensitive. Thus, one would feel much more confident making inferences about treatment differences at 12 weeks than about the presence or absence of change over time within each group. However, with approximately 50% of the data missing, all conclusions about the differences in the FACT-Lung TOI should be made cautiously. It is also reassuring that the estimated variance of the parameters increases as the dependence shifts from the observed data (Y_{i1}) to the missing data (Y_{i2}). For the estimated group differences at 12 weeks, the standard error more than doubles from 2.22 to 4.82.

8.3 Monotone dropout

Next we extend the possibilities for missing data patterns to longitudinal studies with monotone dropout. Three sets of restrictions have been proposed for monotone missing data patterns. The first is an extension of Little's CCMV restriction described in the previous section. The second is the available case missing value (ACMV) restriction. The third is the neighboring case missing value (NCMV) restriction.

Table 8.7. NSCLC patients with monotone dropout patterns by treatment.

Pattern	Observation				No Taxol		Taxol	
	1	2	3	4	N	%	N	%
1	X	X	X	X	56	30.6	131	36.1
2	X	X	X		42	23.0	80	22.0
3	X	X			30	16.4	75	20.7
4	X				55	30.0	77	21.2

NSCLC study

In the NSCLC study, patients with one of the four patterns of data conforming exactly to a monotone dropout pattern account for 82% of the patients. In practice, one is reluctant to omit 18% of the subjects from the analysis. However, for the purpose of illustration, we will use only the patients with a monotone dropout pattern. Note that each pattern has approximately one fourth of the patients, so that no pattern contains fewer than 30 subjects (Table 8.7).

Complete-case missing value restriction

In the CCMV restriction, the data from the subjects in pattern 1 are used to impute the means for the missing observations in the remaining patterns.

$$\theta^{\{2\}}_{[4\cdot 123]} = \theta^{\{1\}}_{[4\cdot 123]}, \tag{8.24}$$

$$\theta^{\{3\}}_{[34\cdot 12]} = \theta^{\{1\}}_{[34\cdot 12]}, \tag{8.25}$$

$$\theta^{\{4\}}_{[234\cdot 1]} = \theta^{\{1\}}_{[234\cdot 1]}, \tag{8.26}$$

where $\theta^{\{1\}}_{[34\cdot 12]}$ denotes the parameters from the regression of Y_3 on Y_1 and Y_2 and the regression of Y_4 on Y_1 and Y_2 using the complete cases in pattern 1. As a practical note, this restriction is feasible only when the number of cases in pattern 1 is sufficient to estimate these parameters reliably.

The CCMV restrictions result in six equations that must be solved for the unknown means and variance parameters. Although this is burdensome, solving the equations for the unknown parameters is straightforward. However, deriving the appropriate variance for the pooled estimates is very complex. Curren [23] suggests an analytic technique using multiple imputation to avoid this problem. The procedure is as follows:

1. Pattern 2 (Equation 8.24): Impute missing values at T4 using cases in pattern 1.

2. Pattern 3 (Equation 8.25): Impute missing values at T3 and T4 using cases in pattern 1.

3. Pattern 4 (Equation 8.26): Impute missing values at T2, T3, and T4 using cases in pattern 1.

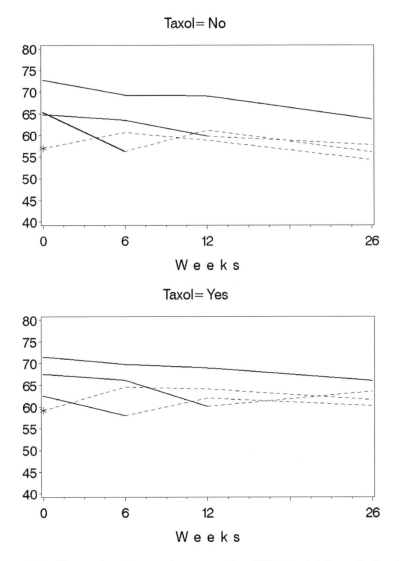

Figure 8.2. Observed and imputed means under CCMV restrictions displayed by pattern of dropout. Observed means indicated by solid line. Imputed means indicated by dashed lines.

4. Analyze each set of imputed data and combine estimates as previously described in Chapter 7.

The resulting estimates for the NSCLC patients are displayed in Figure 8.2. Note that the imputed values under the CCMV restriction tend to increase initially after the last observed FACT-Lung TOI score, especially for patients who had only the initial assessments. This illustrates the consequences of the implicit assumption with the CCMV restriction. Obviously, in the setting of the NSCLC study, we do not believe that the HRQoL of the individuals who drop out early is likely to be similar to that of individuals who have all four assessments.

Available case missing value restriction

In the ACMV restriction, available data from subjects in all the patterns are used to impute the means for the missing observations in the remaining patterns. The restrictions for the patterns in Table 8.7 are

$$\theta^{\{2\}}_{[4\cdot 123]} = \theta^{\{1\}}_{[4\cdot 123]}, \tag{8.27}$$

$$\theta^{\{3\}}_{[3\cdot 12]} = \theta^{\{1,2\}}_{[3\cdot 12]}, \quad \theta^{\{3\}}_{[4\cdot 123]} = \theta^{\{1\}}_{[4\cdot 123]}, \tag{8.28}$$

$$\theta^{\{4\}}_{[2\cdot 1]} = \theta^{\{1,2,3\}}_{[2\cdot 1]}, \quad \theta^{\{4\}}_{[3\cdot 12]} = \theta^{\{1,2\}}_{[3\cdot 12]}, \quad \theta^{\{4\}}_{[4\cdot 123]} = \theta^{\{1\}}_{[4\cdot 123]}, \tag{8.29}$$

where $\theta^{\{1,2\}}_{[3\cdot 12]}$ denotes the parameters from the regression of Y_3 on Y_1 and Y_2 using the cases in patterns 1 and 2. As a practical note, this restriction is a bit more feasible than the CCMV restriction, as more observations are used to estimate some of these parameters.

Using the same multiple imputation approach, the procedure is as follows:

1. Pattern 2 (Equation 8.27): Impute missing values at T4 using cases in pattern 1.
2. Pattern 3 (Equation 8.28): Impute missing values at T3 using cases in patterns 1 and 2. Impute missing values at T4 using cases in pattern 1 and the imputed values at T3 in pattern 3.
3. Pattern 4 (Equation 8.29): Impute missing values at T2 using cases in patterns 1, 2, and 3. Impute missing values at T3 using cases in patterns 1 and 2 and the imputed values at T2 in pattern 4. Impute missing values at T4 using cases in pattern 1 and the imputed values at T2 and T3 in pattern 4.
4. Analyze each set of imputed data and combine estimates as previously described in Chapter 7.

The resulting estimates for the NSCLC patients are displayed in Figure 8.3. Note that the imputed values under the ACMV restriction no longer tend to increase but rather tend to remain at the same level as the last observed FACT-Lung TOI measure. This is a slight improvement over the CCMV but still seems to overestimate the HRQoL of patients who drop out.

Neighboring case missing value restriction

In the NCMV restriction, available data from subjects in the neighboring pattern are used to impute the means for the missing observations.

$$\theta^{\{2\}}_{[4\cdot 123]} = \theta^{\{1\}}_{[4\cdot 123]}, \tag{8.30}$$

$$\theta^{\{3\}}_{[3\cdot 12]} = \theta^{\{2\}}_{[3\cdot 12]}, \quad \theta^{\{4\}}_{[2\cdot 1]} = \theta^{\{3\}}_{[2\cdot 1]}, \tag{8.31}$$

$$\theta^{\{4\}}_{[4\cdot 123]} = \theta^{\{1\}}_{[4\cdot 123]}, \quad \theta^{\{4\}}_{[3\cdot 12]} = \theta^{\{2\}}_{[3\cdot 12]}, \quad \theta^{\{3\}}_{[4\cdot 123]} = \theta^{\{1\}}_{[4\cdot 123]}. \tag{8.32}$$

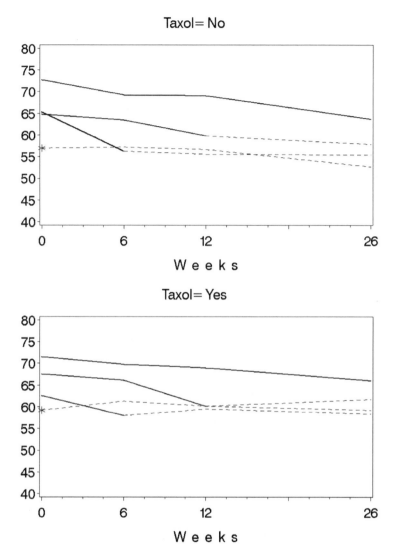

Figure 8.3. Observed and imputed means under ACMV restrictions displayed by pattern of dropout. Observed means indicated by solid line. Imputed means indicated by dashed lines.

Using the same multiple imputation approach, the procedure is as follows:

1. Pattern 2 (Equation 8.30): Impute missing values at T4 using cases in pattern 1.
2. Pattern 3 (Equation 8.31): Impute missing values at T3 using cases in pattern 2. Impute missing values at T4 using cases in pattern 1 and the imputed values at T3 in pattern 3.
3. Pattern 4 (Equation 8.32): Impute missing values at T2 using cases in pattern 3. Impute missing values at T3 using cases in pattern 2 and the

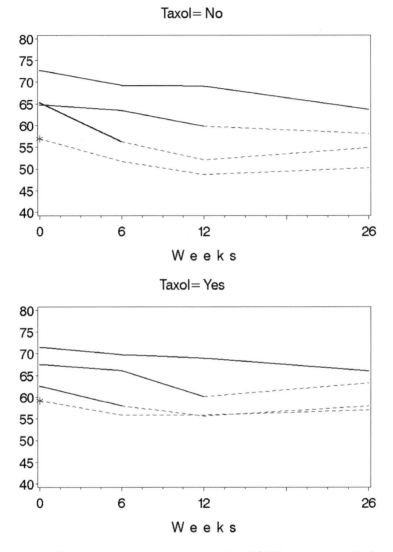

Figure 8.4. Observed and imputed means under NCMV restrictions displayed by pattern of dropout. Observed means indicated by solid line. Imputed means indicated by dashed lines.

imputed values at T2 in pattern 4. Impute missing values at T4 using cases in patterns 1 and the imputed values at T2 and T3 in pattern 4.
4. Analyze each set of imputed data and combine estimates as previously described in Chapter 7.

The resulting estimates for the NSCLC patients are displayed in Figure 8.4. Note that the imputed values under the NCMV restriction tend to fall initially

Table 8.8. Sensitivity of estimates of change between the initial and 12-week assessments for the hth treatment group with CCMV, ACMV, NCMV, and REML of available data.

	No Taxol		Taxol		Difference	
	Est	(S.E.)	Est	(S.E.)	Est	(S.E.)
CCMV	−1.7	(2.7)	−1.5	(1.1)	0.2	(3.0)
ACMV	−3.9	(1.8)	−2.9	(1.1)	1.0	(2.0)
NCMV	−7.3	(2.3)	−4.6	(1.3)	2.7	(2.4)
MLE	−2.9	(1.8)	−2.9	(1.2)	−0.2	(2.1)

over time, especially for subjects who dropped out early. This would seem to be the most appropriate of the three restrictions for the NSCLC study, but it may still overestimate the HRQoL of subjects who drop out of the study.

Comparison of CCMV, ACMV, and NCMV estimates

Figure 8.5 and Table 8.8 displays the overall estimates for the three restrictions. Table 8.9 summarizes the three sets of restrictions used to generate estimates. Notice the sensitivity of the estimates to the assumptions, particularly the decreasing estimates for the 12-week scores. The upward trend in the patients not receiving Taxol is clinically counterintuitive but not surprising, as these estimates rely on the 26-week data from patients who completed all assessments.

8.4 Parametric models

Another approach is to fit growth curve models to the data in each pattern, extrapolating past the point of dropout [23, 66]. Polynomial models can be fit within each of the P patterns where there are sufficient observations over time to estimate the parameters.

$$Y_{hij}^{\{p\}} = \beta^{\{p\}} X_{hij}^{\{p\}} + \epsilon_{hij}^{\{p\}}. \tag{8.33}$$

Note that the fixed effects and the covariance parameters may differ across the patterns. The pooled parameter estimates are

$$\hat{\beta}_k = \sum^P \hat{\pi}^{\{p\}} \hat{\beta}^{\{p\}}. \tag{8.34}$$

In practice, it may be necessary to pool some of the patterns with a small number of subjects. It may also be necessary to make some additional restrictions to estimate all the parameters.

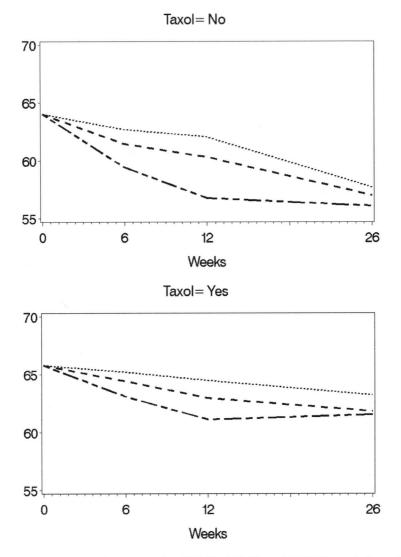

Figure 8.5. Estimated means under CCMV, ACMV, and NCMV restrictions. Curves, from highest to lowest, correspond to CCMV, ACMV, and NCMV.

Linear trends

In a limited number of studies, it is reasonable to believe that the change in HRQoL is linear over time (t).

$$Y_{hij}^{\{p\}} = \beta_0^{\{p\}} + \beta_1^{\{p\}} t_{hij}^{\{p\}} + \epsilon_{hij}^{\{p\}}. \tag{8.35}$$

However, even with this simple model, we can immediately see the challenges. The two fixed-effects parameters (intercept and slope) can be estimated only in the patterns with at least two observations per subject. Thus, we need to

Table 8.9. Contrast of CCMV, ACMV, and NCMV restrictions.

Pattern	Week 0 (Y_1)	Week 6 (Y_2)	Week 12 (Y_3)	Week 26 (Y_4)
CCMV				
1				
2				$\hat{\theta}^{\{1\}}_{[4\cdot123]} Y_{1,2,3}$
3			$\hat{\theta}^{\{1\}}_{[3\cdot12]} Y_{1,2}$	$\hat{\theta}^{\{1\}}_{[4\cdot12]} Y_{1,2}$
4		$\hat{\theta}^{\{1\}}_{[2\cdot1]} Y_1$	$\hat{\theta}^{\{1\}}_{[3\cdot1]} Y_1$	$\hat{\theta}^{\{1\}}_{[4\cdot1]} Y_1$
ACMV				
1				
2				$\hat{\theta}^{\{1\}}_{[4\cdot123]} Y_{1,2,3}$
3			$\hat{\theta}^{(1,2)}_{[3\cdot12]} Y_{1,2}$	$\hat{\theta}^{\{1\}}_{[4\cdot123]} Y_{1,2}, Y_3^{(m)}$
4		$\hat{\theta}^{(1,2,3)}_{[2\cdot1]} Y_1$	$\hat{\theta}^{(1,2)}_{[3\cdot12]} Y_1, Y_2^{(m)}$	$\hat{\theta}^{\{1\}}_{[4\cdot123]} Y_1, Y_{2,3}^{(m)}$
NCMV				
1				
2				$\hat{\theta}^{\{1\}}_{[4\cdot123]} Y_{1,2,3}$
3			$\hat{\theta}^{\{2\}}_{[3\cdot12]} Y_{1,2}$	$\hat{\theta}^{\{1\}}_{[4\cdot123]} Y_{1,2}, Y_3^{(m)}$
4		$\hat{\theta}^{\{3\}}_{[2\cdot1]} Y_1$	$\hat{\theta}^{\{2\}}_{[3\cdot12]} Y_1, Y_2^{(m)}$	$\hat{\theta}^{\{1\}}_{[4\cdot123]} Y_1, Y_{2,3}^{(m)}$

For example, $\hat{\theta}^{\{1\}}_{[4\cdot123]} Y_1, Y_{2,3}^{(m)}$ in the last column of the fourth row of the AMCV or NCMV sections indicates that data from pattern 1 will be used to estimate the regression parameters and the observed data (Y_1) and the imputed data ($Y_{2,3}^{(m)}$) from pattern 4 will be used to estimate Y_4 in pattern 4.

impose an additional restriction to estimate the parameters for the remaining patterns. Consider the four dropout patterns observed in the NSCLC study after collapsing the 15 observed patterns by time of dropout (see Table 8.7). The slope is not estimable in pattern 4 without additional assumptions. One reasonable restriction is to assume that the slope for subjects in pattern 4 is the same as the slope for subjects in pattern 3:

$$\hat{\beta}_1^{\{4\}} = \hat{\beta}_1^{\{3\}}. \tag{8.36}$$

The plots in the upper half of Figure 8.6 illustrate this for the NSCLC example.

An alternative approach is to place parametric assumptions on the parameters using the time of dropout as a covariate [23, 100]. For example, one might assume that there was an interaction between the time of dropout ($d^{\{p\}}$) and

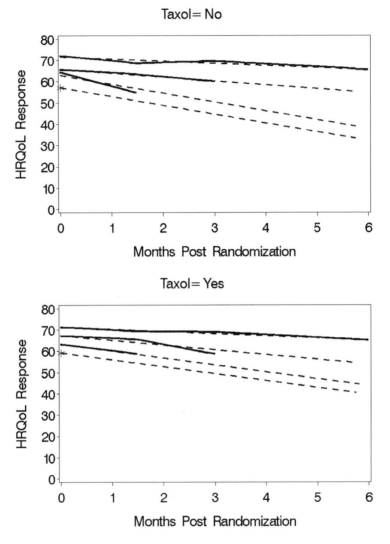

Figure 8.6. Extrapolation of linear trends in patterns defined by the time of the last observation. Dashed lines in upper plots are based on Equations 8.35 and 8.36. Dashed lines in the lower plots are based on Equation 8.37. Solid lines are based on MLE of available data using a piecewise linear regression model.

the intercept and slope in each pattern. With both linear and quadratic terms for the time of dropout, the model might appear as

$$Y_{hij}^{\{p\}} = \underbrace{\beta_0^{\{p\}} + \beta_1^{\{p\}} d^{\{p\}} + \beta_2^{\{p\}} d^{\{p\}2}}_{\text{Intercept}}$$
$$+ \underbrace{\beta_3^{\{p\}} t_{hij} + \beta_4^{\{p\}} t_{hij} d^{\{p\}} + \beta_5^{\{p\}} t_{hij} d^{\{p\}2}}_{\text{Slope}} + \epsilon_{hij}^{\{p\}}. \qquad (8.37)$$

PARAMETRIC MODELS

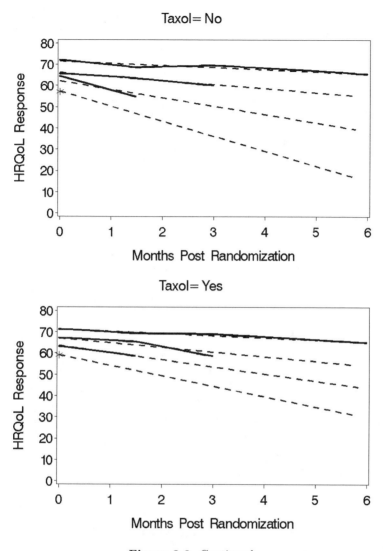

Figure 8.6. Continued

Pattern-specific estimates using this approach are illustrated in the plots in the lower half of Figure 8.6. Examination of all plots suggests that both approaches reasonably approximate the observed data. This is indicated by the close approximation of the curves to estimates of change obtained using MLE with a piecewise linear regression model. Table 8.10 summarizes both the pattern-specific estimates and the pooled parameter estimates. Not surprisingly, the major difference between the two methods of extrapolation occurs for subjects who have only a baseline observation (pattern 4). The estimates of the slopes for the smaller treatment group not receiving Taxol are also unstable, especially for the second approach. Note that there are almost 200

Table 8.10. Pattern-specific estimates for two approaches for the estimation of a linear model for changes in the FACT-Lung TOI. Model 1 is described by Equations 8.35 and 8.36. Model 2 is described by Equation 8.37.

Pattern	Group	Model 1		Model 2	
		Intercept	Slope	Intercept	Slope
1	No Taxol	71.6	−1.01	71.1	−0.97
	Taxol	71.3	−1.01	71.3	−1.02
2	No Taxol	65.7	−1.80	66.7	−0.26
	Taxol	67.3	−2.68	67.3	−2.58
3	No Taxol	62.9	−6.33	62.6	−1.73
	Taxol	63.3	−2.67	63.7	−2.98
4	No Taxol	57.2	−6.33	57.4	−11.3
	Taxol	59.2	−2.67	58.9	−3.13
Pooled	No Taxol	64.6	−3.62	64.6	−5.02
	Taxol	66.2	−2.06	66.0	−2.15

subjects in that group. This is a relatively large sample size for many clinical trials, but when we start dividing subjects into patterns, the number of subjects per pattern may decline rapidly. The sensitivity of the results to different, but reasonable, assumptions is further illustrated in Table 8.8. The differences in the 12-week means range from 0.5 to 6.0 points, bracketing the estimates obtained from the CCMV, ACMV, and NCMV restrictions. Although the differences remain statistically nonsignificant, the wide range is of concern.

Variance estimation

To describe the estimation of the variance of the pooled parameter estimates, we need to introduce some matrix notation [23]. In this notation, Equation 8.34 for the pooled parameter estimates is

$$\hat{\beta}_k = \sum^P \hat{\pi}^{\{p\}} \hat{\beta}^{\{p\}} = (\hat{\pi}^P)' A_k \hat{\beta}^P. \tag{8.38}$$

$\hat{\pi}^P$ and $\hat{\beta}^P$ are the stacked vectors of the r estimates of $\pi^{\{p\}}$ and the c estimates of $\beta^{\{p\}}$ from all P patterns. A_k is an $r \times c$ matrix of known constants (usually 0s and 1s) derived from the partial derivatives of Equation 8.34 with respect to π^P and β^P:

$$A_k = \left[\frac{\partial^2 \sum^P \hat{\pi}^{\{p\}} \hat{\beta}^{\{p\}}}{\partial \pi^{\{p\}} \partial \beta^{\{p\}}} \right]. \tag{8.39}$$

For example, consider the first approach for the linear patterns where the slopes of the third and fourth patterns are constrained to be equal, $\beta_{h1}^{\{4\}} = \beta_{h1}^{\{3\}}$.

PARAMETRIC MODELS

Thus,

$$\begin{aligned}\beta_{h1} &= \pi_h^{\{1\}}\beta_{h1}^{\{1\}} + \pi_h^{\{2\}}\beta_{h1}^{\{2\}} + \pi_h^{\{3\}}\beta_{h1}^{\{3\}} + \pi_h^{\{4\}}\beta_{h1}^{\{4\}} \\ &= \pi_h^{\{1\}}\beta_{h1}^{\{1\}} + \pi_h^{\{2\}}\beta_{h1}^{\{2\}} + \pi_h^{\{3\}}\beta_{h1}^{\{3\}} + \pi_h^{\{4\}}\beta_{h1}^{\{3\}}.\end{aligned} \quad (8.40)$$

If $\beta^{\{p\}} = [\beta_{h0}^{\{1\}}, \beta_{h1}^{\{1\}}, \ldots, \beta_{h0}^{\{4\}}, \beta_{h1}^{\{4\}}]$, the first derivative with respect to β_{h1} is

$$\frac{\partial \beta_{h1}}{\partial \beta^{\{p\}}} = \begin{bmatrix} \frac{\partial \hat{\beta}_{h1}}{\partial \hat{\beta}_{h0}^{\{1\}}} \\ \vdots \\ \frac{\partial \hat{\beta}_{h1}}{\partial \hat{\beta}_{h1}^{\{4\}}} \end{bmatrix} = \left(0, \pi_h^{\{1\}}, 0, \pi_h^{\{2\}}, 0, \pi_h^{\{3\}} + \pi_h^{\{4\}}, 0, 0\right).$$

Notice that the columns that correspond to the intercept parameters are all zero, as these parameters are not used in the estimate of the slope. Then, if $\pi^{\{p\}} = [\pi_h^{\{1\}}, \pi_h^{\{2\}}, \pi_h^{\{3\}}, \pi_h^{\{4\}}]$, the second derivative with respect to π is

$$\frac{\partial^2 \beta_{h1}}{\partial \pi^{\{p\}} \partial \beta^{\{p\}}} = \begin{bmatrix} \left(0, \pi_h^{\{1\}}, 0, \pi_h^{\{2\}}, 0, \pi_h^{\{3\}} + \pi_h^{\{4\}}, 0, 0\right)/\partial \pi_h^{\{1\}} \\ \left(0, \pi_h^{\{1\}}, 0, \pi_h^{\{2\}}, 0, \pi_h^{\{3\}} + \pi_h^{\{4\}}, 0, 0\right)/\partial \pi_h^{\{2\}} \\ \left(0, \pi_h^{\{1\}}, 0, \pi_h^{\{2\}}, 0, \pi_h^{\{3\}} + \pi_h^{\{4\}}, 0, 0\right)/\partial \pi_h^{\{3\}} \\ \left(0, \pi_h^{\{1\}}, 0, \pi_h^{\{2\}}, 0, \pi_h^{\{3\}} + \pi_h^{\{4\}}, 0, 0\right)/\partial \pi_h^{\{4\}} \end{bmatrix}$$

$$= \begin{bmatrix} 0 & 1 & 0 & 0 & 0 & 0 & 0 & 0 \\ 0 & 0 & 0 & 1 & 0 & 0 & 0 & 0 \\ 0 & 0 & 0 & 0 & 0 & 1 & 0 & 0 \\ 0 & 0 & 0 & 0 & 0 & 1 & 0 & 0 \end{bmatrix}.$$

This is more work than one needs to do to derive the pooled estimates, but it greatly facilitates the estimation of the variance that follows.

When the proportions are known (and not estimated), the variance of $\hat{\beta}_k$ is solely a function of the variance of the parameter estimates:

$$\text{Var}[\hat{\beta}_k] = \hat{\pi}^{P\prime} A_k \ \text{Var}[\hat{\beta}^P] A_k' \hat{\pi}^P. \quad (8.41)$$

However, because the proportions are also estimates, we use the delta method (Taylor series approximation) to approximate the variance of the pooled estimates:

$$\text{Var}[\hat{\beta}_k] = \hat{\pi}^{P\prime} A_k \ \text{Var}[\hat{\beta}^P] A_k' \hat{\pi}^P + \hat{\beta}^{P\prime} A_k' \ \text{Var}[\hat{\pi}^P] A_k \hat{\beta}^P, \quad (8.42)$$

where $\text{Var}[\hat{\pi}_h^P] = [\text{diag}(\hat{\pi}_h^P) - \hat{\pi}_h^P \hat{\pi}_h^{P\prime}]/N_h$ and

$$\text{Var}[\hat{\pi}^P] = \begin{bmatrix} \text{Var}[\hat{\pi}_1^P] & & \\ & \ddots & \\ & & \text{Var}[\hat{\pi}_H^P] \end{bmatrix}$$

for the H independent groups (treatment arms). This approximation is appropriate for large samples, but with small samples a bootstrap procedure may be necessary. In very large samples, $\text{Var}(\hat{\pi}_h^{\{p\}})$ is very small and, for all practical purposes, ignorable.

SAS example of a pattern mixture model

In the NSCLC study, the datafile EXAMPLE2 has a unique record for each quality of life assessment and the datafile PATIENT2 has one record for each patient. CASEID identifies the patient, TAXOL identifies the treatment arm, and MONTHS identifies the time of the assessment. The pattern is defined by LAST_QoL, which is the follow-up number of the last HRQoL assessment. For example, pattern 1 contains subjects with only the first HRQoL assessment. Thus, the order of the patterns in the example is reversed from that shown above.

Step 1: Estimates of π_h^P

The first step is to obtain estimates for proportions in each pattern by treatment group. This is done using the SAS FREQ procedure. We will need both the proportions and the number in each treatment group, so we use SAS macro variables &p1, &p2, &n1, and &n2 to store the information.

```
* Row=Treatment Group, Column=Pattern Identifier *;
PROC FREQ DATA=PATIENT2;
  TABLE TAXOL*LAST_QoL/NOPERCENT NOCOL;
  RUN;
%LET P1=.3043, .1576, .2283, .3098; %LET N1=184;
%LET P2=.2110, .2082, .2137, .3671; %LET N2=365;
```

Step 2: Estimates of β_h^P

The second step is to obtain the parameter estimates for the linear regression equations in each pattern. The CLASS statement defines TAXOL and LAST_QoL as categorical variables so that the term TAXOL*LAST_QoL in the MODEL statement, combined with the NOINT option, defines a design matrix for unique intercepts within each pattern and treatment group. The term TAXOL*LAST_QoL*MONTHS defines a design matrix for unique slopes within each pattern and treatment group. The SOLUTION and COVB options will allow us to create new data sets containing estimates of β_h^P and its variance.

```
PROC MIXED DATA=WORK.MERGED NOCLPRINT COVTEST;
  CLASS TAXOL LAST_QoL;
  MODEL FACT_T2=TAXOL*LAST_QoL TAXOL*LAST_QoL*MONTHS
       /NOINT SOLUTION COVB;

  RANDOM INTERCEPT MONTHS/SUBJECT=CASEID TYPE=UN;
```

PARAMETRIC MODELS   175

In this example, we assume a mixed-effects model with two random effects, INTERCEPT and MONTHS, similar to that described in Chapter 3. We also assume that the covariance structure is the same across all patterns and treatments. In theory, the covariance of each pattern may be different. However, in practice some restrictions are required for estimation of the variance parameters in patterns with a limited number of repeated assessments. Estimates of variance parameters in small samples lack the precision of estimates from larger samples. Thus, pooling across treatments and patterns will also stabilize the estimates of the variance parameters.

The addition of two statements creates data sets containing the estimates of the parameters and their variances. The statements would appear as

ODS OUTPUT SOLUTIONF=WORK.BETA COVB=WORK.VARBETA;

We also create another macro variable, &NBETA, equal to the number of estimated parameters for use later in the program.

%LET NBETA=16;

Note that if we needed only estimates and not the variance of the pooled intercept (I) and slope (S) parameters, these could be obtained with ESTIMATE statements using the estimated proportion of subjects in each stratum. However, because the proportions are also estimates, the standard errors and other test statistics reflect an underestimation of the true variance of the pooled estimates.

```
ESTIMATE 'No  I' TAXOL*LAST_QoL            .30  .16  .23  .31
                                           .00  .00  .00  .00;
ESTIMATE 'Yes I' TAXOL*LAST_QoL            .00  .00  .00  .00
                                           .21  .21  .21  .37;
ESTIMATE 'No  S' TAXOL*LAST_QoL*MONTHS     .00  .46  .23  .31
                                           .00  .00  .00  .00;
ESTIMATE 'Yes S' LAST_QoL*TAXOL*MONTHS     .00  .00  .00  .00
                                           .00  .42  .21  .37;
```

Step 3: Pooling estimates and computing variance

The next step is to pool the estimates and calculate the variance of the pooled estimates. To accomplish this, the SAS IML procedure is used for matrix manipulation. First, we import the estimates and variance of β^P obtained from the second step. Then, we create the matrices P_BETA and P_COVB:

```
PROC IML;
   USE WORK.BETA;        * Input Estimates of Beta *;
   READ ALL VAR{ESTIMATE} INTO P_BETA[ROWNAME=EFFECT];
   USE WORK.VARBETA;     * Input Variance of Beta *;
   READ ALL VAR("COL1":"COL&NBETA") INTO P_COVB[ROWNAME=EFFECT];
```

Then the variances of the proportions are estimated using the SAS macro variables created in the first step. Note that the variance of the proportion is calculated for each treatment group separately and then combined into a block diagonal matrix. The matrix VAR_PI is created as follows:

```
P_PATTRN={&P1}//{&P2};                    * Vector of proportions *;
VAR1=(DIAG({&P1})-{&P1}*{&P1}')/&N1;      * No Taxol *;
VAR2=(DIAG({&P2})-{&P2}*{&P2}')/&N2;      * Taxol *;
VAR_PI=BLOCK(VAR1,VAR2);
```

It is easier to identify A_k and then compute the quantities $\hat{\beta}_k$, $\hat{\pi}^{P\prime} A_k$, and $\hat{\beta}^{P\prime} A'_k$ separately for each β_k; thus, we use a short macro. Note that the number of rows of A_k should equal the number of patterns times the number of groups (treatment arms), which is also the dimension of VAR_PI. The number of columns should equal the number of elements in P_BETA.

```
%MACRO POOL(A,A_PI,A_BETA,BETA);
  &BETA=P_PATTRN'*&A*P_BETA;
  &A_PI=(&A*P_BETA)';
  &A_BETA=P_PATTRN'*&A;
%MEND POOL;

* No Taxol - Itercept *;
C1={1 0 0 0  0 0 0 0  0 0 0 0  0 0 0 0,
    0 1 0 0  0 0 0 0  0 0 0 0  0 0 0 0,
    0 0 1 0  0 0 0 0  0 0 0 0  0 0 0 0,
    0 0 0 1  0 0 0 0  0 0 0 0  0 0 0 0,
    0 0 0 0  0 0 0 0  0 0 0 0  0 0 0 0,
    0 0 0 0  0 0 0 0  0 0 0 0  0 0 0 0,
    0 0 0 0  0 0 0 0  0 0 0 0  0 0 0 0,
    0 0 0 0  0 0 0 0  0 0 0 0  0 0 0 0};
%pool(C1,AP1,AB1,Beta1);

* No Taxol - Slope *;
C2={0 0 0 0  0 0 0 0  0 1 0 0  0 0 0 0,
    0 0 0 0  0 0 0 0  0 1 0 0  0 0 0 0,
    0 0 0 0  0 0 0 0  0 0 1 0  0 0 0 0,
    0 0 0 0  0 0 0 0  0 0 0 1  0 0 0 0,
    0 0 0 0  0 0 0 0  0 0 0 0  0 0 0 0,
    0 0 0 0  0 0 0 0  0 0 0 0  0 0 0 0,
    0 0 0 0  0 0 0 0  0 0 0 0  0 0 0 0,
    0 0 0 0  0 0 0 0  0 0 0 0  0 0 0 0};
%pool(C2,AP2,AB2,Beta2);

* Taxol - Itercept *;
C3={0 0 0 0  0 0 0 0  0 0 0 0  0 0 0 0,
    0 0 0 0  0 0 0 0  0 0 0 0  0 0 0 0,
    0 0 0 0  0 0 0 0  0 0 0 0  0 0 0 0,
    0 0 0 0  0 0 0 0  0 0 0 0  0 0 0 0,
    0 0 0 0  1 0 0 0  0 0 0 0  0 0 0 0,
    0 0 0 0  0 1 0 0  0 0 0 0  0 0 0 0,
    0 0 0 0  0 0 1 0  0 0 0 0  0 0 0 0,
    0 0 0 0  0 0 0 1  0 0 0 0  0 0 0 0};
%pool(C3,AP3,AB3,Beta3);
```

PARAMETRIC MODELS 177

```
* Taxol - Slope *;
C4={ 0 0 0 0  0 0 0 0  0 0 0 0  0 0 0 0,
     0 0 0 0  0 0 0 0  0 0 0 0  0 0 0 0,
     0 0 0 0  0 0 0 0  0 0 0 0  0 0 0 0,
     0 0 0 0  0 0 0 0  0 0 0 0  0 0 0 0,
     0 0 0 0  0 0 0 0  0 0 0 0  0 1 0 0,
     0 0 0 0  0 0 0 0  0 0 0 0  0 1 0 0,
     0 0 0 0  0 0 0 0  0 0 0 0  0 0 1 0,
     0 0 0 0  0 0 0 0  0 0 0 0  0 0 0 1};
%pool(C4,AP4,AB4,Beta4);
```

The estimates $\hat{\beta}_k$, $\hat{\pi}^{P\prime}A_k$, and $\hat{\beta}^{P\prime}A'_k$ are concatenated and $\mathrm{Var}(\hat{\beta})$ is calculated.

```
BETA=BETA1//BETA2//BETA3//BETA4;
A_PI=AP1//AP2//AP3//AP4;
A_BETA=AB1//AB2//AB3//AB4;
VAR_BETA=A_BETA*P_COVB*A_BETA'+A_PI*VAR_PI*A_PI';
SE_BETA=SQRT(VECDIAG(NEW_VAR));
PRINT 'Estimates' BETA[FORMAT=6.3] 'Std Err' [FORMAT=5.3];
```

Step 4: Hypothesis testing

A SAS macro (TEST) is created to facilitate multiple hypothesis tests:

```
START TEST(BETA,VARBETA,C,C_NAME);
  THETA=C*BETA;
  VAR_TH=C*VARBETA*C';
  SE_TH=SQRT(VECDIAG(VAR_TH));
  Z=THETA/SE_TH;
  P_VAL=(1-PROBNORM(ABS(Z)))*2;
  CHISQ=THETA'*INV(VAR_TH)*THETA;
  DF=NROW(C);
  P_VAL2=(1-PROBCHI(CHISQ,DF));
  PRINT 'Estimates of Theta and Univariate Tests (2-sided)',
        C_NAME THETA[FORMAT=5.2] SE_TH[FORMAT=5.2]
        Z[FORMAT=5.2] P_VAL[FORMAT=6.4];
  PRINT 'Wald Chi2 Test of Theta=0',
        CHISQ[FORMAT=5.2] DF[FORMAT=2.] P_VAL2[FORMAT=6.4];
FINISH;
```

We then estimate the means at 12 weeks (or 2.77 months) and test the difference.

```
PRINT 'TWELVE WEEK ESTIMATES';
C={1 2.77 0 0, 0 0 1 2.77};
C_NAME={'NO TAXOL', 'TAXOL'};
RUN TEST(NEW_BETA,NEW_VAR,C,C_NAME);
C={-1 -2.77 1 2.77};
C_NAME={'NO VS YES'};
RUN TEST(NEW_BETA,NEW_VAR,C,C_NAME);
```

8.5 Additional reading

Extensions of bivariate case

Little and Wang [93] extend the bivariate case for normal measures to a more general case for multivariate measures with covariates. However, their extension is still limited to cases where there are only two patterns of missing data, one of which consists of complete cases. For the nonignorable missing data, the multivariate analogue of the restriction is used ($\Theta_{[1.2]}^{\{2\}} = \Theta_{[1.2]}^{\{1\}}$). The model is *just* identified when the number of missing observations exactly equals the number of nonmissing observations in the second pattern. Explicit expressions can be derived for the maximum likelihood estimates. When the number of nonmissing observations exceeds the number of missing observations, the model is *overidentified*. Little and Wang recommend an EM algorithm to obtain estimates. Finally, if the number of missing observations is greater than the number of nonmissing observations, additional restrictions are required.

Extensions of the sensitivity analysis

Small-sample Bayesian inference is described by Little [91] for the bivariate case described in Section 8.2. Daniels and Hogan [26] describe an extension of the sensitivity analysis to a more general missing-data pattern. They illustrate the extension with a study that has three repeated measures and monotone dropout. The sensitivity analysis is no longer a function of a single parameter, λ, but of multiple parameters. The attraction of their approach is that by reparameterizing the restriction, the unknown parameters are interpretable as the between-pattern differences in means and variances.

Nonparametric analyses

Yao et al. [170] describe an extension of a nonparametric analysis of longitudinal data with nonignorable dropout. The advantage of the proposed method is that it can be applied to settings where the HRQoL assessments do not follow the planned timing of the assessments and the distribution of the HRQoL scores is non-normal. There is, however, a strong assumption made in this extension. Specifically, this approach assumes that the differences in HRQoL between the two treatment arms do not vary over time. This assumption severely limits the settings where the method is useful.

8.6 Algebraic details

Simple linear regression of Y on X

$$\hat{\beta}_{1[Y \cdot X]} = \frac{\sum (X_i - \bar{X})(Y_i - \bar{Y})}{\sum (X_i - \bar{X})^2} = \frac{\hat{\sigma}_{XY}}{\hat{\sigma}_X^2},$$

$$\hat{\beta}_{0[Y \cdot X]} = \bar{Y} - \hat{\beta}_{1[Y \cdot X]} \bar{X} = \bar{Y} - \frac{\hat{\sigma}_{XY}}{\hat{\sigma}_X^2} \bar{X},$$

where $\hat{\sigma}_X^2 = \sum (X_i - \bar{X})^2/(n-1)$ and $\hat{\sigma}_{XY} = \sum (X_i - \bar{X})(Y_i - \bar{Y})/(n-1)$.

ALGEBRAIC DETAILS

Complete-case missing variable restriction

Equation 8.9

$$\hat{\mu}_2^{\{2\}} = \hat{\beta}_{0[2\cdot 1]}^{\{1\}} + \hat{\beta}_{1[2\cdot 1]}^{\{1\}} \bar{Y}_1^{\{2\}}$$

$$= \underbrace{\bar{Y}_2^{\{1\}} - \frac{\hat{\sigma}_{12}^{\{1\}}}{\hat{\sigma}_{11}^{\{1\}}} \bar{Y}_1^{\{1\}}}_{\hat{\beta}_{0[2\cdot 1]}^{\{1\}}} + \underbrace{\frac{\hat{\sigma}_{12}^{\{1\}}}{\hat{\sigma}_{11}^{\{1\}}}}_{\hat{\beta}_{1[2\cdot 1]}^{\{1\}}} \bar{Y}_1^{\{2\}}$$

$$= \bar{Y}_2^{\{1\}} - \frac{\hat{\sigma}_{12}^{\{1\}}}{\hat{\sigma}_{11}^{\{1\}}} \left(\bar{Y}_1^{\{1\}} - \bar{Y}_1^{\{2\}} \right).$$

Equation 8.11

$$\hat{\mu}_2 = \hat{\pi}^{\{1\}} \hat{\mu}_2^{\{1\}} + \hat{\pi}^{\{2\}} \hat{\mu}_2^{\{2\}}$$

$$= \hat{\pi}^{\{1\}} \bar{Y}_2^{\{1\}} + \hat{\pi}^{\{2\}} \underbrace{\left(\bar{Y}_2^{\{1\}} - \frac{\hat{\sigma}_{12}^{\{1\}}}{\hat{\sigma}_{11}^{\{1\}}} \left(\bar{Y}_1^{\{1\}} - \bar{Y}_1^{\{2\}} \right) \right)}_{\text{Equation 8.9}}$$

$$= \underbrace{(\hat{\pi}^{\{1\}} + \hat{\pi}^{\{2\}})}_{1} \bar{Y}_2^{\{1\}} + \frac{\hat{\sigma}_{12}^{\{1\}}}{\hat{\sigma}_{11}^{\{1\}}} \left(-\hat{\pi}^{\{2\}} \bar{Y}_1^{\{1\}} + \hat{\pi}^{\{2\}} \bar{Y}_1^{\{2\}} \right)$$

$$= \bar{Y}_2^{\{1\}} + \frac{\hat{\sigma}_{12}^{\{1\}}}{\hat{\sigma}_{11}^{\{1\}}} \left(-\hat{\pi}^{\{2\}} \bar{Y}_1^{\{1\}} \underbrace{- \hat{\pi}^{\{1\}} \bar{Y}_1^{\{1\}}}_{\text{Subtracted}} + \underbrace{\hat{\pi}^{\{1\}} \bar{Y}_1^{\{1\}}}_{\text{Added}} + \hat{\pi}^{\{2\}} \bar{Y}_1^{\{2\}} \right)$$

$$= \bar{Y}_2^{\{1\}} + \frac{\hat{\sigma}_{12}^{\{1\}}}{\hat{\sigma}_{11}^{\{1\}}} \left(\underbrace{-\hat{\pi}^{\{2\}} \bar{Y}_1^{\{1\}} - \hat{\pi}^{\{1\}} \bar{Y}_1^{\{1\}}}_{-\bar{Y}_1^{\{1\}}} + \underbrace{\hat{\pi}^{\{2\}} \bar{Y}_1^{\{2\}} + \hat{\pi}^{\{1\}} \bar{Y}_1^{\{1\}}}_{\bar{Y}_1 \text{ or } \hat{\mu}_1} \right)$$

$$= \bar{Y}_2^{\{1\}} + \frac{\hat{\sigma}_{12}^{\{1\}}}{\hat{\sigma}_{11}^{\{1\}}} \left(\hat{\mu}_1 - \bar{Y}_1^{\{1\}} \right).$$

Brown's protective restriction

Equation 8.17

$$\hat{\mu}_2^{\{2\}} = \left(\bar{Y}_1^{\{2\}} - \hat{\beta}_{0[1\cdot 2]}^{\{1\}} \right) / \hat{\beta}_{1[1\cdot 2]}^{\{1\}}$$

$$= \left(\bar{Y}_1^{\{2\}} - \underbrace{[\bar{Y}_1^{\{1\}} - \frac{\hat{\sigma}_{12}^{\{1\}}}{\hat{\sigma}_{22}^{\{1\}}} \bar{Y}_2^{\{1\}}]}_{\hat{\beta}_{0[1\cdot 2]}^{\{1\}}} \right) \Big/ \underbrace{\frac{\hat{\sigma}_{12}^{\{1\}}}{\hat{\sigma}_{22}^{\{1\}}}}_{\hat{\beta}_{1[1\cdot 2]}^{\{1\}}}$$

$$= \frac{\hat{\sigma}_{22}^{\{1\}}}{\hat{\sigma}_{12}^{\{1\}}} \bar{Y}_1^{\{2\}} - \frac{\hat{\sigma}_{22}^{\{1\}}}{\hat{\sigma}_{12}^{\{1\}}} \bar{Y}_1^{\{1\}} + \bar{Y}_2^{\{1\}}$$

$$= \bar{Y}_2^{\{1\}} - \frac{\hat{\sigma}_{22}^{\{1\}}}{\hat{\sigma}_{12}^{\{1\}}} \left(\bar{Y}_1^{\{1\}} - \bar{Y}_1^{\{2\}} \right).$$

Equation 8.19

$$\hat{\mu}_2 = \hat{\pi}^{\{1\}} \hat{\mu}_2^{\{1\}} + \hat{\pi}^{\{2\}} \hat{\mu}_2^{\{2\}}$$

$$= \hat{\pi}^{\{1\}} \bar{Y}_2^{\{1\}} + \hat{\pi}^{\{2\}} \underbrace{\left(\bar{Y}_2^{\{1\}} - \frac{\hat{\sigma}_{22}^{\{1\}}}{\hat{\sigma}_{12}^{\{1\}}} \left(\bar{Y}_1^{\{1\}} - \bar{Y}_1^{\{2\}} \right) \right)}_{\text{Equation 8.17}}$$

$$= \underbrace{\hat{\pi}^{\{1\}} \bar{Y}_2^{\{1\}} + \hat{\pi}^{\{2\}} \bar{Y}_2^{\{1\}}}_{\bar{Y}_2^{\{1\}}} + \frac{\hat{\sigma}_{22}^{\{1\}}}{\hat{\sigma}_{12}^{\{1\}}} \left(\hat{\pi}^{\{2\}} \bar{Y}_1^{\{2\}} - \hat{\pi}^{\{2\}} \bar{Y}_1^{\{1\}} \right)$$

$$= \bar{Y}_2^{\{1\}} + \frac{\hat{\sigma}_{22}^{\{1\}}}{\hat{\sigma}_{12}^{\{1\}}} \left(\hat{\pi}^{\{2\}} \bar{Y}_1^{\{2\}} + \underbrace{\hat{\pi}^{\{1\}} \bar{Y}_1^{\{1\}}}_{\text{Added}} - \underbrace{\hat{\pi}^{\{1\}} \bar{Y}_1^{\{1\}}}_{\text{Subtracted}} - \hat{\pi}^{\{2\}} \bar{Y}_1^{\{1\}} \right)$$

$$= \bar{Y}_2^{\{1\}} + \frac{\hat{\sigma}_{22}^{\{1\}}}{\hat{\sigma}_{12}^{\{1\}}} \left(\underbrace{\hat{\pi}^{\{2\}} \bar{Y}_1^{\{2\}} + \hat{\pi}^{\{1\}} \bar{Y}_1^{\{1\}}}_{\bar{Y}_1 \text{ or } \hat{\mu}_1} - \underbrace{\hat{\pi}^{\{1\}} \bar{Y}_1^{\{1\}} - \hat{\pi}^{\{2\}} \bar{Y}_1^{\{1\}}}_{\bar{Y}_1^{\{1\}}} \right)$$

$$= \bar{Y}_2^{\{1\}} + \frac{\hat{\sigma}_{22}^{\{1\}}}{\hat{\sigma}_{12}^{\{1\}}} \left(\hat{\mu}_1 - \bar{Y}_1^{\{1\}} \right).$$

Other

$$\hat{\mu}_1 - \bar{Y}_1^{\{1\}} = \underbrace{\left(\hat{\pi}^{\{1\}} \bar{Y}_1^{\{1\}} + \hat{\pi}^{\{2\}} \bar{Y}_1^{\{2\}} \right)}_{\hat{\mu}_1} - \bar{Y}_1^{\{1\}}$$

$$= \underbrace{\left(\hat{\pi}^{\{1\}} - 1 \right)}_{\hat{\pi}^{\{2\}}} \bar{Y}_1^{\{1\}} + \hat{\pi}^{\{2\}} \bar{Y}_1^{\{2\}}$$

$$= -\hat{\pi}^{\{2\}} \bar{Y}_1^{\{1\}} + \hat{\pi}^{\{2\}} \bar{Y}_1^{\{2\}}$$

$$= \hat{\pi}^{\{2\}} \left(\bar{Y}_1^{\{2\}} - \bar{Y}_1^{\{1\}} \right).$$

8.7 Summary

- Pattern mixture models have the advantage that a model for the dropout mechanism does not need to be specified.
- This advantage is balanced by the need to specify a set of restrictions to estimate all of the parameters.
- The validity of these restrictions cannot be tested and the results may be sensitive to the choice of restrictions.
- It is, however, easy to display the underlying assumptions by plotting the trajectories for each pattern.
- A large number of patterns and small sample sizes will limit the application of pattern mixture models.

CHAPTER 9

Random-Effects Mixture, Shared-Parameter, and Selection Models

9.1 Introduction

In this chapter, we examine three more models for nonignorable missing data. They represent a small subset of all those that have been proposed. However, these three models clearly illustrate the following:

1. All models for nonignorable data require the analyst to make strong assumptions.

2. These assumptions cannot be formally tested. Defense of the assumptions must be made on a clinical basis rather than a statistical basis.

3. Lack of evidence of nonignorable missing data for any particular model does not prove that the missing data are ignorable.

4. Estimates are not robust to model misspecification.

Mixture models

The term *mixture model* originates from the concept of mixing the distributions $f(\mathbf{Y}|\mathbf{M})$ or, more formally, integrating over $f(\mathbf{M})$ to obtain the marginal distribution of the longitudinal outcome. M_i denotes a vector of variables representing the missing data process. Often $M_i = R_i$, where R_i denotes a vector of binary indicators of whether a particular HRQoL score was observed ($r_{ij} = 1$) or missing ($r_{ij} = 0$), but it can also denote the time to dropout, an associated event (T_i^D), or a random coefficient (β_i). The specific form of $\mathbf{M}$ distinguishes the various mixture models. When $M_i = R_i$, the missingness can be classified into patterns (see Chapter 8). In the special case where missing data are due to dropout, the distributions may be a function of the time to dropout or an associated event.

Pattern mixture	$M_i = R_i$	$f(Y_i|R_i).$	(9.1)
Time-to-event mixture	$M_i = T_i^D$	$f(Y_i|T_i^D).$	(9.2)
Random-effects mixture	$M_i = \beta_i$	$f(Y_i|\beta_i).$	(9.3)

Finally, in the random-effects mixture, $f(Y_i|\beta_i)$ is a mixed-effects model where the random-effects model includes the dropout time T_i^D. Both the *conditional linear model* proposed by Wu and Bailey [167] and the *joint model* proposed by Schluchter [133] are random-effects mixture models (see Sections 9.2 and 9.3).

Selection models

The term *selection model* was originally used to classify models with a univariate response y_i, where the probability of being *selected* into a sample depended on the response.

In the above sections we have used the notation $f(\mathbf{M}|\mathbf{Y}^{\text{obs}}, \mathbf{Y}^{\text{mis}}, \mathbf{X})$. We can expand this definition to differentiate among selection models. Specifically, in *outcome-dependent* [67] selection models the mechanism depends directly on the elements of $\mathbf{Y}$, and in *random-effects* [67] or *random-coefficient* [92] selection models missingness depends on $\mathbf{Y}$ through the subject-specific random effects β_i or d_i.

$$\text{Outcome-dependent selection} \quad f\left(M_i | Y_i^{\text{obs}}, Y_i^{\text{mis}}\right) \quad (9.4)$$
$$\text{Random-effects-dependent selection} \quad f(M_i|\beta_i) \quad (9.5)$$

An example of an outcome-dependent selection model is the model proposed by Diggle and Kenward [36] (see Section 9.4), and an example of a random-effects selection model is the joint model proposed by Schluchter [133] and DeGruttola and Tu [30] (see Section 9.3).

In addition to adjusting the estimates for the missing data, these models allow the investigator to explore possible relationships between HRQoL and explanatory factors causing missing observations. This is particularly interesting, for example, if death or disease progression was the cause of dropout. The criticism of selection models is that the validity of the models for the missing data mechanism is untestable because the model includes the missing values (Y_i^{mis}) as an explanatory variable. The major concern is that the estimates of the primary parameters ($\boldsymbol{\Theta}$) describing changes in HRQoL are very sensitive to misspecification of the missing data model.

Overview

In some trials, it is reasonable to believe that the rate of change in HRQoL is associated with the length of time a subject remains on the study. This is typical of patients with rapidly progressing disease, where more rapid decline in HRQoL is associated with earlier termination of the outcome measurement. The first two models are based on that principle. The first model is the *conditional linear model* proposed by Wu and Bailey [167] (see Section 9.2). Each individual's rate of change in HRQoL is assumed to depend on covariates and the time to an event associated with dropout. The second model is the *joint mixed-effects and time to dropout-event model* proposed by Schluchter [133] and DeGruttola and Tu [30]. These first two models are appropriate to settings where simple growth curve models describe the changes in the outcome and there is variation in the rates of change among the individual subjects (Table 9.1). Further distinctions between these two models are discussed in more detail later in the chapter.

The third model is a logistic selection model proposed by Diggle and Kenward [36] for a repeated measures design. This model is appropriate to

Table 9.1. General requirements of the conditional linear model, joint mixed-effects model, and logistic selection model.

Model characteristic	Conditional linear	Joint mixed-effects	Logistic selection
Repeated measures	No	No	Yes
Growth curve model	Linear[a]	Yes	Possible
Slope random-effect	Required[b]	Required[c]	No[d]
Baseline missing	Not allowed[e]	Allowed	Not allowed
Mistimed observations	Allowed	Allowed	Not allowed
Monotone dropout	Yes	Yes	Required
Intermittent pattern	Yes if MAR	Yes if MAR	Not allowed
Censoring of T_i^D	Not allowed	Yes	

[a] Higher-order polynomials possible but challenging.
[b] Random intercept is unrelated to dropout.
[c] Variation of slope is required.
[d] Random intercept only.
[e] Not allowed if baseline value included as a covariate in the model.

settings where there are equally spaced repeated measures and the missing data patterns are strictly monotone. Other assumptions are described later in the chapter.

9.2 Conditional linear model

Wu and Bailey [167] proposed a *conditional linear model* for studies where the primary interest focuses on estimating and comparing the average rate of change of an outcome over time (slope). The basis of their models is the assumption that the slope depends on covariates, the baseline value of the outcome, and the time of dropout T_i^D. Consider a model where each individual's HRQoL can be described by a linear function of time:

$$Y_i = X_i \beta_i + \epsilon_i, \qquad X_i' = \begin{bmatrix} 1 & 1 & \cdots & 1 \\ t_{i1} & t_{i2} & \cdots & t_{iJ} \end{bmatrix}, \qquad \beta_i = [\beta_{i1} \ \beta_{i2}] \quad (9.6)$$

with random variation of the intercept β_{i1} and rate of change (slope) β_{i2}.*

$$\beta_i \sim N(\beta_h, D) \quad \beta_h' = [\beta_{h1} \ \beta_{h2}] \tag{9.7}$$

$$\epsilon_i \sim N(0, \sigma^2 \mathbf{I}) \tag{9.8}$$

Each individual's slope may depend on M covariates (V_{mi}), the initial value of the outcome (Y_{i1}), as well as a polynomial function of the time of dropout (T_i^D). The form of the relationship is allowed to vary across the h

* Note that the model is equivalent to a mixed-effects model, $X_i \beta_i = X_i \beta + Z_i d_i$, when $X_i = Z_i$ and $\beta_i = \beta + d_i$.

treatment groups. The expected slope for the ith individual is

$$E[\beta_{i2}|T_i^D, V_{mi}, Y_{i1}] = \sum_{l=0}^{L} \gamma_{hl}(T_i^D)^l + \sum_{m=1}^{M} \gamma_{h(L+m)}V_{mi} + \gamma_{h(L+M+1)}Y_{i1}, \quad (9.9)$$

where $\gamma_{h0}, \ldots, \gamma_{h(L+M+1)}$ are the coefficients for the hth group and L is the degree of the polynomial. The intercept for the ith individual, β_{i1}, is not dependent on covariates or the time of dropout; thus, the expected intercept is

$$E[\beta_{i1}] = \beta_{h1}. \quad (9.10)$$

By substituting Equations 9.9 and 9.10 into Equation 9.6,

$$Y_{ij} = E[\beta_{i1}] + E[\beta_{i2}]t_{ij} + \epsilon_{ij}$$
$$= \beta_{h1} + \left(\sum_{l=0}^{L} \gamma_{hl}(T_i^D)^l + \sum_{m=1}^{M} \gamma_{h(L+m)}V_{mi} + \gamma_{h(L+M+1)}Y_{i1} \right)t_{ij} + \epsilon_{ij}.$$
$$(9.11)$$

The mean slope in the hth group is the expected value of the individual slopes of the subjects in the hth group ($i \in h$):

$$\beta_{h2} = E_{i \in h}\left[\beta_{i2}|T_i^D, V_{mi}, Y_{i1}\right]. \quad (9.12)$$

One of the estimates proposed by Wu and Bailey is referred to as the *linear minimum variance unbiased estimator* (LMVUB):

$$\beta_{h2} = \sum_{l=0}^{L} \hat{\gamma}_{hl}(\bar{T}_h^D)^l + \sum_{m=1}^{M} \hat{\gamma}_{h(L+m)}\bar{V}_{hm} + \hat{\gamma}_{h(L+M+1)}\bar{Y}_{h1}, \quad (9.13)$$

where $\bar{T}_h^D$ is the mean dropout time in the hth group, $\bar{V}_{hm}$ is the mean of the mth covariate in the hth group, and $\bar{Y}_{h1}$ is the mean of the baseline measure in the hth group. In a randomized trial, prerandomization characteristics are theoretically the same in all treatment groups. To avoid introducing differences that are the result of random differences in these baseline characteristics, $\bar{V}_{hm}$ and $\bar{Y}_{h1}$ are estimated using all randomized subjects ($\bar{V}_m$ and $\bar{Y}_1$).

There are several practical consequences and assumptions of this model:

1. Changes over time are assumed to be roughly linear.

2. There is enough variation in the rate of change among subjects to allow modeling of the variation.

3. All subjects must have a baseline measurement and complete data for the selected covariates (V) or they will be excluded.

4. The time of dropout is known for all subjects. All subjects have been followed until they either dropped out or completed the final assessment.

5. Subjects with an assessment at the last follow-up behave as if they dropped out immediately after that point in time. Basically, there is no way to distinguish between subjects who would have continued to have assessments and those who would have dropped out before the next assessment if the follow-up extended.

Testing MAR vs. MNAR under assumptions of conditional linear model

Note that if the slopes were dependent only on covariates, we would consider the data to be MCAR and Equation 9.9 would reduce to

$$E[\beta_{i2}|V_{mi}] = \gamma_{h0} + \sum_{m=1}^{M} \gamma_{hm} V_{mi}. \tag{9.14}$$

If the slopes were dependent on the baseline measure of the outcome but not the time of dropout, we would consider the data to be MAR. In this case, Equation 9.9 would reduce to

$$E[\beta_{i2}|V_{mi}, Y_{i1}] = \gamma_{h0} + \sum_{m=1}^{M} \gamma_{hm} V_{mi} + \gamma_{h(M+1)} Y_{i1}. \tag{9.15}$$

When the terms involving functions of the time of dropout T_i^D remain in the model, there is evidence that the data are MNAR. Thus, testing the hypothesis $\gamma_{hl} = 0$ vs. $\gamma_{hl} \neq 0$, $l = 1, \ldots, L$ is a test of the MAR assumption against MNAR. If it is rejected, there is evidence that missingness is nonignorable. However, if the test is not rejected, one can only conclude that the missingness is ignorable only if this particular model is correct. Unfortunately, we cannot test or prove that the model is correctly specified. Thus, failing to reject the hypothesis cannot be considered proof that the data are MAR.

NSCLC example

Previous examination of the NSCLC data suggests that the change in the FACT-Lung TOI scores over time is approximately linear. Assuming that the endpoint of interest is comparison of the slopes of patients not receiving Taxol to those receiving Taxol, one might proceed as follows:

1. Estimate the slopes in a simple mixed-effects model.

$$\text{Model 1:} \quad Y_{ij} = \beta_{hi1} + \gamma_{h0} t_{ij} + \epsilon_{ij}. \tag{9.16}$$

The SAS statements are as follows:

```
PROC MIXED DATA=WORK.MERGED METHOD=ML COVTEST;
  CLASS TAXOL;
  MODEL FACT_T2=TAXOL TAXOL*MONTHS/NOINT SOLUTION;
  RANDOM INTERCEPT MONTHS/SUBJECT=CASEID TYPE=UN;
  ESTIMATE 'NO - SLOPE'    TAXOL*MONTHS 1 0;
  ESTIMATE 'YES - SLOPE'   TAXOL*MONTHS 0 1;
  ESTIMATE 'DIFF - SLOPE'  TAXOL*MONTHS -1 1;
RUN;
```

Check the variance of the random slope effects. If this value is small (i.e., not significantly different from zero), seriously reconsider using a conditional linear model as an analysis strategy. First, it does not make sense to develop a model to explain variation when there is none. Second, models will be very slow to converge (if they do at all) when they include a variance parameter

Table 9.2. Summary of slope estimates based on the conditional linear model.

Model	No Taxol	Taxol	Difference	Variance	$-2 \log L$	χ^2_2
1	−0.74 (0.32)	−0.92 (0.21)	−0.18 (0.38)	1.74 (0.88)	11226.8	
2	−0.85 (0.32)	−0.95 (0.21)	−0.95 (0.38)	1.76 (0.88)	11215.6	11.2
3	−0.97 (0.32)	−0.89 (0.21)	0.07 (0.38)	0.55 (0.70)	10901.1	314.5
4	−1.77 (0.59)	−1.87 (0.35)	−0.10 (0.68)	0.67 (0.75)	10886.4	14.7
5	−3.35 (0.89)	−2.64 (0.51)	0.77 (1.02)	0.46 (0.78)	10876.3	10.1

that is very close to zero. In this example, the variance of the slopes is significant but only moderately different from zero (Table 9.2).

2. Identify baseline covariates that might predict change and test the significance of their interaction with time in a mixed-effects model:

$$\text{Model 2:} \quad Y_{ij} = \beta_{hi1} + \gamma_{h0}t_{ij} + \underbrace{\sum_{m=1}^{M} \gamma_{hm}V_{mi}t_{ij}}_{\text{Addition to Model 1}} + \epsilon_{ij}. \quad (9.17)$$

Symptoms of metastatic disease (SX_MET) were the strongest predictor of the slope among the available demographic* and disease measures prior to treatment.** Note that the term TAXOL*MONTHS*SX_MET has been added to the MODEL statement.

```
PROC MIXED DATA=WORK.MERGED NOCLPRINT METHOD=ML;
  CLASS TAXOL CASEID;
  MODEL FACT_T2=TAXOL TAXOL*MONTHS TAXOL*SX_MET*MONTHS
              /NOINT SOLUTION;
  RANDOM INTERCEPT MONTHS /SUBJECT=CASEID TYPE=UN;
  ESTIMATE 'NO - SLOPE'   TAXOL*MONTHS 1 0
                          TAXOL*SX_MET*MONTHS 0.55 0;
  ESTIMATE 'YES - SLOPE'  TAXOL*MONTHS 0 1
                          TAXOL*SX_MET*MONTHS 0 0.55;
  ESTIMATE 'DIFF - SLOPE' TAXOL*MONTHS -1 1
                          TAXOL*SX_MET*MONTHS -0.55 0.55;
RUN;
```

Prior to running the procedure to estimate the parameters of the mixed-effects model, the mean of SX_MET was estimated in each of the two groups. Because SX_MET was coded as an indicator variable,*** the mean is also the proportion of patients with symptoms of metastatic disease at diagnosis in each group, 58 and 54%, respectively. The means were inserted into the ESTIMATE statement to estimate the group slopes (β_{h2}). Addition of symptoms of metastatic disease prior to treatment explained a significant

---

  * Age and gender.
 ** Stage of disease, Eastern Cooperative Oncology Group (ECOG) performance status, >5% weight loss in last 6 months, primary disease symptoms, metastatic disease symptoms, systemic disease symptoms.
*** 0 = No, 1 = Yes.

proportion of the variability of the slope ($\chi_2^2 = 35.3, p < 0.001$), but it did not affect the estimates of the slopes in the two treatment groups (Table 9.2).

3. Add the baseline measure of the outcome variable to the model and test for an interaction with time.

$$\text{Model 3:} \quad Y_{ij} = \beta_{hi1} + \gamma_{h0}t_{ij} + \sum_{m=1}^{M}\gamma_{hm}V_{mi}t_{ij} + \underbrace{\gamma_{h(M+1)}Y_{i1}t_{ij}}_{\text{Addition to Model 2}} + \epsilon_{ij}.$$

(9.18)

The interaction term TAXOL*BASELINE*MONTHS is added to the MODEL statement. To facilitate the interpretation of the coefficients, BASELINE was calculated as the initial FACT-Lung TOI score minus 65, which was approximately the mean of the baseline scores.

```
PROC MIXED DATA=WORK.MERGED NOCLPRINT METHOD=ML;
  CLASS TAXOL CASEID;
  MODEL FACT_T2=TAXOL TAXOL*MONTHS TAXOL*SX_MET*MONTHS
              TAXOL*BASELINE*MONTHS /NOINT SOLUTION;
  RANDOM INTERCEPT MONTHS /SUBJECT=CASEID TYPE=UN;
  ESTIMATE 'NO - SLOPE'    TAXOL*MONTHS 1 0
                           TAXOL*SX_MET*MONTHS 0.55 0
                           TAXOL*BASELINE*MONTHS 0.582 0;
  ESTIMATE 'YES - SLOPE'   TAXOL*MONTHS 0 1
                           TAXOL*SX_MET*MONTHS 0 0.55
                           TAXOL*BASELINE*MONTHS 0 0.582;
  ESTIMATE 'DIFF - SLOPE'  TAXOL*MONTHS -1 1
                           TAXOL*SX_MET*MONTHS -0.55 0.55
                           TAXOL*BASELINE*MONTHS -0.582 0.582;
RUN;
```

As in the previous case, the average BASELINE value in each group is calculated prior to fitting the mixed-effects model and inserted into the ESTIMATE statement. Addition of the baseline value of the outcome also explained a significant proportion of the variability of the slope ($\chi_2^2 = 314.2, p < 0.001$), but again it did not affect the estimates of the slopes in the two treatment groups (see Table 9.2). This should not be surprising, since Model 2 is unbiased if missingness depends only on the observed baseline data.

4. Finally, the interaction of time of dropout with the slope is added to the model.

$$\text{Models 4 and 5:} \quad Y_{ij} = \beta_{hi1} + \gamma_{h0}t_{ij} + \underbrace{\sum_{l=1}^{L}\gamma_{hl}\left(T_i^D\right)^l t_{ij}}_{\text{Addition to Model 3}}$$

$$+ \sum_{m=1}^{M}\gamma_{h(L+m)}V_{mi}t_{ij} + \gamma_{h(L+M+1)}Y_{i1}t_{ij} + \epsilon_{ij}.$$

(9.19)

There are several possibilities at this point for defining T_i^D, including the planned time of the last assessment and the observed time of the last assessment. In the following illustration, T_i^D was defined as the observed time in months from randomization to the last HRQoL assessment (LAST_MO). Other possibilities are the time to disease progression, termination of therapy, or death. In the NSCLC example, a linear (Model 4: $L = 1$) and a quadratic (Model 5: $L = 2$) model for the time of dropout were tested. The quadratic model provided the best fit:

```
PROC MIXED DATA=WORK.MERGED NOCLPRINT METHOD=ML;
   CLASS TAXOL CASEID;
   MODEL FACT_T2=TAXOL TAXOL*MONTHS TAXOL*SX_MET*MONTHS
            TAXOL*BASELINE*MONTHS TAXOL*MONTHS*LAST_MO
            TAXOL*MONTHS*LAST_MO*LAST_MO
            /NOINT SOLUTION;
   RANDOM INTERCEPT MONTHS/SUBJECT=CASEID TYPE=UN;
   ESTIMATE 'NO TAXOL' TAXOL*MONTHS 1 0
                      TAXOL*SX_MET*MONTHS 0.55 0
                      TAXOL*BASELINE*MONTHS 0.582 0
                      TAXOL*MONTHS*LAST_MO 2.62 0
                      TAXOL*MONTHS*LAST_MO*LAST_MO 13.62 0;
   ESTIMATE 'TAXOL'   TAXOL*MONTHS 0 1
                      TAXOL*SX_MET*MONTHS 0 0.55
                      TAXOL*BASELINE*MONTHS 0 0.582
                      TAXOL*MONTHS*LAST_MO 0 3.04
                      TAXOL*MONTHS*LAST_MO*LAST_MO 0 15.74;
   ESTIMATE 'DIFF' TAXOL*MONTHS -1 1
                   TAXOL*SX_MET*MONTHS -0.55 0.55
                   TAXOL*BASELINE*MONTHS -0.582 0.582
                   TAXOL*MONTHS*LAST_MO -2.62 3.04
                   TAXOL*MONTHS*LAST_MO*LAST_MO 13.62 -15.74;
RUN;
```

Addition of the time of dropout also explained a significant proportion of the variability of the slope (Model 3 vs. 4: $\chi_2^2 = 14.7, p < 0.001$; Model 4 vs. 5: $\chi_2^2 = 10.1, p = 0.005$). In contrast with the previous models, there was a dramatic effect on the estimates of the slopes, with a doubling of the estimated rate of decline in both treatment groups when the linear interaction was added and a tripling of the rates when the quadratic interaction was added (see Table 9.2).

Examination of the coefficients of Model 5 (Table 9.3) suggests that the HRQoL measure decreases about 1 point per month faster in subjects with symptoms of metastatic disease than in those without symptoms prior to randomization (-1.27 and -0.71 in the two groups). It also predicts a faster decline of the same magnitude in a subject who scored 16 points lower at baseline than another subject ($1/0.061$ and $1/0.064$). The rate of decline is slower in those who stay on therapy longer; initially, the relative increase will range from 1 to 1.6 points per month for each additional month of follow-up (positive linear terms). However, the benefit will diminish with

Table 9.3. Summary of coefficients from the conditional linear model 5.

Effect	Taxol	Estimate	S.E.
Intercept	No	64.9	1.17
	Yes	66.3	0.82
Slope	No	−4.18	2.05
	Yes	−3.79	1.29
Slope * metastic disease[a]	No	−1.23	0.61
	Yes	−0.71	0.38
Slope * baseline[b]	No	−0.064	0.021
	Yes	−0.064	0.013
Slope * time of dropout[a]	No	1.64	0.49
	Yes	1.02	0.34
Slope * time of dropout[c]	No	−0.116	0.047
	Yes	−0.051	0.024

[a]0 = No, 1 = Yes.
[b]Score = 65.
[c]Last HRQoL assessment (months).

Table 9.4. Comparison of estimates of change in FACT-Lung TOI per month from selected models where change over time is assumed to be linear.

Method	No Taxol	Taxol	Difference
Ignorable (MLE)	−0.75 (0.32)	−0.91 (0.21)	−0.16 (0.39)
Conditional linear model 4	−1.91 (0.91)	−1.98 (0.38)	0.06 (0.91)
Conditional linear model 5	−3.72 (1.14)	−2.83 (0.60)	0.90 (1.23)
Pattern-mixture 1	−3.63 (0.96)	−2.06 (0.53)	1.57 (1.10)
Pattern-mixture 2	−5.03 (1.75)	−2.21 (0.85)	2.82 (1.94)

time (negative quadratic terms). For example, a subject on the control arm with no metastatic disease and a baseline score of 65 is expected to decline at a rate of 4.2 points per month if the subject's last HRQoL assessment was at baseline at a rate of 2.7 points per month if the subject dropped out at 1 month,* and almost not at all if the subject's last HRQoL assessment was at 3 months.** It is reassuring that all of these trends are in the expected directions.

Table 9.4 contrasts the results of the conditional linear model with the two pattern-mixture models described in the previous chapter. The estimates of change are between those estimated under the MAR assumptions and the pattern-mixture models.

* 1 month: $-4.18 + 1.64 * 1 - 0.12 * 1^2 = -2.7$.
** 3 months: $-4.18 + 1.64 * 3 - 0.12 * 3^2 = -0.3$.

Table 9.5. Comparison of naive and bootstrap estimates of the variance.

Model	Method	No Taxol	Taxol	Difference
Linear	Naive	−1.82 (0.61)	−1.93 (0.35)	0.11 (0.70)
	Bootstrap	−1.91 (0.91)	−1.98 (0.38)	0.06 (0.91)
Quadratic	Naive	−3.50 (0.91)	−2.72 (0.52)	−0.77 (1.05)
	Bootstrap	−3.72 (1.14)	−2.83 (0.60)	−0.90 (1.23)

Naive estimate assumes that means of covariates, baseline, and time to dropout are fixed and have no variance.

Estimation of the standard errors

Computations of the standard errors reported in the output associated with ESTIMATE statements are made with the assumption that the means of the covariates, baseline scores, and time to dropout are fixed and known. Because they are estimates, the standard errors will underestimate the true variance of the slopes. Wu and Bailey [167] provide corrected estimates of the variance for a special case. Bootstrapping is a more useful tool to handle all models, especially with small or moderately sized samples (Table 9.5).

Assumptions

There are two major conditions that must be true to implement the conditional linear model. The first condition is a linear pattern of change in the HRQoL measures over time. Although it is theoretically possible to extend this model to more complex growth curves, the models are very complex and difficult to estimate unless the size of the sample is very large. In small studies, there may be more parameters than observations. Even in moderate studies, there will be insufficient information to obtain precise estimates of the parameters. The second condition is that there is random variation in the slopes among subjects ($\text{Var}[d_{i2}] \gg 0$). Of practical note, this random effect may exist in Model 1 but disappear as more variation of the slopes is explained. In the NSCLC example, there was significant variation among the slopes in models 1 and 2, but the addition of baseline as an interaction explained approximately 70% of the variability of the slopes. Although all variance parameters were estimable in this example, it is likely that as the variance approaches zero problems with convergence of the algorithm will develop and the second random effect will need to be dropped from the model.

Random-coefficient mixture model

The conditional linear model has been described as a *random-coefficient pattern mixture model* [92] and a *random-effects mixture model* [67]. Each subject has a unique pattern defined by the dropout time, covariates, and the baseline measure. The restrictions placed on the model are defined by the conditional linear model (Equation 9.12).

9.3 Joint mixed-effects and time to dropout

To begin, consider the same basic mixed-effects model described by Equations 9.6 through 9.8, where changes in HRQoL are described by a simple two-stage mixed-effects model. Each individual's HRQoL is described by a linear function of time, with random variation among subjects of the intercept, β_{i1}, and the linear rate of change (slope), β_{i2}. The time of an event associated with the discontinuation of HRQoL measurement ($\mathcal{T}_i^D$) is incorporated into the model by allowing some function of the time to discontinuation ($f(\mathcal{T}_i^D)$) to be correlated with the random effects of the longitudinal model for HRQoL [30, 122, 133, 134].

$$\begin{bmatrix} \beta_i \\ f(\mathcal{T}_i^D) \end{bmatrix} \sim N\left(\begin{bmatrix} \beta \\ \mu_T \end{bmatrix}, \begin{bmatrix} D & \sigma_{bt} \\ (\sigma_{bt})' & \tau^2 \end{bmatrix} \right). \tag{9.20}$$

It is important to note that $\mathcal{T}_i^D$ does not have to be the time after which no HRQoL assessments were made but can, instead, be the time to any event associated with dropout. This is helpful when some of the dropout is unrelated to the outcome. For example, if the event were termination of therapy due to toxicity or lack of efficacy, then individuals who drop out for unrelated reasons would not be treated as if they experienced a negative outcome.

The first implication of this model is that the expected changes in HRQoL are a function of the dropout time. This is illustrated in Figure 9.1. Note that the patients with earlier dropout start with lower FACT-Lung TOI scores and decline more rapidly than subjects who remain longer. In the model (Equation 9.20), both the intercepts (β_{i1}) and the slopes (β_{i2}) are positively

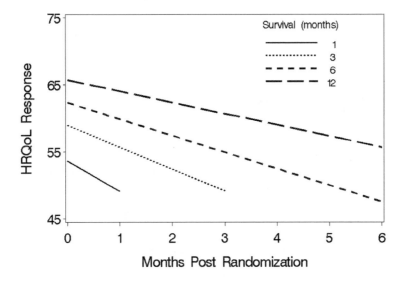

Figure 9.1. Expected change in FACT-Lung TOI among NSCLC patients given death occurred at 1, 3, 6, and 12 months.

correlated with longer survival ($\sigma_{bt} > 0$). More formally, the conditional expectation of the random effects is a function of the dropout time.

$$E[\beta_i|T_i^D] = \beta + \sigma_{bt}\tau^{-2}(f(T_i^D) - \mu_t). \qquad (9.21)$$

In the example presented in Figure 9.1, the expected intercept for a subject surviving to T_i^D is

$$E[\beta_{i1}|T_i^D] = 65.3 + 8.381 * 1.721^{-1}(\ln(T_i^D) + 0.088)$$
$$= 65.7 + 4.870 * \ln(T_i^D).$$

Thus, the average baseline score is 59.0 for a patient who survives 3 months ($\ln(0.25 \text{ years}) = -1.386$) and 65.7 for a patient surviving 12 months ($\ln(1.00 \text{ years}) = 0.00$). The expected change over time is

$$E[\beta_{i2}|T_i^D] = -1.78 + 1.974 * 1.721^{-1}(\ln(T_i^D) + 0.088)$$
$$= -1.77 + 1.147 * \ln(T_i^D).$$

The predicted decline is 3.4 points per month for a patient who survives 3 months but only 1.8 points per month for a patient surviving 12 months.

This model differs from the *conditional linear model* in several respects.

1. The joint model allows the intercept and slope to be related to the time of dropout.
2. There is an added restriction that the relationships are linear functions of $f(T_i^D)$.

$$E[\beta_i|T_i^D] = \beta + \sigma_{bt}\tau^{-2}(f(T_i^D) - \mu_t)$$
$$= \underbrace{\beta - \sigma_{bt}\tau^{-2}\mu_t}_{\gamma_{h0}} + \underbrace{\sigma_{bt}\tau^{-2}}_{\gamma_{h1}} f(T_i^D). \qquad (9.22)$$

3. The algorithms developed by Schluchter [133] and DeGruttola and Tu [30] allow censoring of T_i^D. This allows us to differentiate a subject who completes the 6-month evaluation but dies shortly thereafter (e.g., $T_i^D = 8$ months) from a subject who remains alive (e.g., $T_i^D > 8$ months). This frees the analyst from assigning an arbitrary dropout time to subjects who complete the study.

The second implication of the joint model is that the expected time of dropout is a function of the initial HRQoL scores as well as the rate of change over time. More formally, the conditional distribution of the dropout times is a function of the random effects.

$$E[f(T_i^D)|\beta_i] = \mu_t + \sigma'_{bt}D^{-1}\beta_i. \qquad (9.23)$$

Testing MAR vs. MNAR under the assumptions of the joint model

Under this model, the missing data are nonignorable if the random effects (particularly the slope) are correlated with the time of dropout ($\sigma_{bt} \neq 0$). For example, if patients with more rapid rates of decline in their HRQoL scores failed earlier (and thus were more likely to miss subsequent assessments), the random effect corresponding to the rate of change is positively correlated with the failure time.

Again, it should be emphasized that the lack of significant correlation implies the the missing data are ignorable *only if the model for dropout is correct*. If dropout was the result of a sudden change in the outcome rather than a gradual change (as measured by slopes), then the dropout model is misspecified and would not identify the nonignorable process.

Selection or mixture model?

Little [92] classifies this model as a *random-coefficient selection model* with nonignorable random-coefficient-based dropout ($[T_i^D|X_i,\beta_i]$). In contrast, Hogan and Laird [67] describe this model as a random-effects mixture model. This model has also been referred to as a *shared-parameter model* [51, 67, 155, p. 326]. We considered the *observed data* to include the observed HRQoL responses (Y_i^{obs}) as well as the time to dropout (T_i^D). The assumption is that the data are missing at random (MAR) conditional on the augmented *observed data*. In this framework, the choice of the event that defines T_i^D might not be strictly the time of dropout but, rather, a more specific event related to both discontinuation of HRQoL assessment and HRQoL itself. For example, the event might be a specific cause of dropout such as the lack of efficacy. Other causes of dropout that are not associated with the treatment would be treated as if T_i^D were censored for administrative reasons.

NSCLC example

A practical requirement of the joint model is nonzero variation in the random effects. If the variance of the random effects is close to zero, it is difficult, if not impossible, to estimate the covariance between the random effects and the time to dropout. Prior to embarking on analyses using the joint model, it is wise to check the estimates of variance in the simpler mixed-effects model. The COVTEST option in the MIXED procedure statement generates these estimates and their estimated standard errors.

```
PROC MIXED DATA=BOOK.EXAMPLE2 COVTEST;
   CLASS TAXOL;
   MODEL FACT_T2=TAXOL TAXOL*MONTHS\NOINT;
   RANDOM INTERCEPT MONTHS\SUBJECT=CASEID TYPE=UN;
RUN;
```

The estimated variances of the random effects for all subscales of the FACT-Lung are summarized in Table 9.6. The results suggest that there are no problems estimating the covariance of the random intercepts with time to dropout, but problems will definitely occur with the social and physical well-being subscale and possibly for the emotional well-being subscale.

In the NSCLC study, the protocol specified that HRQoL was to be collected until the final follow-up, regardless of disease progression or discontinuation

Table 9.6. Estimates of variance of random effects for subscales of the FACT-Lung in the NSCLC study.

Subscale	Intercept			Slope		
	Var	(S.E.)	p	Var	(S.E.)	p
Functional well-being	264.8	(28.0)	<0.001	4.46	(1.81)	0.006
Lung CA specific issues	154.1	(16.0)	<0.001	2.21	(0.97)	0.01
Emotional well-being	203.8	(19.3)	<0.001	1.26	(0.91)	0.08
Physical well-being	177.0	(24.6)	<0.001	1.13	(1.43)	0.22
Social well-being	110.8	(12.5)	<0.001	No estimate		
FACT-Lung TOI	148.6	(15.3)	<0.001	1.81	(0.89)	0.02

No estimate: Note in log `G not positive definite`.

Table 9.7. Joint model for FACT-Lung TOI and various measures of the time to dropout $(\mathcal{T}^D)$.

Dropout event $(\mathcal{T}^D)$	Correlation $(\beta_i, \mathcal{T}^D)$		Change in TOI	
	Intercept	Slope	Estimate	S.E.
None (MLE)			−0.86	0.17
End of therapy	0.41	0.22	−1.24	0.13
Last HRQoL assessment	0.40	0.35	−1.76	0.13
ln(event free survival)	0.43	0.58	−1.44	0.13
ln(survival) long follow-up	0.46	0.73	−1.78	0.13
ln(survival) short follow-up	0.52	0.82	−1.78	0.16

Estimates of correlation between time $(\mathcal{T}^D)$ and random effects (β_i) and linear change in FACT-Lung TOI $(\hat{\beta}_2)$.

of treatment. Thus, theoretically, death is the event that censored the measurement of HRQoL. In practice, it became difficult to follow patients after disease progression for various reasons. In addition to time to death, one might consider time to the last HRQoL measurement as a candidate for the joint model. Finally, there is the possibility that the rate of change in HRQoL depends on other clinical events, such as time to disease progression.

Table 9.7 summarizes the results from a number of joint models for the NSCLC study and compares the estimates to the corresponding mixed-effects model. First, visual examination of the distribution of the dropout-event times $(\mathcal{T}_i^D)$ suggested that the times of the last HRQoL measurement and the end of therapy had roughly symmetric (although not strictly normal) distributions, while the times to disease progression and death were skewed to the right. As a result, a log transformation was used for time to death (survival) and time to disease progression (event-free survival). We also considered a model with survival measured with a short follow-up of only 6 months and a model with extended follow-up (>5 years), where 90% of the deaths were observed. All the events were moderately correlated with the intercept (ρ in the range of 0.4 to 0.5). The correlation with the slopes was weakest for the time to treatment discontinuation ($\rho \approx 0.2$) and last HRQoL assessment ($\rho \approx 0.35$). The weaker correlations are expected, as there are a wide range of reasons for these events. There was a stronger correlation with death than disease progression ($\rho \approx 0.6$). One explanation for this is that disease progression is often determined with radiological imaging, before disease progression produces symptoms that would impact the subject's HRQoL. The strong correlations ($\rho > 0.7$) of change with time to death fit with the observation that deterioration in physical and functional well-being accelerate in the months prior to death. It is also likely that events distant from the period of the study are not correlated with the changes in the FACT-Lung TOI during the 6 months of the study.

Initial estimates

The algorithms for estimation of the joint model require initial estimates of the parameters. Good starting estimates speed up the convergence of the program, decrease the chance of finding a local minimum, and, for some algorithms, avoid nonpositive definite covariance matrices. The following procedure is suggested.

1. Fit a mixed-effects model for the HRQoL data, assuming the data are MAR. Use these estimates for β, D, and σ^2.
2. Estimate the distribution of $f(T_i^D)$. To estimate μ_T and τ^2 when a natural log transformation is used and T_i^D is censored for some subjects:

```
PROC LIFEREG;
   MODEL TSURV*FAIL(0)= / DISTRIBUTION=LNORMAL;
RUN;
```

When the times (T^D) are assumed to be normally distributed, the estimates can be obtained using

```
PROC LIFEREG;
   MODEL TSURV*FAIL(0)= /DISTRIBUTION=NORMAL;
RUN;
```

3. Assume that the random effects are weakly correlated ($\rho \approx 0.2$) with $f(T_i^D)$. Thus,

$$\sigma_{1bt} = 0.2\sqrt{\sigma_{11}\tau^2},$$
$$\sigma_{2bt} = 0.2\sqrt{\sigma_{22}\tau^2},$$

where σ_{11} and σ_{22} are the diagonal elements of D.

Extension to more complex mixed-effects models

The joint model can be extended to more complex models [41, 42, 122]. Consider the more general mixed-effects model for the HRQoL outcome:

$$Y_i = X_i\beta + Z_i d_i + e_i. \tag{9.24}$$

The marginal model ($X_i\beta$) does not need to be constrained to be linear over time but could contain polynomial or piecewise regression terms. Further, the random effects do not have to have a one-to-one correspondence with the fixed effects ($X_i \neq Z_i$). In this more general model, the distribution displayed in Equation 9.20 is modified by replacing β_i with d_i and β with 0.

$$\begin{bmatrix} d_i \\ f(T_i) \end{bmatrix} \sim N\left(\begin{bmatrix} 0 \\ \mu_T \end{bmatrix}, \begin{bmatrix} D & \sigma_{bt} \\ (\sigma_{bt})' & \tau^2 \end{bmatrix} \right). \tag{9.25}$$

Renal cell carcinoma example

This extension to more complex models is illustrated in the renal cell carcinoma example, where the change in the FACT-TOI was not linear over time. Recall that a piecewise linear model with changes in the slope at 2, 8, and 17 weeks was used to describe change in HRQoL over time. One might consider adding additional random effects corresponding to these terms in the piecewise linear model. Algorithms for estimating models with more random effects often fail to converge unless there is sufficient information in the data to estimate the variance of these random effects. This will not be the case unless there is extended follow-up in a large number of subjects.

In the renal cell carcinoma study, the follow-up on most subjects is relatively short and we are limited to a model with only two random effects. In this study, both the intercepts and slopes are correlated with the log transformed time of death. The expected changes in the FACT-BRM TOI for patients surviving 8, 17, and 52 weeks are displayed in Figure 9.2. As seen in the previous example, subjects with longer survival tend to start with higher FACT-BRM TOI scores. A little less obvious in this figure, because of the shapes of the curves, are the increased initial rates of decline of the subjects with shorter survival. The overall estimates in the two treatment groups are displayed in Figure 9.3. Although the shapes of the curves are very similar, the estimates of the rate of change in the FACT-BRM TOI scores change in the later phase of the study. Under the MAR assumption, HRQoL appears to be improving after week 17, whereas under the joint model assumptions the profiles have flattened.

9.4 Selection model for monotone dropout

Diggle and Kenward [36] proposed a selection model for monotone missing data. They defined the dropout process in terms that correspond to MCAR, MAR, and MNAR. *Completely random dropout* (CRD) corresponds to MCAR, where dropout is completely independent of measurement. *Random dropout* (RD) corresponds to MAR, where dropout depends on only observed

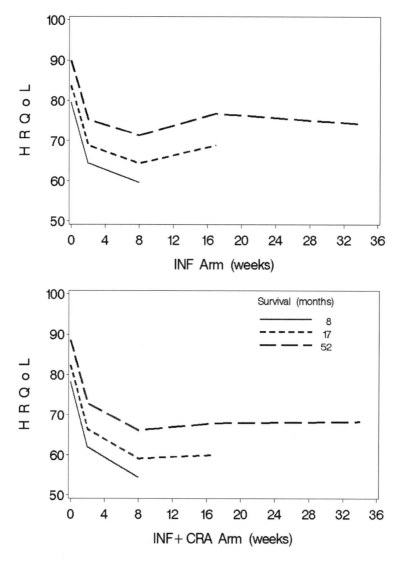

Figure 9.2. Expected change in FACT-BRM TOI among renal cell carcinoma patients given that death occurred at 8, 17, or 52 weeks. Upper figure corresponds to interferon arm (IFNα) and lower figure corresponds to interferon plus cis-retinoic acid (IFNα+CRA) arm of trial.

measurements (prior to dropout). *Informative dropout* (ID) corresponds to MNAR, where dropout depends on unobserved measures. The *response model* is the same multivariate linear regression model that we have used throughout, $f(Y_i|\Theta)$. For the *dropout model* they assume a logistic regression, $f(R_i|Y_i,\Gamma)$, which may depend on covariates $\mathcal{X}_i$ (CRD), previous observations (RD), or the unobserved measurement at the time of dropout (ID). The conditional

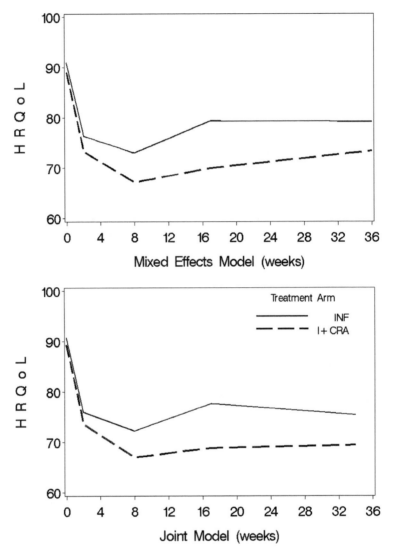

Figure 9.3. Expected change in FACT-TOI among patients with renal cell carcinoma. Solid line corresponds to interferon arm; dashed line corresponds to interferon plus cis-retinoic acid arm of trial.

probability of dropout at time j, given the history through time $j-1$, is denoted by

$$P_j = Pr(T_i^D = t_j | Y_{i1}, \ldots, Y_{ij-1}). \qquad (9.26)$$

The logistic linear model for the dropout process takes the form

$$\text{logit}[P_j] = \gamma_0 \mathcal{X}_i + \gamma_1 y_{ij} + \gamma_2 y_{ij-1}. \qquad (9.27)$$

If $\gamma_2 \neq 0$, then dropout depends on the previously observed response (y_{ij-1}), and if $\gamma_1 \neq 0$, then dropout depends on the current unobserved response (y_{ij}). Therefore, if $\gamma_1 = \gamma_2 = 0$, the dropout process is completely random (CRD). If $\gamma_1 = 0$ and $\gamma_2 \neq 0$, then dropout depends only on the previously observed responses and the process is RD. If $\gamma_1 \neq 0$, then dropout depends on the current data (y_{ij}) and the process is informative (ID). If the dropout process is CRD or RD, the *response model* and the *dropout model* can be estimated separately. However, if the dropout process is ID, Θ and Γ must be estimated jointly.

Outcome-dependent selection model

Little [92] classifies this model as a *random coefficient selection model* with nonignorable outcome-based dropout $([R_i|X_i, Y_i^{\text{obs}}, Y_i^{\text{mis}}])$.

NSCLC example

The NSCLC study is used to illustrate this approach. Note that this is for illustrative purposes only, as there are some constraints imposed by the model and the estimation procedure. First, we will have to exclude 15% of the patients who have intermittent missing data as well as 6% who have no data. This leaves 471 subjects. Second, we will have to assume that the interval between the third and fourth measurements is equivalent to the intervals between the first, second, and third with respect to the dropout model. In practice, we would not use a model that excludes such a large portion of the data, nor would we assume equal spacing of the assessments.

In the following example, we use the Oswald library of functions written for S-Plus. A full discussion of the software is presented in the next section. The first step is to explore models describing the dropout process under the CRD assumption. In model 1 (CRD1), we assume that the probability of dropout is the same for the second, third, and fourth assessment $(\mathcal{X}_{i1} = 1)$.

$$\text{logit}[P_j|\mathcal{X}_i] = \gamma_{01} \tag{9.28}$$

$$Pr(T_i^D = t_j) = \frac{e^{\gamma_{01}}}{1 + e^{\gamma_{01}}}, \quad j = 2, 3, 4. \tag{9.29}$$

The estimated parameters for the model are displayed in Table 9.8. The estimated probability of dropout (Table 9.9) at each follow-up visit is

$$\hat{P}_j = e^{-0.806}/(1 + e^{-0.806}) = 0.31.$$

This implies that 31% of the remaining subjects drop out at each of the follow-up visits. The probability of completing the HRQoL assessment at the final visit is the product of the probability of remaining in the study at each follow-up. Thus, the model predicts that 69% of the subjects will have an assessment at 6 weeks $[(1 - \hat{P}_2) = 0.69]$, 48% at 12 weeks $[(1 - \hat{P}_2)(1 - \hat{P}_3) = 0.48]$, and 33% at 26 weeks $[(1 - \hat{P}_2)(1 - \hat{P}_3) \times (1 - \hat{P}_4) = 0.33]$. The estimated probabilities of dropout and of remaining in the study are compared to the observed probabilities in Tables 9.9 and 9.10.

Table 9.8. Diggle and Kenward models assuming completely random dropout.

Parameter		CRD1	CRD2	CRD3	CRD4
$\hat{\beta}_1$	Intercept	63.9	63.9	63.9	63.9
$\hat{\beta}_2$	Group	1.69	1.69	1.69	1.69
$\hat{\beta}_3$	Time	−0.266	−0.266	−0.266	−0.266
$\hat{\beta}_4$	Group:time	0.073	0.073	0.073	0.073
$\hat{\gamma}_0$	Intercept	−0.806	−0.597	−0.933	−0.549
				−0.954	−1.005
				−0.399	−0.198
	Group		−0.307		−0.592
					0.071
					−0.285
	−2 log L	16179.39	16174.77	16166.90	16158.19
	Comparison		CRD1	CRD1	CRD3
	LR statistic		$\chi_1^2 = 4.62$	$\chi_2^2 = 13.53$	$\chi_3^2 = 8.69$
	p-value		0.032	0.0012	0.034

Table 9.9. Probability of dropout at the jth assessment if observed at $j-1$ ($Pr[R_{ij} = 0|R_{ij-1} = 1]$).

Group	Weeks	Obs	CRD1	CRD2	CRD3	CRD4
No Taxol	6	0.37	0.31	0.35	0.28	0.37
	12	0.27	0.31	0.35	0.28	0.27
	26	0.45	0.31	0.35	0.40	0.45
Taxol	6	0.24	0.31	0.29	0.28	0.24
	12	0.28	0.31	0.29	0.28	0.28
	26	0.38	0.31	0.29	0.40	0.38

In model 2 (CRD2), we allow the probability to differ across the two treatments by adding an indicator for the Taxol group ($\mathcal{X}_{i2} = 0$ if No Taxol, $\mathcal{X}_{i2} = 1$ if Taxol).

$$\text{logit}[P_j, \mathcal{X}_i] = \gamma_{01} + \gamma_{02}\mathcal{X}_{i2}, \tag{9.30}$$

$$Pr(T_i^D = t_j | \mathcal{X}_{i2} = 0) = \frac{e^{\gamma_{01}}}{1 + e^{\gamma_0}}, \tag{9.31}$$

$$Pr(T_i^D = t_j | \mathcal{X}_{i2} = 1) = \frac{e^{\gamma_{01}+\gamma_{02}}}{1 + e^{\gamma_{01}+\gamma_{02}}}. \tag{9.32}$$

The estimated probability of dropout is higher among the subjects not assigned to the Taxol therapy ($\hat{P}_k = 0.35$) than among those assigned to the Taxol therapy ($\hat{P}_k = 0.29$).

In model 3 (CRD3), we assume that the probability is the same across the two treatments but differs by time ($\mathcal{X}_{i1} = 1$ if t_2, $\mathcal{X}_{i2} = 1$ if t_3, $\mathcal{X}_{i3} = 1$

Table 9.10. Probability of a subject remaining on study at the jth assessment $(Pr[R_{ij} = 1])$.

Group	Weeks	j	Obs	CRD1	CRD2	CRD3	CRD4
No Taxol	6	2	0.63	0.69	0.65	0.72	0.63
	12	3	0.41	0.48	0.42	0.52	0.46
	26	4	0.25	0.33	0.27	0.31	0.25
Taxol	6	2	0.76	0.69	0.71	0.72	0.76
	12	3	0.54	0.48	0.51	0.52	0.54
	26	4	0.34	0.33	0.36	0.31	0.34

if t_4, 0 otherwise).

$$\text{logit}[P_j, \mathcal{X}_i] = \gamma_{01}\mathcal{X}_{i1} + \gamma_{02}\mathcal{X}_{i2} + \gamma_{03}\mathcal{X}_{i3} \tag{9.33}$$

$$Pr(T_i^D = t_2) = \frac{e^{\gamma_{01}}}{1 + e^{\gamma_{01}}} \tag{9.34}$$

$$Pr(T_i^D = t_3) = \frac{e^{\gamma_{02}}}{1 + e^{\gamma_{02}}} \tag{9.35}$$

$$Pr(T_i^D = t_4) = \frac{e^{\gamma_{03}}}{1 + e^{\gamma_{03}}} \tag{9.36}$$

The predicted dropout rate at 6 weeks ($\hat{P}_k = 0.28$) is very similar to that at 12 weeks ($\hat{P}_k = 0.28$) and increases at 26 weeks ($\hat{P}_k = 0.40$). This model fits the observed data better than the model where we assume a constant dropout rate (see Table 9.8).

Finally, in model 4 (CRD4), we allow the probability to differ across the two treatments by adding indicators for the Taxol group at each time ($\mathcal{X}_{i4} = \mathcal{X}_{i5} = \mathcal{X}_{i6} = 0$ if No Taxol, $\mathcal{X}_{i2} = \mathcal{X}_{i5} = \mathcal{X}_{i6} = 1$ if Taxol).

$$\text{logit}[P_j, \mathcal{X}_i] = \gamma_{01}\mathcal{X}_{i1} + \gamma_{02}\mathcal{X}_{i2} + \gamma_{03}\mathcal{X}_{i3} + \gamma_{04}\mathcal{X}_{i4}$$
$$+ \gamma_{05}\mathcal{X}_{i5} + \gamma_{06}\mathcal{X}_{i6}, \tag{9.37}$$

$$Pr(T_i^D = t_2 | \mathcal{X}_{i4} = 0) = \frac{e^{\gamma_{01}}}{1 + e^{\gamma_{01}}}, \tag{9.38}$$

$$Pr(T_i^D = t_2 | \mathcal{X}_{i4} = 1) = \frac{e^{\gamma_{01}+\gamma_{04}}}{1 + e^{\gamma_{01}+\gamma_{04}}}, \tag{9.39}$$

$$Pr(T_i^D = t_3 | \mathcal{X}_{i5} = 0) = \frac{e^{\gamma_{02}}}{1 + e^{\gamma_{02}}}, \tag{9.40}$$

$$Pr(T_i^D = t_3 | \mathcal{X}_{i5} = 1) = \frac{e^{\gamma_{02}+\gamma_{05}}}{1 + e^{\gamma_{02}+\gamma_{05}}}, \tag{9.41}$$

$$Pr(T_i^D = t_4 | \mathcal{X}_{i6} = 0) = \frac{e^{\gamma_{03}}}{1 + e^{\gamma_{03}}}, \tag{9.42}$$

$$Pr(T_i^D = t_4 | \mathcal{X}_{i6} = 1) = \frac{e^{\gamma_{03}+\gamma_{06}}}{1 + e^{\gamma_{03}+\gamma_{06}}}. \tag{9.43}$$

This model fits the observed data better than either of the previous two models (see Table 9.8). Note that none of the parameter estimates for the HRQoL data changes. This is to be expected, as the longitudinal model and the dropout model are estimated separately.

Building on the best CRD model, we fit the corresponding RD model by allowing dropout to depend on the value of the previous observation (Y_{ij-1}). Note that this model assumes that this relationship is the same for each follow-up assessment and the previous measurement. Thus, the relationship between dropout at 6 weeks and the baseline value of the FACT-Lung TOI is assumed to be the same as between dropout at 26 weeks and the 12-week value of the FACT-Lung TOI.

$$\text{logit}[P_j, \mathcal{X}_i] = \gamma_{01}\mathcal{X}_{i1} + \gamma_{02}\mathcal{X}_{i2} + \gamma_{03}\mathcal{X}_{i3} + \gamma_{04}\mathcal{X}_{i4}$$
$$+ \gamma_{05}\mathcal{X}_{i5} + \gamma_{06}\mathcal{X}_{i6} + \gamma_2 Y_{ij-1}, \quad (9.44)$$

$$Pr(T_i^D = t_2 | \mathcal{X}_{i4} = 0) = \frac{e^{\gamma_{01}+\gamma_2 Y_{ij-1}}}{1 + e^{\gamma_{01}+\gamma_2 Y_{ij-1}}}, \quad (9.45)$$

$$Pr(T_i^D = t_2 | \mathcal{X}_{i4} = 1) = \frac{e^{\gamma_{01}+\gamma_{04}+\gamma_2 Y_{ij-1}}}{1 + e^{\gamma_{01}+\gamma_{04}+\gamma_2 Y_{ij-1}}}, \quad (9.46)$$

and so forth. This RD model fits the data much better than the CRD model, with strong evidence to reject the CRD assumption (Table 9.11). As expected, there is still no change in the mean and variance parameters for the

Table 9.11. Diggle and Kenward models contrasting completely random dropout (CRD), random dropout (RD), and informative dropout (ID).

Parameter		CRD4	RD4	ID4
$\hat{\beta}_1$	Intercept	63.9	63.9	63.9
$\hat{\beta}_2$	Group	1.69	1.69	1.70
$\hat{\beta}_3$	Time	−0.266	−0.266	−0.254
$\hat{\beta}_4$	Group:Time	0.073	0.073	0.068
$\hat{\gamma}_0$	Time2	−0.549	1.872	1.810
	Time3	−1.005	1.377	1.317
	Time4	−0.198	2.286	2.228
	Time2 ∗ group	−0.592	−0.574	−0.577
	Time3 ∗ group	0.071	0.134	0.002
	Time4 ∗ group	−0.285	−0.274	−0.281
$\hat{\gamma}_1$				0.0022
$\hat{\gamma}_2$			−0.0386	−0.0397
−2 log L		16158.19	16078.13	16078.11
Comparison			CRD4	RD3
LR statistic			$\chi_1^2 = 80.1$	$\chi_1^2 = 0.018$
p-value			<0.001	0.89

longitudinal HRQoL data. The RD model predicts that the probability of dropout will decrease with increasing FACT-Lung TOI scores during the previous assessment. Thus, in the patient assigned to the treatment that did not include Taxol, the predicted probabilities of dropout at 6 weeks are 44, 35, and 27% for subjects with baseline scores of 55, 65, and 75, respectively.

$$\hat{P}_2 = \frac{e^{\hat{\gamma}_{01}+\hat{\gamma}_2 Y_{ij-1}}}{1+e^{\hat{\gamma}_{01}+\hat{\gamma}_2 Y_{ij-1}}} = \frac{e^{1.872-0.0385*55}}{1+e^{1.872-0.0385*55}} = 0.44, \quad \mathcal{X}_{i4}=0, Y_{i1}=55,$$

$$\hat{P}_2 = \frac{e^{\hat{\gamma}_{01}+\hat{\gamma}_2 Y_{ij-1}}}{1+e^{\hat{\gamma}_{01}+\hat{\gamma}_2 Y_{ij-1}}} = \frac{e^{1.872-0.0385*65}}{1+e^{1.872-0.0385*65}} = 0.35, \quad \mathcal{X}_{i4}=0, Y_{i1}=65,$$

$$\hat{P}_2 = \frac{e^{\hat{\gamma}_{01}+\hat{\gamma}_2 Y_{ij-1}}}{1+e^{\hat{\gamma}_{01}+\hat{\gamma}_2 Y_{ij-1}}} = \frac{e^{1.872-0.0385*75}}{1+e^{1.872-0.0385*75}} = 0.27, \quad \mathcal{X}_{i4}=0, Y_{i1}=75.$$

It is also possible to let dropout depend on the observed scores lagging back two observations. However, to do this in the current study, we would have had to restrict the data to subjects with the first two observations; less than half of the subjects would remain. Thus, in this study, we are limited to a single lag.*

Finally, we examine the ID model by adding the term that allows dropout to depend on the current unobserved FACT-Lung TOI measure (Y_{ij}).

$$\text{logit}[P_j, \mathcal{X}_i)] = \gamma_{01}\mathcal{X}_{i1} + \gamma_{02}\mathcal{X}_{i2} + \gamma_{03}\mathcal{X}_{i3} + \gamma_{04}\mathcal{X}_{i4}$$
$$+ \gamma_{05}\mathcal{X}_{i5} + \gamma_{06}\mathcal{X}_{i6} + \gamma_1 Y_{ij} + \gamma_2 Y_{ij-1}, \qquad (9.47)$$

$$Pr(T_i^D = t_2 | \mathcal{X}_{i4}=0) = \frac{e^{\gamma_{01}+\gamma_1 Y_{ij}+\gamma_2 Y_{ij-1}}}{1+e^{\gamma_{01}+\gamma_2 Y_{ij-1}}}, \qquad (9.48)$$

$$Pr(T_i^D = t_2 | \mathcal{X}_{i4}=1) = \frac{e^{\gamma_{01}+\gamma_1 Y_{ij}+\gamma_{04}+\gamma_2 Y_{ij-1}}}{1+e^{\gamma_{01}+\gamma_{04}+\gamma_2 Y_{ij-1}}}, \qquad (9.49)$$

and so forth. The ID model was not significantly different from the RD model. This is rather surprising, as there was evidence of nonignorable missing data for all other models considered in this and the previous chapter. This illustrates a very important point. The failure to reject a hypothesis of informative dropout (ID vs. RD) is not conclusive proof that the dropout is ignorable (RD). *The assumption of random dropout (RD) is acceptable only if the ID model was the correct alternative and the parametric form of the ID process is correct.* If, for example, either the logistic model was inappropriate or the assumption that the relationship between dropout and Y_{ij} is the same at 6, 12, and 26 weeks is incorrect, then the failure to reject the RD model may be incorrect. It may also be the case, in this study, that the omission of the second random effect** corresponding to variation in the rates of change among individuals may be the critical difference.

---

* The Oswald routine will run without error messages other than the note that the algorithm failed to converge. The resulting parameters describing dropout at 6 weeks make no sense.
** Oswald (Version 3.4) does not allow this option.

Oswald program

For this example, I have used S-Plus (Version 4.5) with the Oswald (Version 3.4) library of functions [109] and have reset the S default parameterization, which uses Helmert contrasts, to the more familiar reference cell design matrices.

```
> library(oswald)
> options(contrasts=c("contr.treatment","contr.poly"))
```

First, two data sets are imported into S-Plus. The first data set, patient, has one record per subject and contains the CASEID in column 1 and a treatment indicator for Taxol (TAXOL) in column 2. The second data set, assmnt, consists of four rows for each subject corresponding to the four planned assessments. It contains the CASEID in column 1, the FUNO in column 2, the FACT-Lung TOI score (FACT.T2)* in column 4 and the planned time of the assessment (0, 6, 12, or 26 weeks) in column 6. An ldamat object FACT is created from three data objects, fact.t2, time, and caseid.

```
> fact.t2 <- assmnt[,4]    # Reads FACT_T2 into FACT.T2
> time    <- assmnt[,6]
> caseid  <- assmnt[,1]
> fact <- conv.ldamat(fact.t2,time,caseid)
```

The next S-Plus statement creates a full-rank reference cell design matrix for GROUPS such that when GROUPS is included in the model the intercept corresponds to the patients in the "No Taxol" group and the GROUP parameter to the difference between the two groups.

```
> groups(fact) <- patient[,2]   # Reads TAXOL and creates GROUP
```

Finally, a design matrix (DT) is created that has indicators for the different times of dropout.

```
> temp <- assmnt[,2]        # Reads FUNO into TEMP
> temp[temp==1] <- 0        # Replaces values of 1 with 0
> dt <- as.factor(temp)     # Creates design matrix DT
```

Note that if there were no dropout at either baseline or 6 weeks, we would set both the rows corresponding to the first and second visit to 0.

```
> temp[temp==1|temp==2] <- 0   # Replaces values of 1 or 2 by 0
```

Longitudinal model

The pcmid function in the Oswald library fits a *parametric correlation model with informative dropout*. It consists of several parts. The longitudinal model $(E[Y_i] = X_i\beta, \mathrm{Var}[Y_i] = \nu^2 J + \varsigma^2 H + \tau^2 I)$ is defined by formula, vparms,

---
* S-Plus converts FACT_T2 to FACT.T2 when imported from the SAS data set.

Table 9.12. Output from pcmid function for a longitudinal model with compound symmetry.

```
Longitudinal Data Analysis Model assuming completely random dropout

Call: pcmid(formula=fact~group*time,vparms=c(0,120,0),correxp = 1)

Analysis Method: Maximum Likelihood(ML)
Correlation structure: exp(- phi*|u| ^ 1 )

Maximized log-likelihood: [1] -7438.93

Mean Parameters:
          (Intercept)     group      time   group:time
PARAMETER  63.875429  1.694745  -0.2662796  0.07277491
STD.ERROR   1.114316  1.344469   0.1108001  0.13124155

Variance Parameters:
 nu.sq  sigma.sq   tau.sq  phi
     0  148.1602  120.2703    0

Maximization converged after 48 iterations.
```

and correxp. I is a diagonal matrix of 1s, J is a matrix of 1s, and H is a correlation matrix where the elements are $\rho_{rc} = e^{-\phi|r-c|}$.

formula	Defines structure of the longitudinal model
vparms=c(#,#,#)	Initial estimates of the variance parameters ν^2, τ^2, and ϕ
correxp=#	Exponent in the correlation function

For example, if # indicates a nonzero value, the command

> pcmid(formula=fact~group*time, vparms=c(0,#,0), correxp=1)

defines a model with fixed-effect parameters labeled as (Intercept), group, time, and group:time (Table 9.12). These correspond to the intercept in the No Taxol group, the difference between the intercepts for the two groups, the slope in the No Taxol group, and the effect of Taxol on the slope. Setting the first and third numbers in the vparms arguments to zero constrains ν^2 and ϕ to be zero. Thus, $\rho = e^{-\phi|r-c|} = e^0 = 1$, $H = J$, and $\text{Var}[Y_i] = \varsigma^2 J + \tau^2 I$. This results in a variance structure with compound symmetry (Table 9.12). Although any positive number could be used as an initial estimate of τ^2, a close guess will reduce the computing time and decrease the possibility of convergence to a local maximum. One might also assume a random subject effect where the residual errors have a serial correlation (AR(1)).

> pcmid(formula=fact~group*time, vparm=c(#,0,#), correxp=1)

In this model, τ^2 is constrained to zero; thus, $\text{Var}[Y_i] = \nu^2 J + \varsigma^2 H$.

Dropout model

The dropout model is defined by the dropmodel, drop.cov.parms, and drop.parms arguments of the pcmid function.

dropmodel	A model defining the covariate part of the dropout model (the parameters of γ_0)
drop.cov.parms	Initial estimates of the parameters of γ_0; initial estimate of 0 will constrain parameter to be 0
drop.parms	Initial estimates of γ_1, γ_2, etc.; initial estimate of 0 will constrain the parameter to be 0

When drop.parms is omitted or defined as drop.parms=c(0,0), both γ_1 and γ_2 are constrained to zero and a completely random dropout (CRD) model is assumed. Table 9.13 illustrates this by showing the coefficients under y.d and y.d-1 to be zero. Providing an initial estimate of γ_2 assumes a random dropout (RD) model drop.parms=c(0,#) dependent on the previous observation. The output (Table 9.14) now displays the estimate of γ_2. Similarly,

Table 9.13. Output from pcmid function assuming completely random dropout (CRD).

```
Longitudinal Data Analysis Model
assuming random dropout based on 1 previous observations

Call: pcmid(formula=fact~group*time, vparms=c(0,120,0), correxp=1,
dropmodel=~1+dt*group,drop.cov.parms=c(0,-.5,-1,-.2,0,-.5,-.1,-.3),
drop.parms=c(0,0), reqmin = 1e-012)

Analysis Method: Maximum Likelihood(ML)
Correlation structure: exp(- phi*|u| ^ 1 )

Maximized log-likelihood: [1] -8079.097

Mean Parameters:
          (Intercept)     group       time    group:time
PARAMETER   63.875429   1.694745   -0.2662796  0.07277491
STD.ERROR    1.114316   1.344469    0.1108001  0.13124155

Variance Parameters:
nu.sq  sigma.sq    tau.sq   phi
    0  148.1602  120.2703    0

Dropout parameters:
(I)      dt2       dt3      dt4  group  dt2grp  dt3grp  dt4grp  y.d  y.d-1
  0  -0.5493   -1.0046  -0.1978      0 -0.5916  0.0708 -0.2854    0      0

Maximization converged after 2688 iterations.
```

Table 9.14. Output from `pcmid` function assuming random dropout (RD).

```
Longitudinal Data Analysis Model
assuming random dropout based on 1 previous observations

Call: pcmid(formula=fact~group*time,vparms=c(0,120,0),correxp=1,
dropmodel=~1+dt*group,drop.cov.parms=c(0,1.9,1.4,2.3,0,-.6,.1,-.3),
drop.parms = c(0, -0.04), reqmin = 1e-012)

Analysis Method: Maximum Likelihood (ML)
Correlation structure: exp(- phi *|u| ^ 1 )

Maximized log-likelihood: [1] -8039.064

Mean Parameters:
          (Intercept)     group         time  group:time
PARAMETER   63.875423  1.694822   -0.2662785    0.0727742
STD.ERROR    1.114316  1.344469    0.1108001    0.1312415

Variance Parameters:
nu.sq sigma.sq   tau.sq phi
    0 148.1605 120.2702   0

Dropout parameters:
(I)   dt2    dt3    dt4  group dt2grp  dt3grp  dt4grp  y.d  y.d-1
  0 1.872  1.377  2.286      0 -0.5736 0.1345 -0.2735    0 -0.0385

Maximization converged after 2779 iterations.
```

providing initial estimates of both γ_2 and γ_3 assumes a random dropout (RD) model `drop.parms=c(0,#)` dependent on the two previous observations. Finally, including an initial estimate of γ_1 allows an informative dropout (ID) model `drop.parms=c(#,#)`.

The arguments `dropmodel` and `drop.cov.parms` define the part of the dropout model described by γ_0. For example, the model labeled CRD1 in the preceding example is specified as

> pcmid(..., dropmodel~1, drop.cov.parms=c(\#))

Model CRD2 includes the covariate `group`:

> pcmid(..., dropmodel~1+group, drop.cov.parms=c(\#,\#))

Model CRD3 allows a different dropout rate at each of the follow-up visits and constrains the intercept to be zero. This is equivalent to using a `CLASS DT;` statement and a `NOINT` option in the model statement when using SAS.

> pcmid(..., dropmodel~1+dt, drop.cov.parms=c(0,\#,\#,\#))

Finally, the model CRD4 is specified as follows, with two parameters constrained to be zero to obtain a full rank model.

```
..., dropmodel~1+dt*group, drop.cov.parms=c(0,\#,\#,\#,0,\#,\#,\#))
```

Oswald warnings

The Oswald documentation states the need to double-check the convergence of each model by changing the parameter estimates and modifying the convergence criteria. This is absolutely critical, as the routine is very prone to find local maxima and print a message that the 'Maximization converged ...'. For the CRD and RD models, one way to check is to ensure that the HRQoL mean and variance parameters in each model are converging to the same values. This does not guarantee that the maximum is found, but if they differ, one or more of the models have not been maximized.

9.5 Advanced readings

Intermittent missing data

In addition to these monotone patterns of missing data due to dropout, non-monotone patterns may exist. Troxel [151] describes a likelihood method with Markovian correlation structure in which the missingness follows a logistic model. It is an extension of the model proposed by Diggle and Kenward [36] and utilizes numerical integration to solve the problem.

More selection models

Heckman probit stochastic dropout model

This model assumes that nonresponse occurs when response crosses a threshold.

$$Pr(r_{i2} = 0|y_{i1}, y_{i2}, \Psi) = \Phi(\psi_0 + \psi_1(y_{i1} + \psi_2 y_{i2})), \quad (9.50)$$

where $\Phi(\cdot)$ is the normal cumulative distribution function and ψ_0, ψ_1, ψ_2 are unknown parameters. If $\psi_1 = 0$, then the data are MCAR and non-ignorable if both $\psi_1 \neq 0$ and $\psi_2 \neq 0$. Estimation relies heavily on normal assumptions.

Wu and Carroll

Wu and Carroll [168] propose a selection model that is applicable to growth curve models with the individual slope parameters related to nonresponse for later observations (right censoring) through a probit model.

Mori

Mori et al. [103] propose empirical Bayes estimates of the individual subject slopes that adjust for informative dropout. When a patient is censored early, the time of censoring dominates the estimate of the change in HRQoL, whereas when dropout occurs later, the ordinary least-squares estimate of the individual's slope dominates the estimate.

Nonparametric analyses

Yao et al. [170] describe an extension of a nonparametric analysis of longitudinal data with nonignorable dropout. The advantage of the proposed method is that it can be applied to settings where the HRQoL assessments do not follow the planned timing of the assessments and the distribution of the QoL scores is non-normal. There is, however, a strong assumption made in this extension. Specifically, this approach assumes that the difference in QoL between the two treatment arms does not vary over time. This assumption severely limits the settings where this method is useful.

9.6 Summary

- All these models require the analyst to make strong assumptions.
- These assumptions cannot be formally tested. Defense of the assumptions must be made on a clinical basis rather than statistically.
- Lack of evidence of nonignorable missing data for any particular model does not prove that the missing data are ignorable.
- Estimates are not robust to model misspecification; thus, more than one model should be considered, which is a sensitivity analysis.

CHAPTER 10

Summary Measures

10.1 Introduction

In most clinical trials, investigators assess HRQoL longitudinally over the period of treatment and, in some trials, subsequent to treatment. Each assessment involves multiple scales that measure the general and disease-specific domains of HRQoL. For example, in the NSCLC study, there are three treatment arms, four assessments, and five subscales of the FACT-L. Thus, most studies entail multiple HRQoL measures that are assessed periodically. As a result, addressing the problem of multiple comparisons is one of the analytic challenges in these trials [79]. Not only are there concerns about Type I errors, but large numbers of statistical tests generally result in a confusing picture of HRQoL that is difficult to interpret [31].

Addressing multiplicity of endpoints

There are three general approaches to reduce the impact of multiplicity:

1. *A priori* specification of a limited number of *confirmatory* tests
2. Multiple comparison procedures including alpha adjustments (e.g., Bonferroni) and closed multiple testing
3. The use of summary measures or statistics

In practice, a combination of focused hypotheses, summary measures, and multiple comparison procedures is necessary in most clinical trails. In this chapter, the computations of summary measures and statistics are presented with details concerning how their derivation is affected by missing data. Selected multiple comparison procedures are presented in the following chapter.

Summary measures vs. summary statistics

The terms *summary measures* and *summary statistics* are often interchanged. The following definitions are used in this chapter. A *summary measure* reduces the repeated observations on each individual to a single number (see Table 10.1). The procedure is first to summarize the data within an individual subject by calculating a single value (summary measure) for each individual and then to perform an analysis of the summary measures. For example, we can estimate the rate of change experienced by each individual using ordinary

Table 10.1. Comparison of summary measures and summary statistics for combining information across time.

Method	Summary measures ($S_i = \sum_{j=1}^{J} w_j f(Y_{ij})$)
Strategy	1. Summarize data within ith patient (over J repeated evaluations)
	2. Univariate analysis of S_i
Advantage	Easy to describe and interpret
Disadvantages	Often difficult to develop strategy for handling every missing value on an individual basis; some measures are biased, depending on pattern and reasons for missing data
Method	Summary statistics ($S_h = \sum_{j=1}^{J} w_j g(\beta_{hj})$)
Strategy	1. Fit multivariate model, estimating means (or parameters) for repeated measures or mixed-effects model
	2. Compute summary statistic (generally linear combination of parameters)
	3. Test hypothesis (H_0: $S_j = S_{j'}$ or $S_j - S_{j'} = 0$)
Advantage	Strategies for handling missing data are model based
Disadvantage	Harder to describe procedure

least squares (OLS) and then apply a two-sample t-test to compare the estimates in two treatment groups. Other examples of summary measures include the average of the within-subject post-treatment values [31, 54, 97], last value minus baseline [54], average rate of change over time (or slope) [97], maximum value [31, 97, 117], area under the curve [20, 97], and time to reach a peak or prespecified value [97, 117].

In contrast, a *summary statistic* reduces the measurements on a group of individuals to a single value. Data are initially analyzed using multivariate techniques for longitudinal models and summary statistics are constructed from the estimates of the parameters. For example, the mean rate of change (or slope) for each treatment group is estimated using a mixed-effects model and the differences in the slopes between the two treatment groups are tested. Other examples include the average of the group means during the post-treatment period and area under the mean HRQoL vs. time curve.

Missing data are dealt with differently in the construction of summary measures and statistics [39]. For summary measures (see Section 10.3), we must develop a procedure to handle missing data at the subject level, possibly by using interpolation and extrapolation or by imputing missing observations. For summary statistics (see Section 10.4), missing data handled by the selection of the analytic model is described in Chapters 5, 8, and 9.

Strengths and weaknesses

Easier interpretation

There are several motivations for the use of summary measures in the analysis of a longitudinal study of HRQoL [39]. The primary advantage of summary measures is that they facilitate interpretation. Not only is the number of comparisons reduced, but measures such as the rate of change and the area under the curve are familiar concepts in clinical medicine.

Increased power

Summary measures and statistics also have greater power to detect small but consistent differences that may occur over extended periods of time or multiple domains of HRQoL. In contrast to the Bonferroni correction or a general multivariate test (Hotelling's T), these summary statistics are more sensitive to the settings where there are consistent differences over time. To illustrate, consider the two hypothetical examples displayed in Figure 10.1. In the first example (Figure 10.1A), the measure of HRQoL is consistently better in one treatment during all four post-baseline assessments. In the second example (Figure 10.1B), the second treatment has a negative impact (toxicity) 1 month postdiagnosis, but this difference almost disappears by the third month and begins to reverse by the ninth month. Although the differences between the groups in both examples are of clinical interest, in most clinical trials one would wish to have test procedures that are more sensitive to (or have greater power to detect) the consistent differences displayed in Figure 10.1A.

Weakness

The primary weakness of summary measures or statistics is that differences in specific domains of HRQoL or transient differences at specific points in time may be obscured. Investigations that are confirmatory, designed to test the question of differences in overall HRQoL, may benefit from the use of summary measures. This is especially useful in studies where early toxicity in one treatment group may be balanced by later improvements in disease control. In contrast, studies that have more exploratory objectives of identifying which aspects of HRQoL are impacted by the disease or a particular therapy may not benefit from the use of summary measures or statistics.

10.2 Choosing a summary measure

The selection of a summary measure as the endpoint in a clinical trial depends on the objective of the investigation. The summary measure should have a clear clinical relevance and ideally should be determined prior to data collection [22, 97]. Posing the research question simply (e.g., "How do the groups differ?") is too vague to indicate the correct measure. The process of identifying the appropriate summary measure often requires the investigators to decide

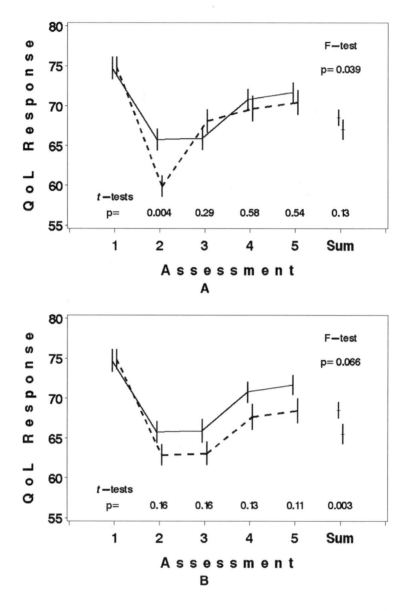

Figure 10.1. Hypothetical studies with (A) consistent differences in HRQoL over time or (B) a large difference at a single point in time. Summary measure is the mean of the post-baseline assessments. Means are joined by horizontal line. Vertical lines indicate 1 standard error. F-test indicates multivariate test of group differences at assessments 2, 3, 4, and 5. t-tests indicate test of group difference at that assessment or for the summary measure.

what specific questions the HRQoL data are expected to answer. For example, Curren et al. [22] describe a hypothetical trial where the objective is to reduce toxicity and maintain acceptable HRQoL. In this setting one might want to study the worst (minimum) HRQoL score that occurred for each individual.

The selection also depends on the expected pattern of change across time and patterns of missing data. Consider several possible patterns of change in HRQoL across time (Figure 10.2). One profile is a steady rate of change over time, reflecting either a constant decline in HRQoL (Figure 10.2A) or a constant improvement (Figure 10.2B). The first pattern is typical of patients with progressive disease where standard therapy is palliative rather than curative. This is the pattern observed in the NSCLC study (Example 2). This pattern of change suggests that the rate of change or slope is a possible choice of a summary measure. In contrast, measures such as the change from baseline to the last measure might not be desirable if patients who fail earlier and thus drop out of the study earlier have smaller changes than those patients with longer follow-up.

An alternative profile is an initial rapid change with a subsequent plateau after the maximum therapeutic benefit is realized (Figure 10.2D). This might occur for therapies where the dose needs to be increased slowly over time or where there is a lag between the time when therapy is initiated and the time when maximal benefit is achieved. This profile illustrates the importance of identifying the clinically relevant question *a priori*. If the objective is to identify the therapy that produces the most rapid improvement in HRQoL, the time to reach a peak or prespecified value is good choice. If, in contrast, the ultimate level of benefit is more important than the time to achieve the benefit, then a measure such as the post-treatment mean or mean change relative to baseline is desirable. More than one summary measure can be constructed to investigate different questions. It is rare that more than two are clinically relevant.

A third pattern of change could occur with a therapy that has transient benefits or toxicity (Figures 10.2E and F). For example, individuals may experience transient benefits and then return to their baseline levels after the effect of the therapy has ceased. Alternatively, a toxic therapy for cancer may significantly reduce HRQoL during therapy but ultimately result in a better HRQoL following therapy than the patient was experiencing at the time of diagnosis [48, 86]. For these more complex patterns of change over time, a measure such as the area under the curve might be considered as a summary of both early and continued effects of the therapy.

10.3 Constructing summary measures

The approach for constructing summary measures is to reduce the repeated measures from each individual to a single value. This approach is popular because simple univariate tests (e.g., t-tests) can be used for the analysis. For example, one might compute the slope of the scores observed for each subject and test the hypothesis that the slopes differed among the experimental groups.

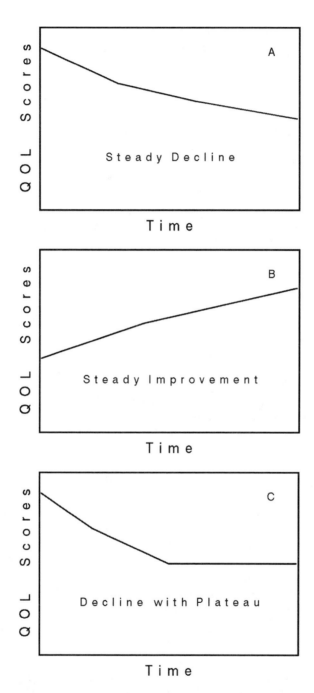

Figure 10.2. Patterns of change in HRQoL over time. (From Fairclough, D.L., in Quality of Life Assessment in Clinical Trials: Methods and Practice, Staquet, M.J. et al., Eds., Oxford University Press, New York, 1998, Chap. 13. With permission.)

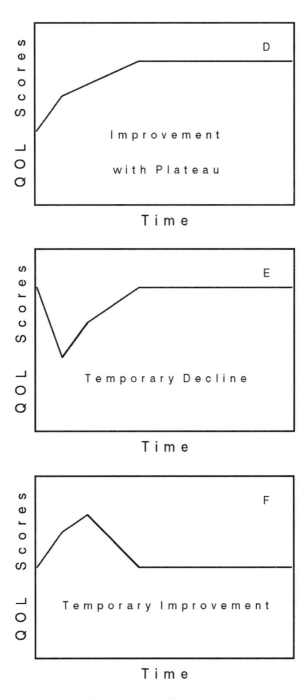

Figure 10.2. Continued

When the period of observation varies widely among subjects or data collection stops for some reason related to the outcome, this construction of summary measures is challenging. Easy fixes without careful thought only hide the problem. Many of the procedures for constructing summary measures assume data are missing completely at random (MCAR) [110] and are inappropriate in studies of HRQoL.

Notation

The construction of a summary measure that reduces the set of J measurements (Y_{ij}) on the ith individual to a single value (S_i) can be described as a weighted sum of the measurements (Y_{ij}) or a function of the measurements $(f(Y_{ij}))$. The general form is

$$S_i = \sum_{j=1}^{J} w_j \, f(Y_{ij}). \tag{10.1}$$

Table 10.2 illustrates how this applies to a number of examples. Although in some cases, such as the average rate of change (slope), there are easier ways of constructing the summary measures, the table illustrates the common structure of all summary measures [39].

Missing data

The calculation of summary measures is straightforward in the absence of missing and mistimed observations. It becomes much more challenging when there are missing data or the length of follow-up differs by individual. Strategies for handling missing data often need to be developed on a case-by-case basis. All of the following approaches make assumptions that may or may not be

Table 10.2. Examples of summary measures constructed within individuals across time: $S_i = \sum_{j=1}^{n} w_j f(Y_{ij})$.

Description	$f(Y_{ij})$	Weights (w_j)
Average rate of change	$Y_{ij} - \bar{Y}_i$	$(t_i - \bar{t})/(\sum t_i - \bar{t})^2$
Mean of r follow-up observations	Y_{ij}	$0, \ldots, \dfrac{1}{r}, \ldots, \dfrac{1}{r}$
Mean of r follow-up, baseline	Y_{ij}	$-1, \ldots, \dfrac{1}{r}, \ldots, \dfrac{1}{r}$
Area under the curve	Y_{ij}	$\dfrac{t_2 - t_1}{2}, \ldots, \dfrac{t_{j+1} - t_{j-1}}{2}, \ldots, \dfrac{t_n - t_{n-1}}{2}$
Average of ranks	$\text{Rank}(Y_{ij})$	$1/n, \ldots, 1/n$
Minimum value	$\text{Min}(Y_i)$	1

Table 10.3. Possible strategies for handling missing data in the calculation of summary measures.

Problem	Solution	Assumptions/limitations
Intermittent missing values	Interpolation	Change approximately linear over period; t_{ij-1} and t_{ij+1} measured under similar conditions
Mistimed last observation $(t_{iJ} \neq T)$	Estimate Y_{iT}	$Y_{iT} = \dfrac{(T - t_{iJ-1})Y_{iJ} + (T - t_{iJ})Y_{iJ-1}}{t_{iJ} - t_{iJ-1}}$
Incomplete follow-up	Extrapolation or LVCF	Potential bias favoring early dropout
Death	Minimum value	Potential bias favoring early death
	Zero	Mimics survival analysis

reasonable in specific settings, and it is advisable to examine the sensitivity of the conclusions to the various assumptions (Table 10.3).

For example, if intermediate observations are missing, one could interpolate between observations. This approach assumes that these intermediate missing values are random and that the previous and following measures are taken under similar conditions. Interpolation is reasonable when the expected pattern of change over time is roughly linear (see Figures 10.2A and B) or constant. Interpolation would not make sense in the design used for the adjuvant breast cancer study (Example 1) for missing assessments during therapy. Interpolation between the pre- and post-therapy assessments would obviously overestimate the HRQoL of subjects during therapy. Also, interpolation during the early phase of the renal cell carcinoma study (Example 3) would not make sense given the rapid drop in HRQoL followed by recovery. Even in the NSCLC study, interpolation assumes that the missingness is not the result of some event, such as an episode of acute toxicity, that would cause the patient to miss the assessment and have poorer HRQoL.

Dropout and other causes of differences in the length of follow-up among individuals are another challenge. For a patient who dropped out, the last measurement could be imputed by (1) carrying the last value forward, (2) extrapolating from the last two observations, or (3) implementing one of the imputation techniques described in Chapters 6 and 7. The most popular approach is to carry the value of the last observation forward. Unfortunately, this strategy is often implemented without careful thought. This is a reasonable strategy if the expected pattern of change within individuals is either a steady improvement (Figure 10.2B) or improvement with a plateau (Figure 10.2D). However, with other patterns of change (Figures 10.2A, C, and E), this strategy would bias the results in favor of interventions with early dropout.

Assigning zero is a valid approach for HRQoL scores that are explicitly anchored at zero for the health state of death. These are generally scores measured using time trade-off (TTO) or standard gamble (SG) techniques to produce *utility* measures. However, the majority of HRQoL instruments are developed to maximize discrimination among patients. In these instruments a value of zero would correspond to the worst possible outcome on every question. Assigning zero also has some statistical implications. If the proportion of deaths is substantial, the observations may mimic a binomial distribution and the results approximate a Kaplan–Meier analysis of survival. When the number of deaths is small, the zero values will violate the multivariate normal distribution assumptions of the analysis methods.

Average rate of change (slopes)

When the changes over time are approximately linear, the average rate of change (or slope) may provide an excellent summary of the effect of an intervention. When there is virtually no dropout during the study or the dropout occurs only during the later part of the study, it is feasible to fit a simple regression model to the available data on each individual. This is often referred to as the ordinary least-squares slope (OLS slope). $\hat{\beta}_{i2}$ is the estimated slope from a simple linear regression:

$$\hat{\beta}_i^{\text{OLS}} = \sum^J \frac{(X_{ij} - \bar{X}_i)(Y_{ij} - \bar{Y}_i)}{(X_{ij} - \bar{X}_i)^2} = (X_i'X_i)^{-1}X_i'Y_i. \qquad (10.2)$$

NSCLC example

At first glance, estimating individual slopes might seem to be an approach for the NSCLC study. But recall that a fourth of the subjects had only a single HRQoL assessment and would contribute nothing to the analysis. Further, less than half of the subjects had three or more observations, so that a substantial proportion of the subjects is likely to have unstable estimates of their slopes. Finally, there is a suspicion that the data are MNAR. As a practical design issue, it is advisable to plan frequent assessments during the early phase of a trial if one is intending to use this approach and dropout is likely.

Missing data

Obviously, slopes for each individual can be estimated if all subjects have two or more observations. However, the estimates of the slopes will have a large associated error when the available observations span a short period of time relative to the entire length of the study. The wide variation in slopes estimated with OLS is displayed in Figure 10.3; note the wide range of estimates for subjects with only two measures. If there is a substantial proportion of subjects with only one or two observations, it may be necessary to use either

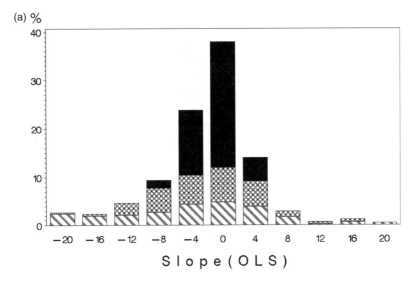

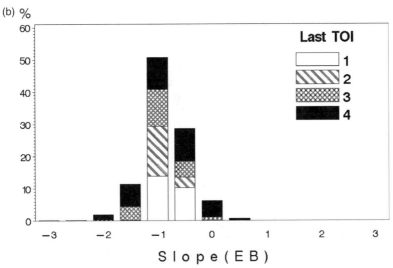

Figure 10.3. Distribution of summary measures using different methods of estimating the slope. (a) Ordinary least squares (OLS); (b) empirical Bayes (EB); (c) last value carried forward (LVCF), (d) multiple imputation (MI).

imputed values for later missing values or the empirical Bayes (EB) estimates from a mixed-effects model. Because this second estimate also uses information from other individuals, it is more stable, especially with highly unbalanced longitudinal studies where some individuals have only a few observations. The EB slopes display shrinkage toward the average slope, as the estimator is a weighted average of the observed data and the overall average slope [82] (see Section 5.6). For individuals with only a few observations, the EB slope is

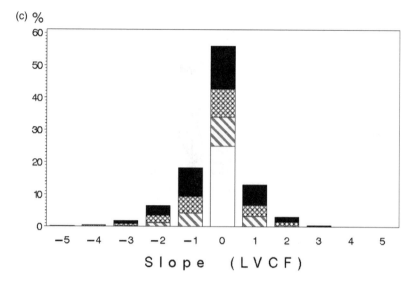

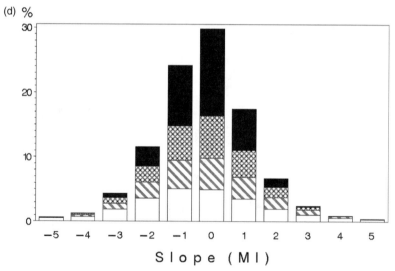

Figure 10.3. Continued

very close to the overall average. This is illustrated by the narrow distribution of estimates displayed in Figure 10.3. Note that both approaches assume the data are missing at random (MAR). The distribution of the slopes derived using LVCF illustrates the tendency of these values to center around zero. This is by definition for those who drop out after the first observation. Finally, the distribution of slopes is displayed from the multiply imputed data. Values are more widely distributed than for either the EB or LVCF strategies. Clearly, the distribution of the summary measures can be sensitive to the method used to handle the missing data.

CONSTRUCTING SUMMARY MEASURES

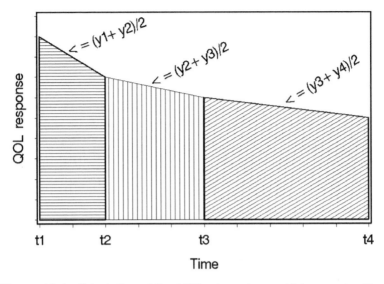

Figure 10.4. Calculation of the AUC using a trapezoidal approximation.

Area under the curve

Another measure summarizing HRQoL over time is the area under the curve (AUC) of the HRQoL scores (Y_{ij}) plotted against time (t) [19, 94]. The AUC for the ith individual can be estimated using a trapezoidal approximation from the observed scores (Figure 10.4). The area of each trapezoid is equal to the product of the height at the midpoint $((Y_{ij} + Y_{i(j-1)})/2)$ and the width of the base $(t_j - t_{j-1})$. The total area is calculated by adding areas of a series of trapezoids

$$S_i = \text{AUC}_i = \sum_{j=2}^{J}(t_j - t_{j-1})\frac{Y_{ij} + Y_{i(j-1)}}{2}. \tag{10.3}$$

With a little algebraic manipulation, this calculation can also be expressed as a weighted function of the HRQoL scores, where the weights are determined by the spacing of the assessments over time:

$$\text{AUC}_i = \frac{t_2 - t_1}{2}Y_{i1} + \sum_{j=2}^{J-1}\frac{t_{j+1} - t_{j-1}}{2}Y_{ij} + \frac{t_J - t_{J-1}}{2}Y_{iJ}. \tag{10.4}$$

Missing data

There are a number of options for constructing a measure of the AUC in the presence of missing data (see Table 10.3). All have some limitations. The best choice will depend on the objectives and the reasons for missing assessments or dropout.

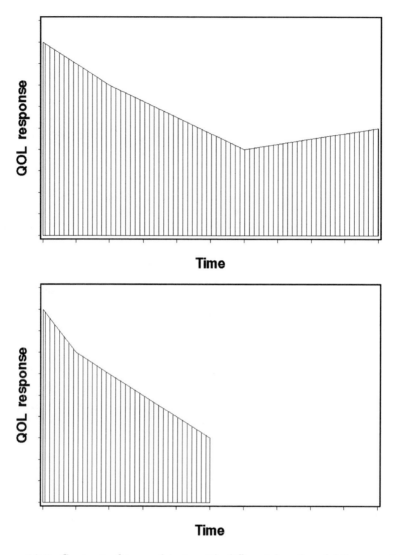

Figure 10.5. Contrast of two subjects with different lengths of follow-up. Both subjects have the same AUC when adjusted by each individual's length of follow-up.

Fayers and Machin [45] describe one alternative, the average AUC, which may be useful in some settings where the length of follow-up varies among subjects. This summary measure is calculated by dividing the total AUC by the total time of observation. $S_i = \mathrm{AUC}_i/T_i$, where T_i is the total time of observation for the ith individual. If the research question concerns the average HRQoL of patients during a limited period such as the duration of a specific therapy, this may be a reasonable approach. However, if early termination due to toxicity or lack of efficacy results in similar or higher summary scores, then the results are biased. This is illustrated in Figure 10.5, where the average areas are the same for the two curves but the scores decline more rapidly in the subject who terminated the study early. As always, the choice between these two approaches depends primarily on the research question.

The issue of selecting a strategy for computing the AUC also occurs when patients die during the study. One strategy is to extrapolate the curve to zero at the time of death. Other proposed strategies include assigning values of (1) the minimum HRQoL score for that individual or (2) the minimum HRQoL score for all individuals [68]. One strategy will not work for all studies. Whichever strategy is chosen, it needs to be justified and the sensitivity of the results to the assumptions examined.

Differences at baseline

A practical problem with the use of the AUC or the mean of post-baseline measures as a summary measure occurs when the baseline HRQoL scores differ among groups. If one group contains more individuals who score their HRQoL consistently higher than other individuals, small (possibly statistically nonsignificant) differences are magnified over time in the summary measure. One possible solution is to calculate the AUC relative to the baseline score.

$$\mathrm{AUC}_i^* = \mathrm{AUC}_i - Y_{i1}(t_J - t_1)$$
$$= \left[\frac{t_2 - t_1}{2} - (t_J - t_1)\right] Y_{i1} + \sum_{j=2}^{J-1} \frac{t_{j+1} - t_{j-1}}{2} Y_{ij} + \frac{t_J - t_{J-1}}{2} Y_{iJ}.$$
(10.5)

Average of ranks

Another method proposed for combining information across repeated measures uses ranks [108]. The measurements on all subjects are ranked at each time point and then the average of the ranks across the n time points is computed for each individual. In the notation of Equation 10.1 and Table 10.2, $f(Y_{ij})$ is the rank of Y_{ij} among all values of the jth measure and S_i is the average of the ranks for the ith individual ($w_j = 1/n$). When the data are complete, this procedure is straightforward.

Missing data

If the reasons for missing data were known and one could make reasonable assumptions about the ranking of HRQoL in patients at each time point, one could possibly adapt this approach to a study with missing data. For example, it would not be unreasonable to assume that the HRQoL of patients who died or left the study due to excessive toxicity was worse than the HRQoL of those patients who remained on therapy. They would then be assigned the lowest possible rank for measurements scheduled after death or during the time of excessive toxicity. Other strategies that might be considered are discussed in Chapter 6 (see Table 6.7).

Univariate analysis of summary measures

After constructing the summary measures, statistical tests (e.g., two-sample t-test, Wilcoxon rank sum test) are used to compare treatment groups. In most cases these tests assume that the observations are independent and identically distributed (i.i.d). The assumption of homogeneity of variance of the summary measures is often violated when the duration of follow-up is vastly different among subjects. For example, slopes estimated for individuals who drop out of the study early will have greater variation than slopes for those who complete the study. One solution is to weight the slopes using their standard errors, giving greater weight to those individuals with the longest follow-up. Unfortunately, unless dropout is MCAR, this will bias the analysis. The alternative procedure is to ignore the possible heterogeneity, giving equal weight to all subjects. This later approach is generally more appropriate in studies of HRQoL where the MCAR assumption is rarely appropriate.

Stratified analysis of summary measures

Dawson and Lagokos [27–29] propose a strategy for handling monotone dropout. First, we identify strata (g) defined by the dropout pattern. Summary measures are then calculated for each individual within the strata using just the observed data. This avoids the need to extrapolate past the point of dropout. Then a standardized test statistic, Z_g, for the two-arm comparison is calculated for each stratum. Dawson and Lagokos [27–29] use the nonparametric van der Waerden scores in their applications. These stratum-specific test statistics are then combined into an overall test statistic $Z = \sum w_g Z_g / \sqrt{\sum w_g^2}$. Dawson uses $w_g = \sqrt{j_g n_{g1} n_{g2}/(n_{g1} + n_{g2})}$ as a general set of weights [29] and $w_g = \sqrt{\sum (x_{gj} - \bar{x}_g)^2 n_{g1} n_{g2}/(n_{g1} + n_{g2})}$ when the summary measures are slopes [28].* Note that these weights will tend to increase the contribution of strata with longer follow-up.

When the data are missing completely at random, this approach will increase the power, since the across-strata variation is removed [28, 29]. However, it is unclear how it will perform when dropout is nonignorable and the pattern of dropout differs by treatment group [22]. For example, there may not be any treatment difference in the summary statistic conditional on dropout: All $Z_g \approx 0 \to Z \approx 0$. However, if the dropout patterns differ and the summary measures differ across the strata, then there are real differences that are not detected. To illustrate, consider a hypothetical example (Table 10.4) where there is extensive early dropout in one arm of the study. Higher scores indicate an improvement in HRQoL. Among those who drop out early ($g = 1$), the average summary measure score is -5, indicating a decline in HRQoL regardless of treatment arm in these subjects. Similarly, among those who remain on the study ($g = 2$), the summary measures average 20 in both groups. If we

---

* n_{gh} is the number of subjects in the gth stratum and the hth treatment arm. j_g is the number of observations used to compute the summary measure in the gth group. x_{gj} denotes the times when subjects in the gth group contribute observations.

Table 10.4. Hypothetical example illustrating problem with stratified analysis of summary measures when dropout rates differ across groups.

Stratum (g)	Treatment	Subjects (n_{gh})	$\hat{S}_{h(g)}$	Z_g
1	A	10	−5	0
	B	40	−5	
2	A	40	20	0
	B	10	20	

Table 10.5. Actual weights (w_j) and relative weights for the NSCLC example. $|w_1|$ is constrained to be 1 for relative weights.

Measure	T1	T2	T3	T4
Actual weights				
Slope	−0.046	−0.020	0.007	0.059
Mean difference	−1.000	0.333	0.333	0.333
AUC	0.125	0.250	0.375	0.250
Relative weights				
Slope	−1.000	−0.429	0.143	1.286
Mean difference	−1.000	0.333	0.333	0.333
AUC	1.000	2.000	3.000	2.000

test for differences within each stratum, we observe none, so the standardized test statistics are both approximately 0 ($Z_g \approx 0$). However, it is clear that in arm A there are more individuals who remained on the study and experienced a greater benefit than on arm B. This example is highly exaggerated, but it illustrates the problem. One could imagine a similar, but less dramatic, scenario on a placebo-controlled trial where there was early dropout among individuals who did not perceive any benefit from the intervention.

NSCLC example

In this example, all five subscales of the FACT-Lung instrument will be analyzed. Three summary measures are examined: the average change (slope), the mean of the post-randomization assessments minus baseline, and the AUC. The weights for the three summary measures are displayed in Table 10.5. Note that the weights for the *slope* and the *mean difference* are similar, weighting early scores negatively and later scores positively. The biggest difference among the three summary measures is the much greater weights for the last assessment when the summary measure is the slope. As approximately $\frac{2}{3}$ of the subjects are missing this assessment, the slope is most sensitive to the manner in which missing values are handled.

To illustrate the sensitivity of the summary measures to the method of handling missing values, two approaches were used. In the first, missing values

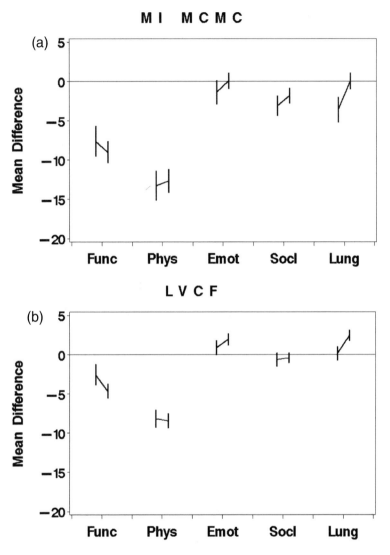

Figure 10.6. Mean difference between postrandomization and prerandomization assessments with missing data handled by multiple imputation (MI MCMC) and LVCF. Pairs display mean ±1 standard error for no Taxol (a) and Taxol (b) groups.

were handled by multiple imputation using the MCMC approach for multivariate normal data described in Chapter 7. All five subscales were jointly modeled with age, log survival, best response, and early progressive disease. In the second, the last value was carried forward (LVCF). The patterns across the five subscales were very similar for all three summary measures. The estimates and their standard errors for the mean difference between postrandomization and baseline are displayed in Figure 10.6.

10.4 Summary statistics across time

In contrast to summary measures, summary statistics are constructed by combining group measures over time. Examples of these group measures are the parameter estimates from growth curve models or means from repeated measures models. In practice, the use of summary statistics rather than summary measures is often preferable because it may be much easier to develop a model-based method for handling missing data than to develop strategies for imputing each individual missing value required to compute the summary measures.

Notation

The general procedure for the construction of summary statistics is to obtain parameter estimates for the hth group $(\hat{\beta}_{hj})$ and then reduce the set of J estimates to a single summary statistic:

$$\hat{S}_h = \sum_{j=1}^{J} w_j g(\hat{\beta}_{hj}). \tag{10.6}$$

In a repeated measures design, $g(\hat{\beta}_{hj})$ is generally a vector of the estimates of the means over time $(\hat{\mu}_{hj})$ adjusted for important covariates [39]. In a growth curve model, $g(\hat{\beta}_{hj})$ contains the parameter estimates of the polynomial or piecewise regression model. $g(\hat{\beta}_{hj})$ may also be a direct estimate of a summary statistic such as the slope or a test statistic such as the ratio of the estimate to its standard error (t_{hj}).

If the data are complete, one can use any multivariate analysis method to estimate β_{hj}. When data are missing, one must use an analytic method that is appropriate for the missing data mechanism as described in Chapter 5, 8, or 9.

Area under the curve

Repeated measures

When the model has been structured as a repeated measures analysis, the AUC can be estimated for each of the H groups by using a trapezoidal approximation.

$$\text{AUC}_h(t_J) = \hat{S}_h = \sum_{j=2}^{J}(t_j - t_{j-1})\frac{\hat{\mu}_{hj} + \hat{\mu}_{h(j-1)}}{2}. \tag{10.7}$$

The equation can be rewritten as a weighted function of the means:

$$\text{AUC}_h(t_J) = \hat{S}_h = \frac{t_2 - t_1}{2}\hat{\mu}_{h1} + \sum_{j=2}^{J-1}\frac{t_{j+1} - t_{j-1}}{2}\hat{\mu}_{hj} + \frac{t_J - t_{J-1}}{2}\hat{\mu}_{hJ}. \tag{10.8}$$

For example, in the NSCLC study, the planned times of the assessments were 0, 6, 12, and 26 weeks. The AUC over 26 weeks for the hth group is

Table 10.6. Examples of summary statistics: $\hat{S}_h = \sum_{j=1}^{p} w_j g(\hat{\beta}_{hj})$.

Description	$g(\hat{\beta}_{hj})$	Weights (w_j)
Mean of r follow-up observations	$\hat{\mu}_{hj}$	$0, \ldots, \frac{1}{r}, \ldots, \frac{1}{r}$
Mean of follow-up first observation	$\hat{\mu}_{hj}$	$-1, \ldots, \frac{1}{r}, \ldots, \frac{1}{r}$
Average rate of change	$\hat{\beta}_{h2}$ (slope)	
Area under the curve	$\hat{\mu}_{hj}$	$\frac{t_2 - t_1}{2}, \ldots, \frac{t_{j+1} - t_{j-1}}{2}, \ldots, \frac{t_J - t_{J-1}}{2}$
Inverse correlation	$\hat{\mu}_{hj} / \hat{\sigma}_{(\hat{\mu}_{hj})}$	$J' R^{-1}$

$J = (1, \ldots, 1)'$, R = correlation of $Y_i = (Y_{i1}, \ldots, Y_{in})'$.

$$\text{AUC}_h(26) = \frac{t_2 - t_1}{2} \hat{\mu}_{h1} + \frac{t_3 - t_1}{2} \hat{\mu}_{h2} + \frac{t_4 - t_2}{2} \hat{\mu}_{h3} + \frac{t_4 - t_3}{2} \hat{\mu}_{h4}$$

$$= \frac{6 - 0}{2} \hat{\mu}_{h1} + \frac{12 - 0}{2} \hat{\mu}_{h2} + \frac{26 - 6}{2} \hat{\mu}_{h3} + \frac{26 - 12}{2} \hat{\mu}_{h4}.$$

As discussed before, dividing this quantity by t_J or scaling time so that $t_J = 1$ has two advantages. First, the statistic is independent of the units of time. Second, the statistic is in the range of values for the scale and has the alternative interpretation of the average score over the period of interest.

Growth curve models

When the model has been structured as a growth curve model, the AUC is computed by integration from 0 to T. If a polynomial model has been used to describe the change in HRQoL over time:

$$\text{AUC}_h(T) = \hat{S}_h = \int_{t=0}^{T} \sum_{j=0}^{J} \hat{\beta}_{hj} t^j \, \partial t = \sum_{j=0}^{J} \frac{T^{j+1}}{j+1} \hat{\beta}_{hj}, \qquad (10.9)$$

where $\hat{\beta}_{h0}$ is the estimate of the intercept for the hth group, $\hat{\beta}_{h1}$ is the linear coefficient for the hth group, etc.

For example, in the renal cell carcinoma study, the AUC is

$$\text{AUC}_h(T) = \sum_{j=0}^{J} \frac{T^{j+1}}{j+1} \hat{\beta}_{hj}$$

$$= \frac{T^1}{1} \hat{\beta}_{h0} + \frac{T^2}{2} \hat{\beta}_{h1} + \frac{T^3}{3} \hat{\beta}_{h2} + \frac{T^4}{4} \hat{\beta}_{h3} + \frac{T^5}{5} \hat{\beta}_{h4} + \frac{T^6}{6} \hat{\beta}_{h5}.$$

If we are interested in the AUC during the initial period of therapy, defined as the first 8 weeks or 1.84 months, the AUC is

$$\text{AUC}_h = \underbrace{\frac{1.84^1}{1}}_{1.84}\hat{\beta}_{h0} + \underbrace{\frac{1.84^2}{2}}_{1.6925}\hat{\beta}_{h1} + \underbrace{\frac{1.84^3}{3}}_{2.076}\hat{\beta}_{h2} + \underbrace{\frac{1.84^4}{4}}_{2.86}\hat{\beta}_{h3}$$
$$+ \underbrace{\frac{1.84^5}{5}}_{4.22}\hat{\beta}_{h4} + \underbrace{\frac{1.84^6}{6}}_{6.46}\hat{\beta}_{h5}.$$

The estimates and their differences for 8 weeks are generated by the ESTIMATE statement as illustrated below:

```
ESTIMATE 'IFN only - AUC 8wks'
         TREAT 1.840 0
         TREAT*MONTHS 1.6925 0
         TREAT*MONTHS*MONTHS 2.076 0
         TREAT*MONTHS*MONTHS*MONTHS 2.86 0
         TREAT*MONTHS*MONTHS*MONTHS*MONTHS 4.22 0
         TREAT*MONTHS*MONTHS*MONTHS*MONTHS*MONTHS 6.46
         /DIVISOR=1.84;
ESTIMATE 'IFN +CRA - AUC 8wks'
         TREAT 0 1.840
         TREAT*MONTHS 0 1.6925
         TREAT*MONTHS*MONTHS 0 2.076
         TREAT*MONTHS*MONTHS*MONTHS 0 2.86
         TREAT*MONTHS*MONTHS*MONTHS*MONTHS 0 4.22
         TREAT*MONTHS*MONTHS*MONTHS*MONTHS*MONTHS 0 6.46
         /DIVISOR=1.84;
ESTIMATE 'Difference - AUC 8wks'
         TREAT -1.840 1.840
         TREAT*MONTHS -1.6925 1.6925
         TREAT*MONTHS*MONTHS -2.076 2.076
         TREAT*MONTHS*MONTHS*MONTHS -2.86 2.86
         TREAT*MONTHS*MONTHS*MONTHS*MONTHS -4.22 4.22
         TREAT*MONTHS*MONTHS*MONTHS*MONTHS*MONTHS -6.46 6.46
         /DIVISOR=1.84;
```

Estimates for longer periods of time, such as 26 and 52 weeks, are generated using the same procedure. In this study, the results would appear as follows where T is rescaled to be equal to 1. The estimates are now on the same scale as the original measure and have the alternative interpretation of the average score over the period from 0 to T.

Label	Estimate	Standard Error	DF	t Value	Pr > |t|
IFN only - AUC 8wks	61.97	1.63	468	38.04	<.0001
IFN +CRA - AUC 8wks	61.30	1.65	468	37.16	<.0001
Difference - AUC 8wks	-0.67	2.32	468	-0.29	0.7739

IFN only - AUC 26wks	64.35	1.66	468	38.65	<.0001
IFN +CRA - AUC 26wks	59.30	1.71	468	34.64	<.0001
Difference - AUC 26wks	-5.05	2.39	468	-2.11	0.0350
IFN only - AUC 52wks	64.73	1.75	468	36.94	<.0001
IFN +CRA - AUC 52wks	61.27	1.82	468	33.61	<.0001
Difference - AUC 52wks	-3.45	2.53	468	-1.37	0.1726

For a piecewise regression model, one could estimate the means at each *knot* and then use a trapezoidal approximation. Integration provides a more direct method:

$$\mathrm{AUC}_h(T) = \hat{S}_h = \int_{t=0}^{T} \sum_{j=0}^{J} \hat{\beta}_{hj} t^{[j]} \partial t$$

$$= \hat{\beta}_{h0} T + \sum_{j=1}^{J} \hat{\beta}_{hj} \frac{\max(T - T^{[j]}, 0)^2}{2}, \qquad (10.10)$$

where $\hat{\beta}_{h0}$ is the estimate of the intercept for the hth group, $\hat{\beta}_{h1}$ is the initial slope, and $\hat{\beta}_{hj}, j > 2$ is the change in slope at each of the knots, $T^{[l]}$. $t^{[0]} = 1$, $t^{[1]} = t$, and $t^{[j]} = \max(t - T^{[j]})$.

In the renal cell carcinoma study, the piecewise regression model has two knots, one at 2 weeks and one at 8 weeks. Thus, the estimated AUC (rescaled to $T = 1$) is

$$\mathrm{AUC}_h(T) = \left(\hat{\beta}_{h0} T + \hat{\beta}_{h1} \frac{T^2}{2} + \hat{\beta}_{h2} \frac{\max(T-2,0)^2}{2} + \hat{\beta}_{h3} \frac{\max(T-8,0)^2}{2} \right) \Big/ T.$$

If we are interested in the early period defined as the first 8 weeks, then

$$\mathrm{AUC}_h(8) = \left(\hat{\beta}_{h0} 8 + \hat{\beta}_{h1} \underbrace{\frac{8^2}{2}}_{=32} + \hat{\beta}_{h2} \underbrace{\frac{\max(8-2,0)^2}{2}}_{=18} + \hat{\beta}_{h3} \underbrace{\frac{\max(8-8,0)^2}{2}}_{=0} \right) \Big/ 8.$$

The ESTIMATE statements follow directly from these equations, as illustrated below for the calculation of the AUC at 8 weeks for each group and their difference.

```
ESTIMATE 'IFN only - AUC 8wks'    TREAT 8 0
                                  TREAT*WEEKS 32 0
                                  TREAT*WEEK2 18 0/DIVISOR=8;
ESTIMATE 'IFN +CRA - AUC 8wks'    TREAT 0 8
                                  TREAT*WEEKS 0 32
                                  TREAT*WEEK2 0 18/DIVISOR=8;
ESTIMATE 'Difference - AUC 8wks'  TREAT -8 8
                                  TREAT*WEEKS -32 32
                                  TREAT*WEEK2 -18 18/DIVISOR=8;
```

Estimates for longer periods of time, such as 26 and 52 weeks, are generated using the same procedure. The results would appear as follows:

```
                                  Standard
Label                  Estimate   Error     DF    t Value  Pr>|t|

IFN only   - AUC 8wks    63.55    1.54     472    41.30    <.0001
IFN +CRA   - AUC 8wks    61.18    1.58     472    38.77    <.0001
Difference - AUC 8wks    -2.37    2.20     472    -1.08    0.2822

IFN only   - AUC 26wks   63.16    1.57     472    40.12    <.0001
IFN +CRA   - AUC 26wks   59.51    1.61     472    36.91    <.0001
Difference - AUC 26wks   -3.66    2.25     472    -1.62    0.1051

IFN only   - AUC 52wks   64.44    1.72     472    37.36    <.0001
IFN +CRA   - AUC 52wks   61.88    1.71     472    36.16    <.0001
Difference - AUC 52wks   -2.70    2.43     472    -1.11    0.2668
```

The interpretation is that there is, on average, a 2- to 4-point difference between the two groups. Although there are consistent differences between the two groups, the magnitude is small. The standard deviation of the FACT-BRM TOI at baseline is approximately 17 points, and differences between 2 and 4 points are not clinically significant.

For the purpose of illustration, we have assumed the data are MAR and estimated the parameters using REML. However, because we suspect that the data are MNAR, these summary measures should be used in the sensitivity analysis as described in Chapters 8 and 9.

10.5 Summarizing across HRQoL domains or subscales

Summarizing across HRQoL domains or subscales is useful when the objective is to obtain increased power to test whether a hypothesis of interest is *consistently* different across scales. However, a change in one domain may be obscured by changes in the opposite direction in another. Alternative methods such as multiple testing procedures (Chapter 11) should be considered when differences among the individual HRQoL domains are of interest. The same two approaches can be used to compute summary measures or statistics across domains or subscales as were used to summarize across time.

Summary measures

Most HRQoL instruments create summary measures. Actually, each subscale is inherently a summary measure constructed by combining the responses to individual items. However, for most instruments, summary measures are also constructed from the subscales. Some options for weighting include

1. Weights proportional to the number of questions for each domain
2. Equal weights for each domain
3. Factor analytic weights

4. Weights derived from patient preferences
5. Statistically derived weights (e.g., correlation among domains)

Weighting proportional to the number of questions

Many HRQoL instruments compute an overall score where domains are weighted in proportion to the number of questions asked about each domain. In the FACT-Lung and FACT-BRM instruments, there are a number of summary measures. For both, a total score is computed by summing all subscales (Table 10.7). Another summary measure, the Trial Outcome Index, is also constructed by summing the physical well-being, functional well-being, and lung cancer–specific items to create the FACT-Lung TOI and by summing the physical well-being, functional well-being, and BRM-specific items to create the FACT-BRM TOI. There is an implicit weighting of the subscales that is dependent on the number of items. For example, because there are only five questions assessing emotional well-being, this domain receives less weight than the other domains of physical, functional, and social well-being (Table 10.7). Similarly, because there are 13 BRM-specific questions and 7 lung cancer–specific questions, the physical and functional well-being subscales have less weight in the FACT-BRM TOI than they do in the FACT-Lung TOI.

Factor analytic weights

The physical component scale (PCS) and the mental component scale (MCS) of the Medical Outcome Study SF-36 are examples of summary scores where weights are derived from factor analysis. These widely used scores present an excellent example of summary scores that need to be carefully examined when interpreting the results of a trial. The weights used to construct the summary

Table 10.7. Summary measures from the FACT-Lung and FACT-BRM Version 2 instruments.

Subscale	Items	Total score		TOI	
		Lung	BRM	Lung	BRM
Physical well-being	7	0.200	0.171	0.333	0.259
Social/family well-being	7	0.200	0.171		
Relationship with doctor	2[a]	0.057	0.049		
Emotional well-being	5[b]	0.143	0.122		
Functional well-being	7	0.200	0.171	0.333	0.259
Lung cancer subscale	7	0.200		0.333	
BRM physical subscale	7		0.171		0.259
BRM mental subscale	6		0.146		0.222

Weights based on number of items used in constructing the total scores and the Trial Outcome Index (TOI).

[a] Dropped from Version 4.

[b] Six items in Versions 3 and 4.

Table 10.8. Factor analytic weights for the PCS and the MCS of the Medical Outcome Study SF-36 from a U.S. general population sample [158].

Component	PF	RP	BP	GH	V	SF	RE	MH
Physical	0.424	0.351	0.318	0.250	0.029	−0.008	−0.192	−0.221
Mental	−0.230	−0.123	−0.097	−0.016	0.235	0.269	0.434	0.486

PF = physical function, RP = role-physical, BP = bodily pain, GH = general health, V = vitality, SF = social function, RE = role-emotional, MH = mental health.

scores were derived from an orthogonal factor rotation. In the resulting scoring algorithms, physical function, role physical, and bodily pain subscales make a modest negative contribution to the MCS, and the mental health and role-emotional subscales make a modest negative contribution to the PCS score (Table 10.8). These negative contributions can produce surprising results. Simon et al. [139] describe this in a study of antidepressant treatment where there were modest positive effects over time on the physical function, role-physical, bodily pain, and general health, but a negative score (nonsignificant) was observed for the PCS because of the very strong positive effects in the remaining scales. The negative contribution of these remaining subscales overwhelmed the smaller contributions of the first four subscales. As a result, the authors suggest very cautious interpretation of these summary scales when the treatment has a strong effect on subscales with negative coefficients.

Patient weights

Weights derived based on patient preferences are currently uncommon, but they have a conceptual lure. For example, it is possible that most patients on adjuvant breast cancer therapy do not consider that physical well-being during a limited treatment period and disease-free survival have equal weight. They are willing to undergo adjuvant therapy with its associated morbidity including severe fatigue, hair loss, and weight gain even after there is no detectable disease to maximize the chance that the disease will never recur. If weights that reflect patient preferences or values are available, they are likely to be more relevant than statistically derived weights.

A series of experimental questions are included in the FACT instruments (Versions 1 to 3) asking the patient to indicate how much the items in each subscale affect the patient's quality of life. For example, following the seven questions asking the patient to comment on energy, pain, nausea, side effects, ability to meet needs of family, feeling ill, and spending time in bed, the following question appears:

Looking at the above 7 questions, how much would you say your PHYSICAL WELL-BEING affects your quality of life?

0 1 2 3 4 5 6 7 8 9 10
Not at all   Very much so

Similar questions appear for the other subscales. Responses to these questions could be used to weight the responses to each of the subscales.

Interestingly, these experimental questions have become optional in Version 4 and are not recommended for use in clinical trials. The developer cites two basic reasons [17]. First, using weighted and unweighted scores produces essentially the same results in all analyses examinined. Second was the concern that the respondents were answering the questions as intended. Although some appeared to answer as a true weight, others seemed to answer the questions as a summary of their response to the items, and as many as 15 to 25% did not seem to understand at all and left the questions blank or responded in rather unusual ways. Other considerations may be (1) a more-complicated scoring system that would preclude hand-scoring of the scale, (2) requirements for additional validation studies, and (3) nonequivalence of scales from study to study.

Statistically derived weights: Inverse correlation

In a procedure proposed by O'Brien [108], the weights are proportional to the inverse of the correlation of the K domains. The result is that the more strongly correlated domains are down-weighted. Two subscales that measure very similar aspects of HRQoL will contribute less to the overall score than two subscales that measure very different aspects of HRQoL. For example, consider the NSCLC results presented previously in this chapter. The subscales measuring the physical/functional aspects of the patient's well-being are more strongly correlated with each other than the emotional and social aspects (Table 10.9). Note that the physical well-being scores have the strongest correlation with the other subscales ($\hat{\rho} = 0.45 - 0.77$) and the social well-being scale has the weakest correlation with the other subscales ($\hat{\rho} = 0.36 - 0.45$). The procedure is first to compute standardized scores (z_{hik}) for each of the K domains or subscales. Then, compute a weighted sum of these standardized scores using the column sum of the inverse of the correlation (Table 10.10). Thus, $\hat{S}_{hi} = J'\hat{R}^{-1}\hat{z}_{hi}$, where $\mathbf{z}_{hi} = (z_{hi1}, \ldots, z_{hiK})'$, $J = (1, \ldots, 1)'$, and R is the estimated common correlation matrix of the observations ($\hat{\Sigma}$).

Summary measures with weights based on the inverse correlation are the most powerful [108, 117] and do not require specification prior to analysis.

Table 10.9. Correlations among the AUC summary measures in the NSCLC study.

	Physical	Functional	Emotional	Social	Lung CA
Physical	1.00	0.77	0.64	0.45	0.65
Functional	0.77	1.00	0.56	0.36	0.68
Emotional	0.64	0.56	1.00	0.41	0.49
Social	0.45	0.36	0.41	1.00	0.36
Lung CA	0.65	0.68	0.49	0.36	1.00

Table 10.10. Inverse correlation (R^{-1}) and weights ($J'R^{-1}$) of the AUC summary measures in the NSCLC study.

	Physical	Functional	Emotional	Social	Lung CA
Physical	3.21	−1.57	−0.76	−0.40	−0.51
Functional	−1.57	2.91	−2.25	0.08	−0.86
Emotional	−0.76	−0.25	1.79	−0.25	−0.12
Social	−0.40	0.08	−0.25	1.30	−0.13
Lung CA subscale	−0.51	−0.86	−0.12	−0.13	2.02
Sum ($J'R^{-1}$)	−0.02	0.31	0.40	0.59	0.40

The disadvantages are that they vary from study to study [20], and they may not reflect the importance that patients place on different domains.

Summary statistics

The weighted average of the individual values proposed by O'Brien [108] also extends to the construction of summary statistics with use of a weighted average of asymptotically normal test statistics such as the two-sample t-statistic.

$$t_{hk} = \frac{\hat{\theta}_{hk}}{\hat{\sigma}_{(\hat{\theta})hk}}, \quad t_h = (t_{h1}, \ldots, t_{hK})', \qquad (10.11)$$

$$\hat{S}_h = J'R^{-1}t_h, \quad J = (1, \ldots, 1)'. \qquad (10.12)$$

R is the estimated common correlation matrix of either the raw data in each treatment group ($\hat{\Sigma}$) or the pooled correlation matrix of the estimated means ($\hat{\mu}_{jk}$). An alternative way to express the summary statistic is

$$\hat{S}_h = \sum_{k=1}^{K} w_k g(\hat{\beta}_{kj}), \qquad (10.13)$$

where $g(\hat{\beta}_{kj}) = \hat{\mu}_{kj}/\hat{\sigma}_{(\hat{\mu}_{kj})}$ and $(w_1, \ldots, w_K) = J'R^{-1}$. Because $\hat{S}_h$ is a linear combination of asymptotically normal parameter estimates, the asymptotic variance of the summary measure is

$$\text{Var}(\hat{S}_h) = W'\text{Cov}[g(\hat{\beta}_{hk})]W. \qquad (10.14)$$

For two treatment groups, we can test the hypothesis $S_1 = S_2$ or $\theta = S_1 - S_2 = 0$ using a t-test with $N-4$ degrees of freedom:

$$t_{N-4} = (\hat{S}_1 - \hat{S}_2)[\text{Var}(\hat{S}_1 - \hat{S}_2)]^{-1/2} = \hat{\theta}[\text{Var}(\hat{\theta})]^{-1/2} \qquad (10.15)$$

for small samples [117]. More generally, for large samples we can test the hypothesis $S_1 = S_2 \cdots = S_k$ using a Wald χ^2 statistic:

$$\chi^2_{k-1} = \hat{\phi}'[\text{Var}(\hat{\phi})]^{-1}\hat{\phi}, \qquad \hat{\phi} = (\hat{S}_2 - \hat{S}_1, \ldots, \hat{S}_n - \hat{S}_1)'. \qquad (10.16)$$

10.6 Advanced notes

Nonparametric procedures

Based on studies of the power and size of the test, O'Brien [108] recommended the nonparametric procedure (Section 10.3) for general use and the inverse correlation procedure for normally distributed data with moderate or large sample sizes.

Combining HRQoL and time to event

Pocock et al. [118] suggest an extension of O'Brien's weighted average z-scores to the combination of any asymptotically normal test statistics, illustrating the concept with the long-rank statistics and a binary endpoint. Fairclough [39] describes an application to repeated assessment of HRQoL and survival where the logarithmic transformation of the survival times is assumed to be normally distributed. Because $\hat{S}_k$ is a linear combination of asymptotically normal parameter estimates, the asymptotic variance of the summary measure is $\text{Var}(\hat{S}_k) = W'\text{Cov}[g(\hat{\beta}_{jk})]W$, where $W = (w_1, \ldots, w_n)$. For two treatment groups, we can test the hypothesis $S_1 = S_2$ using a t-statistic, $t = (\hat{S}_1 - \hat{S}_2)/\text{Var}(\hat{S}_1 - \hat{S}_2)^{1/2}$, with df $= N - 4$ for small samples [118]. More generally, for large samples, we can test the hypothesis $S_1 = S_2 = \cdots = S_K$ using a Wald χ^2 statistic: $\chi^2_{K-1} = \hat{\phi}'[\text{Cov}(\hat{\phi})]^{-1}\hat{\phi}$, where $\hat{\phi} = (\hat{S}_2 - \hat{S}_1, \ldots, \hat{S}_n - \hat{S}_1)$.

Area under the curve

One might be inclined to present the AUC values calculated to the time of censoring, as one would present survival data. This approach would appear to have the advantages of displaying more information about the distribution of the AUC values and accommodating administrative censoring. Unfortunately, administrative censoring is informative on the AUC scale [55, 56, 80] and the usual Kaplan–Meier estimates are biased. Specifically, if the missing data are due to staggered entry and incomplete follow-up is identical for two groups, the group with poorer HRQoL will have lower values of the AUC and is censored earlier on the AUC scale. Knowing when a subject is censored on the AUC scale gives us some information about the AUC score and, thus, the censoring is informative. Korn [80] suggests an improved procedure to reduce the bias of the estimator by assuming that the probability of censoring in short intervals is independent of the HRQoL measures prior to that time. Although this assumption is probably not true, if the HRQoL is measured frequently and the relationship between HRQoL and censoring is weak, the violation may be small enough that the bias in the estimator will also be small.

Latent variable models

The multiple measures of the different aspects of HRQoL can be considered to be measurement of an unobservable latent variable. Latent variable models for longitudinal studies have been used by Zwinderman [174] for dichotomous outcomes and by Busch et al. [12] for continuous normally distributed outcomes. In both applications, the issue of missing assessments was addressed, with the subsequent analyses based on the assumption of MAR.

10.7 Summary

- Summary measures and statistics
  1. Facilitate interpretation by reducing the number of comparisons
  2. Increase the power to detect consistent differences over time or over HRQoL domains
  3. May obscure differences in different directions.
- Selection of a summary measure or statistic should depend on the research question, expected pattern of change over time, and missing-data patterns.
- Statistically derived weights are efficient but have the limitations of varying from study to study and not reflecting patient values.

CHAPTER 11

Multiple Endpoints

11.1 Introduction

The issue of multiple comparisons in clinical trials assessing HRQoL arises from three sources: (1) multiple HRQoL measures (scales or subscales), (2) repeated postrandomization assessments, and (3) multiple (three or more) treatment arms. As a result, the problem of multiple comparisons is one of the major analytic challenges in these trials [79]. For example, in the NSCLC study, there are five major subscales in the FACT-Lung instrument (physical, functional, emotional, and social/family well-being, plus the disease-specific concerns). There are three follow-up assessments, at 6, 12, and 26 weeks, and three treatment arms. If we consider the three possible pairwise comparisons of the treatment arms at each of the three follow-ups for the five primary subscales, we have 45 tests. Not only does this create concerns about Type I error, but reports containing large numbers of statistical tests generally result in a confusing picture of HRQoL.

Although widely used in the analysis of quality of life in clinical trials [132], univariate tests of each HRQoL domain or scale and time point can seriously inflate the Type I (false-positive) error rate for the overall trial such that the analyst is unable to distinguish between the true and false-positive differences. *Post hoc* adjustment is often infeasible because, at the end of analysis, it is impossible to determine the number of tests performed. There are three typical strategies to reduce the problem: (1) *a priori* specification of a limited number of *confirmatory* tests, (2) multiple comparison procedures including alpha adjustments (e.g., Bonferroni) and closed multiple testing, and (3) the use of summary measures or statistics (see Chapter 10). In practice, a combination of focused hypotheses, summary measures, and multiple comparison procedures is necessary.

Limiting the number of confirmatory tests

One recommended solution to the multiple comparison problem is to specify a limited number (≤ 3) of *a priori* endpoints in the design of the trial [59] (Table 11.1). While theoretically improving the overall Type I error rate for the study, in practice investigators are reluctant to ignore the remaining data. Descriptive or graphical comparisons of the remaining scales and/or time points [135] often accompany the formal hypothesis tests. However, these presentations generally include confidence intervals that can be disguised statistical tests. A more important critique of this approach is an ethical question about collection of data that will not be used in the primary analysis.

Table 11.1. General strategies for addressing concerns about multiple comparison issues in HRQoL studies.

Strategy	**Limit confirmatory tests**
Advantage	Does not require any adjustments or special statistical procedures
Disadvantages	Does not strictly control Type I error
	What is done about *exploratory* analyses?
	Ethical issue: What is justification for collection of HRQoL data not required for confirmatory tests?
Strategy	**Summary measures and statistics**
Advantages	Reduce number of comparisons
	Increase power to detect consistent small differences
Disadvantage	Obscure differences in opposite directions
Strategy	**Multiple comparison procedures**
Advantage	Control of Type I errors
Disadvantage	Decreased power

Summary measures and statistics

Well-chosen summary measures or statistics often have greater power to detect patterns of consistent HRQoL differences across time or measures. They also facilitate interpretation, especially when used to summarize information over time. However, they also have the potential to blur differences when components of the summary measure are in opposite directions. Additional details about their advantages and disadvantages are discussed in detail in the previous chapter. In this chapter, we will assume that a summary measure or statistic is used to reduce the the multiplicity of the repeated assessments over time. This is partially to simplify the presentation but also because it is a good strategy.

Multiple comparison procedures

This chapter describes a number of procedures that can be used to control the Type I error rate for K multiple comparisons. Although the procedures can generally be applied to any set of hypotheses, the discussion here is presented for a typical situation of two treatment groups with K distinct measures of HRQoL. Some special cases that are not unique to HRQoL studies, such as designs with three or more ordered treatment arms, will not be addressed. The reader is advised to consult texts on clinical trial design and multiple comparisons.

11.2 Background concepts and definitions

Let $H_{0(1)}, \ldots, H_{0(K)}$ denote the K null hypotheses that are to be tested and let H_0 denote the set of K hypotheses. $T_{(1)}, \ldots, T_{(K)}$ denotes the corresponding K test statistics. The obtained p-value, $p_{(k)}$, denotes the (unadjusted) probability of observing the test statistic, $T_{(k)}$, or a more extreme value if the null hypothesis, $H_{0(k)}$, is true. Finally, $\alpha_{(k)}$ is the significance level for testing the kth hypothesis.

When describing the multiple comparison procedures, it is often useful to order the obtained p-values from smallest to largest: $p_{[1]} \leq \cdots \leq p_{[K]}$ and then to reorder the corresponding hypotheses $H_{0[1]}, \ldots, H_{0[K]}$, test statistics $T_{[1]}, \ldots, T_{[K]}$, and significance levels $\alpha_{[1]} \leq \cdots \leq \alpha_{[k]}$ for the multiple comparison procedures. Note that square brackets are used to indicate the ordered values.

Univariate vs. multivariate test statistics

In this chapter we use the term *univariate* test statistic to refer to the kth test statistic, $T_{[k]}$. In some cases this is a test statistic derived from a longitudinal (multivariate) analysis. For example, a set of five univariate test statistics (t-statistics) could be generated from tests of differences in the slopes from the longitudinal analyses of the five distinct subscales in the lung cancer trial. There is no restriction on whether the K univariate statistics are generated from K separate models or from a joint multivariate model.

In contrast, a *multivariate* test statistic corresponds to the joint test of the K hypotheses, such as an F-test of treatment differences from a MANOVA of summary measures (e.g., AUC) for K subscales. The critical difference is that the multivariate test statistic is a function of the correlation among the subscales and the univariate test statistics are not.

Familywise and experimentwise error rates

There are two ways of controlling the probability of erroneously rejecting at least one null hypothesis. A test or multiple testing procedure controls the *familywise error rate* or *global α-level* if the probability of incorrectly rejecting at least one true null hypothesis does not exceed α when all null hypotheses are simultaneously true. In contrast, a test or multiple testing procedure controls the *experimentwise error rate* or the *multiple α-level* if the probability of incorrectly rejecting at least one true null hypothesis does not exceed α regardless of which (if any) null hypotheses are true. A procedure that controls the multiple α-level also controls the global α-level. The converse is not true. Control of the experimentwise error rate is more important in confirmatory trials or those from which decisions that will affect clinical practice will be made.

Global vs. individual tests

A *global test* generates a single statistic for testing the overall treatment effect and results in the acceptance or rejection of a set of hypotheses.

$$H_0\colon H_{0(1)}, \ldots, H_{0(K)}. \tag{11.1}$$

For example, one might make the decision to approve a drug if the null hypothesis was rejected on the basis of a global test. When the overall test of H_0 has been rejected, the question remains, "Which of the individual hypotheses can be rejected?" A global test does not allow inferences to be made about individual endpoints.

There are a number of strategies for handling the individual tests. The loosest strategies require only that the global test be rejected at α before examining the univariate tests each at α. These strategies control only the global α-level. At the other extreme are formal closed testing procedures designed to control the multiple α-level. A detailed example is shown later. As the testing procedures increase control on the α-level for the worst-case scenario (independent tests), they decrease the power to detect differences for more typical settings (correlated tests).

11.3 Multivariate statistics

Global tests

Examples of multivariate statistics for a global test are the Hotelling–Lawley trace for MANOVA and likelihood ratio tests. Constructing multivariate statistics may be feasible with simple designs (e.g., cross-sectional or pre/postdesigns) with minimal missing data. For purposes of illustration, consider the adjuvant breast cancer study where the Breast Chemotherapy Questionnaire has seven subscales. If our intent is to control the Type I error for testing treatment effects separately for on-therapy and post-therapy, we could perform two multivariate analyses of variance (Table 11.2). By using the change from baseline as the outcome, the global test of treatment effects on the seven BCQ measures is highly significant during therapy($F_{7,135} = 5.73$, $p = 0.0001$) but not significant post-therapy ($F_{7,125} = 0.34$, $p = 0.93$).

Closed multivariate testing procedures

Although the global test allows us to make a decision about the multiple endpoints, we are rarely satisfied with only being able to say that there is a difference for at least one endpoint. The question always follows: "Which endpoints are affected by the intervention?" If we wish to control only the global α-level, we can specify the following procedure. First, perform the multivariate test for the K endpoints, and then if (and only if) that test is significant at α, perform the K univariate tests at α. In the breast cancer trial, no further tests are performed for the post-therapy comparisons. Examination of the univariate

Table 11.2. Results of the multivariate analyses of change from baseline in the adjuvant breast cancer trial.

	During/Pretherapy		Post/Pretherapy	
Global Test	$F_{7,135} = 5.73$, $p = 0.0001$		$F_{7,125} = 0.34$, $p = 0.93$	
Univariate	t	p	t	p
Hair loss	0.13	0.89	NR	NS
Well-being	−1.39	0.17	NR	NS
Symptoms	−4.33	0.0001	NR	NS
Trouble	−1.30	0.20	NR	NS
Fatigue	−4.52	0.0001	NR	NS
Emotional	−0.71	0.48	NR	NS
Nausea	−1.57	0.12	NR	NS

Nominal p-values are reported for univariate tests.
NS = not significant, NR = not reported.

Table 11.3. Breast cancer trial: Correlations between the change scores.

		1	2	3	4	5	6	7
Hair loss	1	—	0.36	0.38	0.07	0.27	0.35	0.16
Well-being	2	0.31	—	0.26	0.01	0.23	0.48	0.12
Symptoms	3	0.36	0.24	—	0.10	0.44	0.28	0.41
Trouble	4	0.10	0.08	0.15	—	0.15	0.14	0.04
Fatigue	5	0.27	0.27	0.33	0.10	—	0.46	0.24
Emotional	6	0.27	0.34	0.35	0.35	0.43	—	0.15
Nausea	7	0.26	0.12	0.42	0.01	0.08	0.16	—

Upper triangle contains the Pearson correlations for during therapy and lower triangle contains the Pearson correlations for post-therapy.

tests reveals significant differences for the symptoms and fatigue subscales (unadjusted $p < 0.05$).

The closed-testing procedure proposed by Marcus et al. [96] for controlling the multiple α-level is more complicated. After rejecting the multivariate test for the K endpoints $H_{0(1)}, \ldots, H_{0(K)}$, a stepdown procedure is used. In this closed-testing procedure, sequentially smaller subsets of the K endpoints are tested only if all the tests containing a subset of the K hypotheses have been previously rejected ($p < \alpha$). Basically, to reject the kth hypothesis $H_{0(k)}$, all possible subsets of hypotheses containing the kth hypothesis must be rejected. In some cases, this could involve the testing of $2^K - 1$ sets of hypotheses.

In the breast cancer example, the multivariate test of differences during therapy for all K scales was first rejected as previously described. The next step was to examine the K multivariate tests for $K-1$ endpoints. All seven multivariate tests of the possible subsets of six subscales were rejected, each at $\alpha = 0.05$. Because all were rejected, all possible $K-2$ combinations were then tested again at $\alpha = 0.05$. Only 1 of the 21 multivariate tests was not rejected, the one not containing the fatigue and symptoms scales. Following the procedure, only hypotheses containing the fatigue and symptoms scales were subsequently tested. The joint test of these two endpoints was rejected, as were the individual univariate tests. The conclusion is that there are significant differences in the endpoints identified as fatigue and symptoms.

Limitations

There are several limitations of these multivariate procedures for HRQoL studies. The first is that describing the sequential method in clinical journals is challenging. Only the p-value for the first global test can be reported; the subsequent test statistics are unadjusted for the conditional tests. This is likely to create confusion for reviewers and readers.

The second is the lack of sensitivity to differences in the same direction across the multiple endpoints. These multivariate statistics test a hypothesis of no treatment differences (H_0) for the K endpoints against a general alternative (H_1) that there is at least one endpoint where there are treatment differences. These tests may sometimes be hard to interpret when the results are counterintuitive [31]. For example, the test may be statistically significant when HRQoL is better in one treatment arm for one endpoint and worse for another endpoint and not significant when one treatment appears to be consistently better over all endpoints [39].

The final limitation is practical. It is very cumbersome (although possible) to set up a full multivariate longitudinal model. In the breast cancer study this would entail 21 repeated measures (7 measures × 3 times). Because of the

Table 11.4. Two testing procedures for identifying individual differences from multivariate tests.

Strategy	**Control of Global α-level**
	1. Test multivariate H_0: $H_{0(1)}, \ldots, H_{0(K)}$
	2. If $p < \alpha \rightarrow$ perform K univariate tests (α)
Advantage	Minimal loss of power
Disadvantage	Controls only global Type I error
Strategy	**Control of Multiple α-level**
	1. Multivariate test: $H_{0(1)}, \ldots, H_{0(K)}$
	2. If multivariate test rejected $p < \alpha \rightarrow$ Sequentially test subsets the K hypotheses
Advantage	Controls multiple and global Type I error
Disadvantages	1. More contrasts to program
	2. Reporting of p-values is complicated

large number of covariance parameters, algorithms are very slow. Implementing procedures and sensitivity analyses for missing data will be even more difficult. Solely for the purposes of illustration, we simplified the example by deciding to control the error rate separately for the comparisons of treatment effects during and after therapy and to ignore the loss of subjects with missing follow-up assessments. In practice we would have to deal with these issues.

11.4 Univariate statistics

In general, multiple comparison procedures using a set of univariate test statistics are much easier to implement and report than those using multivariate test statistics. There are a number of other practical advantages.

1. In the context of HRQoL studies, the major advantage is that any of the analytic methods described in the previous chapters that generate a p-value associated with a test of treatment differences can be used.
2. Another advantage is that the procedures can be adapted to one-sided tests.
3. The univariate analyses do not require that all K endpoints are measured on all subjects (although all issues of nonrandom missing data are still applicable). This is an advantage if a subset of the K endpoints is not measured because a translation is not available for some of the HRQoL measures.
4. Another advantage is the ease of application of nonparametric methods.

NSCLC example

The advantage of the univariate approach is illustrated with the NSCLC example for the summary measures described in Chapter 10. As the missing values were handled using multiple imputation, a multivariate analysis of the M imputed data sets would be complex. In contrast, the univariate analyses are straigtforward, and the results for the AUC summary measure are displayed in Figure 11.1 and Table 11.5.

Alpha adjustments for K univariate tests

Bonferroni adjustment

A traditional method to address the multiple comparison problem is to utilize a procedure such as the Bonferroni correction, which adjusts the test statistics on K endpoints. The global test is based on the smallest p-value, $p_{[1]}$. The global null hypothesis is rejected when

$$p_{[1]} \leq \alpha/K. \tag{11.2}$$

For individual endpoints the procedure is to accept as statistically significant only those tests with p-values that are less than α/K.

The Bonferroni procedure controls the experimentwise error rate but is well known to be quite conservative. If the K outcomes are uncorrelated (the tests

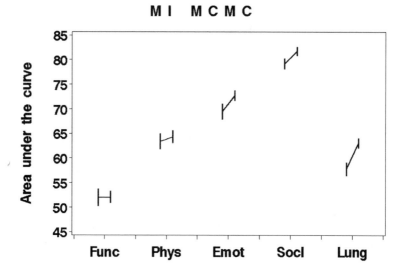

Figure 11.1. Area under the curve (AUC) with missing data handled by multiple imputation (MI MCMC). Pairs display mean ±1 standard error for no Taxol (left) and Taxol (right) groups.

are independent) and the null hypotheses are all true, then the probability of rejecting at least one of the K hypotheses is approximately* αK when α is small. The Bonferroni focuses on the detection of large differences in one or more endpoints and is insensitive to a pattern of smaller differences that are all in the same direction.

Strategy	**Bonferroni Corrections**
	$p < \alpha/K \rightarrow$ reject H_0
Advantage	Well known, simple
Disadvantage	Conservative if K is large and endpoints are correlated

Strategy	**Sequential Rejective Bonferroni Procedure**
	Holm [69]
	Order univariate p-values: $p_{[1]} \leq \cdots \leq p_{[K]}$
	$p_{[1]} \leq \alpha/K$ reject $H_{0[1]}$, else stop
	$p_{[2]} \leq \alpha/(K-1)$ reject $H_{0[2]}$, else stop
	etc.
Advantage	More powerful than Bonferroni when some H_0 are rejected with high probability (large difference for some endpoints)
Disadvantage	Not much gain when most H_0 are approximately true (small differences for all endpoints)

* $Pr[\min(p\text{-value}) \leq \alpha] = 1 - (1-\alpha)^K \approx \alpha K$.

UNIVARIATE STATISTICS

Table 11.5. Summary of univariate test statistics based on analysis of AUC calculated using multiply imputed data for lung cancer study and adjusted α levels for global test of $K = 5$ endpoints.

Univariate analysis	Lung $k=1$	Emotional $k=2$	Social $k=3$	Physical $k=4$	Functional $k=5$
Difference	5.45	3.31	2.50	0.75	−0.08
Standard error	1.63	1.89	1.45	2.02	2.01
T-statistic	3.35	1.75	1.72	0.37	−0.04
$p_{[k]}$	0.0009	0.081	0.087	0.71	0.97

Method	$\alpha_{[k]}$	α Levels for Global Test			
Bonferroni	$\alpha \times 1/K$	0.0100			
Rüger	$\alpha \times K'/K, K' = 3$				
Simes	$\alpha \times k/K$	0.0100	0.0200	0.0300	0.0400	0.0500
Hommel	$\alpha \times k/KC$	0.0044	0.0088	0.0131	0.0175	0.0219
Holms	$\alpha/(K-k+1)$	0.0100	0.0125	0.0167	0.0250	0.0500

Note: $C = \sum_{k=1}^{K}(1/k)$.

Rüger's inequality

Rüger proposed an alternative procedure for situtations where, rather than being interested in only the smallest p-value, one is interested in the K' smallest p-values ($K' \leq K$). For example, one might propose that a general HRQoL benefit is demonstrated by significant improvement in at least half of the measured domains without specifying which domains. The procedure is to order the p-values from smallest to largest:

$$p_{[1]} \leq p_{[2]} \leq \cdots \leq p_{[K]} \tag{11.3}$$

and reject the global test if

$$p_{[K']} < \alpha \frac{K'}{K}. \tag{11.4}$$

If this represents three of the five subscales in the lung cancer study, the critical value for the global test is $\alpha K'/K = 0.05(3/5) = 0.03$ for the third-smallest p-value. If and only if the global test is rejected are the K individual comparisons made. In the lung cancer study, the global test will not be rejected and no further comparisons are made.

Simes' global test

Hommel [70] and Simes [138] both proposed a global test that avoids specifying K'. In the Simes test, the global hypothesis of no treatment differences is rejected if

$$p_{[k]} \leq \alpha \frac{k}{K} \qquad \text{for any } k = 1, \ldots, K. \tag{11.5}$$

This procedure is less conservative than the Bonferroni procedure. However, the procedure does not strictly control the Type I error rate to be less than α except when the tests are independent. For the Hommel procedure, the global hypothesis is rejected if

$$p_{[k]} \leq \alpha \frac{k}{K\left(1 + \frac{1}{2} + \cdots + \frac{1}{K}\right)} \qquad \text{for any } k = 1, \ldots, K. \tag{11.6}$$

Although Hommel's procedure strictly controls the Type I error rate to be less than or equal to α, it does so at the cost of power for the procedure, especially when the tests are expected to be almost independent. However, it is rarely the case (if ever) that the different HRQoL domains are independent (see Table 11.3). Even though the Simes procedure may inflate the Type I error rate two- to three-fold (depending on K) for independent endpoints, it is likely to be very practical (and definitely more powerful) for moderately correlated endpoints typical of HRQoL studies.

UNIVARIATE STATISTICS

Note that both procedures provide only a global test and do not test for the individual endpoints.

Sequential rejective Bonferroni procedure

Holm proposed less conservative alternative to the classical Bonferroni adjustments which allows tests of the individual hypotheses [69]. Again, the univariate p-values are ordered from smallest to largest. Then, in a stepwise procedure, the smallest p-value, $p_{[1]}$, is compared to α/K. If $p_{[1]} \leq \alpha/K$, we reject the corresponding hypothesis and continue with the stepwise procedure, comparing $p_{[k]}$ to $\alpha/(K-k+1)$. If $H_{0[k-1]}$ has been rejected, evaluate

$$p_{[k]} \leq \alpha/(K-k+1). \tag{11.7}$$

At the point where any null hypothesis cannot be rejected, the procedure stops and all remaining null hypotheses are accepted.

When all null hypotheses are approximately true, this procedure does not provide much of an advantage. But when some of the null hypotheses are not true, this procedure substantially increases the power to detect the moderate effects of the treatment.

p-value adjustments

Reporting the results of the individual tests is facilitated by the use of adjusted p-values, $p_{(k)}^{\text{adj}}$. These p-values do not reflect the exact probability of observing the test statistic conditional on the testing procedure but do allow the reader an easy way to evaluate the results relative to the overall significance level, α.

If $\alpha_{[k]} = f_{[k]}\alpha$, then the adjusted p-values can be computed as

$$p_{[k]}^{\text{adj}} = \min(p_{[k]}/f_{[k]}, 1). \tag{11.8}$$

For example, in the lung cancer study, the ordered p-values are

$$p_{[1]} = 0.0009, \quad p_{[2]} = 0.081, \quad p_{[3]} = 0.087, \quad p_{[4]} = 0.71, \quad p_{[5]} = 0.97.$$

For the Simes procedure, $f_{[k]} = k/K$ and the adjusted p-values are

$$p_{[1]}^{\text{adj}} = 0.0045, \quad p_{[2]}^{\text{adj}} = 0.20, \quad p_{[3]}^{\text{adj}} = 0.14, \quad p_{[4]}^{\text{adj}} = 0.89, \quad p_{[5]}^{\text{adj}} = 0.97.$$

This is a bit odd because the adjusted p-values do not reflect the original ordering. An alternative computation corrects this problem. Starting with the largest unadjusted p-value,

$$p_{[K]}^{\text{adj}} = p_{[K]}/f_{[K]}, \tag{11.9}$$

$$p_{[k]}^{\text{adj}} = \min\left(p_{[k]}/f_{[k]}, p_{[k+1]}^{\text{adj}}\right), \quad k = K-1, \ldots, 1. \tag{11.10}$$

In the example, this affects only the second p-value, $p_{[2]}$. The adjusted p-values are

$$p_{[1]}^{\text{adj}} = 0.0045, \quad p_{[2]}^{\text{adj}} = 0.14, \quad p_{[3]}^{\text{adj}} = 0.14, \quad p_{[4]}^{\text{adj}} = 0.89, \quad p_{[5]}^{\text{adj}} = 0.97.$$

11.5 Resampling techniques

The major limitation of all of the previously described global tests is that they were developed to control the Type I error rate under the most conservative condition, K independent tests. However, in most studies of HRQoL, the K endpoints are moderately correlated. As a result, these procedures are very conservative and the power to detect meaningful differences is severely reduced. Application of the *resampling technique* has been proposed as a method to address this problem. The general idea is to obtain an estimate of the distribution of the cut-off test statistics (T_{COT}) for the multiple comparison procedure for endpoints with an unknown correlation structure. A *bootstrap procedure* was first proposed by Westfall and Young [161] for test statistics from binomial distributions and adapted by Reitmeir and Wasser [123] for multiple comparisons of K endpoints between two treatment groups. The procedure is as follows:

1. Identify the statistic for the global test (T_{COT} or p_{COT}) and calculate it from the observed data (Table 11.6).

2. Draw a random sample of subjects with replacement (bootstrap sample) from the pooled sample of the same size as the original sample.

3. Recompute the statistic from the data associated with the subjects drawn in the bootstrap sample, p_{COT}^b.

4. Repeat the previous two steps B times. $B = 10{,}000$ is recommended [123].

Since the bootstrap statistics were calculated under the null hypothesis by generating the bootstrap samples from the pooled sample, the distribution of the test statistic is approximated by the distribution of the p_{COT}^b. The p-value for the global test is the proportion of the B bootstrap statistics that are equal to or more extreme than the observed data statistic ($p_{\text{COT}}^b \leq p_{\text{COT}}$ or $T_{\text{COT}}^b \geq T_{\text{COT}}$). If this proportion is less than α, the global test is rejected.

Table 11.6. Examples of test statistics for resampling procedure.

Technique	Test statistic	
	T_{COT}	p_{COT}
Bonferroni	$T_{[1]}$	$p_{[1]}$
Rüger	$T_{[K']} \times K'$	$p_{[K']} \times K'$
Simes/Hommel	$\max(T_{[k]}/k)$	$\min(p_{[k]}/k)$

11.6 Summary

- Multiple comparisons create a major analytic problem in clinical trials with HRQoL assessments.
- Summary measures and statistics combining information across time are extremely useful for simplifying interpretation, increasing the power to detect differences in the same direction, and reducing the number of comparisons.
- Multiple comparison procedures are most useful for measures of the multiple domains of HRQoL, especially when there is a concern about obscuring effects of components that move in opposite directions with the use of summary measures.
- Combining summary measures or statistics (which tends to increase power) with multiple comparison procedures (which reduce power) is a practical strategy.
- A multiple comparison procedure based on K univariate tests is likely to be easier to report than one based on multivariate tests.
- Selection among the various univariate procedures depends on the research objectives. The Bonferroni procedure will identify a single strong difference, the Rüger procedure will identify a prespecified number of K' moderate effects, and the Simes and Hommel procedures are a compromise.
- Strict control of the α-level for independent endpoints is overly conservative for correlated HRQoL measures and more relaxed procedures are preferable (e.g., Simes is better than Hommel procedure).
- Resampling techniques are especially useful for studies where power is likely to be an issue.

CHAPTER 12

Design: Analysis Plans

12.1 Introduction

The analysis plan is an essential part of any randomized clinical trial. Most statisticians have considerable experience with writing adequate analysis plans for studies that have one or two univariate endpoints. For example, clinical trials of treatments for cancer have a primary and one to two secondary endpoints, which are either the time-to-an-event (e.g., disease progression or death) or a binary outcome such as a complete or partial response (measured as the change in tumor size). The analysis of these univariate outcomes is straightforward.

When multiple measures are assessed repeatedly, the choices for analysis are much more complex. This is true whether the outcome is HRQoL or another set of longitudinal measures. For example, an analgesic trial might include longitudinal patient ratings of the average and worst pain as well as use of additional medication for uncontrolled episodes of pain. Unfortunately, HRQoL is often designated as a secondary endpoint and the development of an analysis is postponed until after the trial begins. Because the analyses are more complex and may require auxiliary information to be gathered, more attention is required during protocol development to ensure an analysis that will answer the research objectives.

At the point that a detailed analysis plan is written, it will become very clear whether the investigators have a clear view of their research objectives. Choices for strategies of handling multiple comparisons will require clarity about the exact role of the HRQoL data. Will it be used in any decision process about the intervention or will it play only an explanatory or supportive role? The choice to use a specific summary measure or to perform tests at each follow-up will require clarity about whether the intent is to explore the patterns of differences over time or to identify a general benefit. The choice of analysis methods and strategies for handling missing data will require clarity about the population of inference. For example, are the conclusions intended for all those started on the intervention (intent-to-treat) or conditional on some criteria (e.g., survival, only while on therapy, etc.).

This chapter focuses on selected issues that are critical to the development of a detailed analysis plan for the HRQoL component of a clinical trial (Table 12.1). Even when it is a policy not to include details of the analysis of secondary endpoints in the protocol, these details should be established before the protocol is finalized. Failure to do so may result in the omission of critical information from the data collection or the ability to make a definitive inference from the data.

Table 12.1. Checklist for statistical analysis plan.

Endpoints
- Definitive research objectives and specific *a priori* hypotheses.
- Superiority vs. equivalence.
- Define primary and secondary endpoints; summary measures.

Scoring of HRQoL instruments
- Specify method (or reference if it contains specific instructions).
- State how missing responses to individual items are handled.

Primary analysis
- Power or sample size requirements.
- Procedures for handling multiplicity of HRQoL measurements:
  - What summary measures are proposed?
  - Adjustment procedures for multiple comparisons.
- What statistical procedure is used to model the repeated measures/ longitudinal data?
- What assumptions are made about the missing data? What are the expected rates of missing data and how do they affect the analysis?

Sensitivity analysis
- What is the plan for sensitivity analyses?
- What models were considered and why were the particular models selected?
- Is the description specific enough for another analyst to implement the analysis?

Secondary analysis
- If some scales are excluded from the primary analysis, what exactly will be reported for these scales?
- What is the justification for including these assessments if they are not part of the primary analysis?
- What exploratory analyses are planned (e.g., psychometric characteristics of HRQoL instrument, relationship between clinical outcomes and HRQoL measures, treatment effects in specific subgroups)?

12.2 General analysis plan—Who is included?

If the data analysis is limited to any subset of the randomized patients, this must be described explicitly and justified by the objectives. One example is the omission of a small proportion of subjects because appropriate translations are not available. At the other extreme is limiting the analysis to those who complete treatment or to survivors. A cautionary note is important at this point. The more the subset of patients included in the analysis deviates from the randomized population, the greater the potential for selection bias. Differences between the two populations may be attributable to selection rather than the effects of treatment. Some exclusions, such as failure to start

12.3 Models for longitudinal data

Missing HRQoL assessments are generally not random. This may introduce bias that cannot be controlled with statistical methods [45] or through imputation [121]. As indicated by the number of chapters in this book, handling missing data is a challenge and requires careful planning. Appropriate strategies will depend on the objectives and the nature and extent of the missing data. No single approach is useful in all settings [6].

Ignorable missing data

With minimal missing data or the expectation that the data will be predominately MAR or MCAR, the recommendation is to use a likelihood-based method that uses all available data (see Chapters 3 and 5). Depending on the design of the study, the proposal can be to use either a repeated measures model (Section 3.3) or a growth curve model (Section 3.4). Even when there is a concern that the data may be MNAR, these models may be proposed for (1) initial analysis to be followed by sensitivity analyses, (2) a means for identifying feasible models for the covariance structure, and (3) generating initial estimates required for other models.

Nonignorable missing data

When there is any suspicion that the missing data will be related to events or outcomes that will affect HRQoL, a strategy for checking the sensitivity of the results should be included in the analysis plan. Because, as we noted in Chapter 9, it is possible a particular model may suggest ignorable missing data when others contradict that finding, the analyst should consider at least two candidate models for the proposed sensitivity analysis.

Event-driven designs and repeated measures models

When the design is event driven or a repeated measures models is appropriate because there will be a limited number of assessments, the following possibilities exist among the methods described in this book. For the simplest design with only two assessments (pre/post) and with missing data limited to follow-up, the sensitivity analysis that includes the CCMV restriction and Brown's protective estimate is a feasible strategy (see Section 8.2). When the analyst has good auxiliary information about the subject's cause of dropout and status after dropout, multiple imputation using MCMC or sequential univariate regression is a possible approach. In the absence of any auxiliary information or as a second strategy in a sensitivity analysis, a pattern mixture model with the NCMV restrictions is a possibility (see Section 8.3). Finally, if the pattern of dropout is monotone, the observations are equally spaced*, and dropout occurs after two or more assessments, the analyst could consider the selection model proposed by Diggle and Kenward (see Section 9.4).

Time-driven designs and growth curve models

A similar logic applies to time-driven designs with growth curve models. Two of the methods proposed in the book rely on the presence of variation in the slopes among subjects. When the change over time is expected to be linear, the conditional linear model is feasible (see Section 9.2). The joint mixed effects model can also be considered when the change over time is linear or has a more complex form (see Section 9.3). The joint model also allows the time to dropout (or other related event) to be censored. If there is no variation of the slopes among the subjects, a pattern mixture model with parametric restrictions is possible (see Section 8.4). The term *pattern mixture model* refers to a large class of models, and it is necessary to specify in the analysis plan what restrictions will be used to overcome the problem of underidentification.

Modification of analysis plan

Most of the analytic methods for nonignorable missing data are dependent on the characteristics of the data. For example, neither the conditional linear model nor the joint mixed-effects/dropout model (Chapter 9) is feasible if there is no random variation in the slopes among subjects. Thus, final decisions about the analytic methods may require preliminary looks at blinded data. Initial analysis plans should consider possible options, followed by an updated plan based on preliminary analyses of blinded data.

12.4 Multiplicity of endpoints

The choice of strategies for handling the multiplicity of endpoints will depend on a number of issues; the most important issues are the intent and objectives of the study.

Primary vs. secondary endpoints

At this point the role of the HRQoL assessments in the clinical trial must be clarified. The intent of the trial could be as strong as demonstrating the efficacy of a drug solely on the basis of HRQoL for the purposes of product registration, advertising claims, or changing practice. At the other extreme, the intent may be solely exploratory with no decisions or claims to be made on the basis of the HRQoL assessments. Most likely, the role of HRQoL will be

---

* May be unequally spaced if the dependence of dropout on previous observations is not a function of the time between measurements.

somewhere between the two extremes. For example, when there are no effective therapies for a life-threatening condition, a decision to declare a drug *effective* might be made solely on the basis of clinical measures. Tumor response (measurable shrinkage of a tumor) and the time to disease progression are typical measures of response for cancer treatments. On the other hand, a decision to declare a drug *beneficial* might be made on the basis of either survival or improvements in a global measure of HRQoL.

If the intent is to make a decision about the efficacy or benefits of the intervention based on the dimensions of HRQoL and other primary endpoints, then HRQoL is taking on the role of a primary endpoint (regardless of the language used in the protocol). This implies a need for an explicit strategy for handling or reducing multiple comparisons. Note that an explicit strategy does not always mean the use of a formal procedure to control the experimentwise error rate simultaneously for all endpoints but may include other options, such as the use of summary measures or controlling error rates within clusters of related endpoints [119]. When the HRQoL assessments are considered supportive of primary endpoints, then HRQoL is taking the role of a secondary endpoint. As secondary endpoints, less stringent criteria are required for controlling error rates. It is still wise to consider options to reduce the multiplicity of endpoints as a means to improve interpretability of the results.

The intent with respect to the multiple dimensions of HRQoL needs to be clarified. Is the intent to claim a generic HRQoL benefit or only benefits in certain dimensions? If generic, what are the criteria that will establish that inference?

Summary measures

As a first step, identify summary measures consistent with the objectives that will reduce multiplicity of data over time. As discussed in detail in Chapter 10, the choice will be determined by the expected pattern of change over time and the period of the study where differences are clinically relevant. Well-chosen summary measures or statistics often have greater power to detect patterns of consistent HRQoL differences across time or measures. This is a particular advantage in smaller studies, where the power to detect meaningful differences is limited.

Multiple comparison procedures

The next step is to consider strategies for controlling the Type I error rate. Consider several scenarios for drugs to treat a fatal disease. In the first scenario, there are no effective drugs. Thus, either extending the duration of survival or the quality of life during survival could be considered a benefit. If this is the first in a series of trials and the decision is only whether to continue development of the drug, then no multiple comparison procedures are mandatory. However, if the intent is to ask for approval of the drug if either survival or HRQoL is improved, then an explicit procedure is necessary.

There are still numerous options. One is based on the argument that because there are no effective drugs, the analyses of survival and HRQoL should each be performed at $\alpha = 0.05$, with multiple comparison procedures for the K HRQoL measures. At worst, the experimentwise error rate is no more than 10%. In a second scenario, there exist current therapies that delay the progression of the disease but do not result in a cure. If the intent was to request approval if either survival or HRQoL was improved, an option is to split the alpha between survival (α_1) and HRQoL (α_2). However, if the intent is to ask for approval only if the drug shows a survival benefit and then examine HRQoL for other reasons, then the analyses of survival and HRQoL would each be performed at $\alpha = 0.05$. If possible, adopt the same procedure used for all other clinical endpoints.

12.5 Sample size and power

Although repeated measures and growth curve models are often used for the analysis of longitudinal studies, it is rare to see sample size calculations for clinical trials that correspond to these analyses. One of the most common approaches is to pick a single point in time (often the last), calculate the sample size for the expected difference in the group means, and inflate that sample size for dropout. Basically, this calculation provides the sample size for a repeated univariate analysis. In most cases, this will provide a conservative (larger than necessary) estimate of the sample size. In this section, a procedure is described for the estimation of the sample size when the analysis is based on MLE of a repeated measures or growth curve model with missing data.

Simple linear combinations of β

First, consider the case where the hypothesis of interest is a univariate test of a linear combination of the parameters:

$$H_0: \theta = C\beta = 0 \quad \text{vs.} \quad H_A: \theta = \delta_\theta,$$

where C is a known $1 \times p$ vector and δ_θ is the value of θ under the alternative hypothesis. The hypothesis can be as simple as: the means at a specific time point are equal across treatment groups. For example, using the cell means model notation, the comparison of the means at the time of the fourth assessment is $H_0: \theta = \mu_{B4} - \mu_{A4} = 0$. When the endpoint is a summary measure, the hypothesis is a linear function of all the parameters.

To illustrate, assume the design for the study includes two groups (A and B) with four repeated measurements of HRQoL: baseline and three follow-ups. We wish to have adequate power to detect differences between the two groups when the true differences are 0.4, 0.5, and 0.6 times the standard deviation at 6, 12, and 26 weeks, respectively. Thus, $\mu_{B1} - \mu_{A1} = 0.0\sigma$, $\mu_{B2} - \mu_{A2} = 0.4\sigma$, $\mu_{B3} - \mu_{A3} = 0.5\sigma$, and $\mu_{B4} - \mu_{A4} = 0.6\sigma$. If the summary measure is the difference between the baseline assessment and the average of the three follow-up assessments, the null hypothesis is

$$\left(\frac{\mu_{B2} + \mu_{B3} + \mu_{B4}}{3} - \mu_{B1}\right) = \left(\frac{\mu_{A2} + \mu_{A3} + \mu_{A4}}{3} - \mu_{A1}\right). \quad (12.1)$$

If the endpoint is the area under the HRQoL vs. time curve (AUC), using a trapezoidal approximation, the null hypothesis is

$$\frac{\mu_{B1} + \mu_{B2}}{2}(6-0) + \frac{\mu_{B2} + \mu_{B3}}{2}(12-6) + \frac{\mu_{B3} + \mu_{B4}}{2}(26-12)$$
$$= \frac{\mu_{A1} + \mu_{A2}}{2}(6-0) + \frac{\mu_{A2} + \mu_{A3}}{2}(12-6) + \frac{\mu_{A3} + \mu_{A4}}{2}(26-12)$$

or

$$3\mu_{B1} + 6\mu_{B2} + 10\mu_{B3} + 7\mu_{B4} = 3\mu_{A1} + 6\mu_{A2} + 10\mu_{A3} + 7\mu_{A4}. \quad (12.2)$$

Secondary endpoints might include the change from baseline to each follow-up assessment:

$$(\mu_{B2} - \mu_{B1}) = (\mu_{A2} - \mu_{A1}), \quad (12.3)$$
$$(\mu_{B3} - \mu_{B1}) = (\mu_{A3} - \mu_{A1}), \quad (12.4)$$
$$(\mu_{B4} - \mu_{B1}) = (\mu_{A4} - \mu_{A1}). \quad (12.5)$$

Rearranging Equations 12.1 through 12.5 in the form $\theta = C\beta$ yields

$$\theta_1 = \left(\frac{\mu_{B2} + \mu_{B3} + \mu_{B4}}{3} - \mu_{B1}\right) - \left(\frac{\mu_{A2} + \mu_{A3} + \mu_{A4}}{3} - \mu_{A1}\right), \quad (12.6)$$
$$\theta_2 = (3\mu_{B1} + 6\mu_{B2} + 10\mu_{B3} + 7\mu_{B4}) - (3\mu_{A1} + 6\mu_{A2} + 10\mu_{A3} + 7\mu_{A4}), \quad (12.7)$$
$$\theta_3 = (\mu_{B2} - \mu_{B1}) - (\mu_{A2} - \mu_{A1}), \quad (12.8)$$
$$\theta_4 = (\mu_{B3} - \mu_{B1}) - (\mu_{A3} - \mu_{A1}), \quad (12.9)$$
$$\theta_5 = (\mu_{B4} - \mu_{B1}) - (\mu_{A4} - \mu_{A1}). \quad (12.10)$$

Under the alternative hypothesis, $\mu_{B1} - \mu_{A1} = 0.0\sigma$, $\mu_{B2} - \mu_{A2} = 0.4\sigma$, $\mu_{B3} - \mu_{A3} = 0.5\sigma$, and $\mu_{B4} - \mu_{A4} = 0.6\sigma$. Thus,

$$\delta_1 = -(\mu_{B1} - \mu_{A1}) + \frac{\mu_{B2} - \mu_{A2}}{3} + \frac{\mu_{B3} - \mu_{A3}}{3} + \frac{\mu_{B3} - \mu_{A3}}{3}$$
$$= -0\sigma + 0.4\sigma/3 + 0.5\sigma/3 + 0.6\sigma/3 = 0.5\sigma, \quad (12.11)$$
$$\delta_2 = 3(\mu_{B1} - \mu_{A1}) + 6(\mu_{B2} - \mu_{A2}) + 10(\mu_{B3} - \mu_{A3}) + 7(\mu_{B4} - \mu_{A4})$$
$$= 3(0\sigma) + 6(0.4\sigma) + 10(0.5\sigma) + 7(0.6\sigma) = 10.5\sigma, \quad (12.12)$$
$$\delta_3 = -(\mu_{B1} - \mu_{A1}) + (\mu_{B2} - \mu_{A2}) = -0 + 0.4\sigma = 0.4\sigma, \quad (12.13)$$
$$\delta_4 = -(\mu_{B1} - \mu_{A1}) + (\mu_{B3} - \mu_{A3}) = -0 + 0.5\sigma = 0.5\sigma, \quad (12.14)$$
$$\delta_5 = -(\mu_{B1} - \mu_{A1}) + (\mu_{B4} - \mu_{A4}) = -0 + 0.6\sigma = 0.6\sigma. \quad (12.15)$$

Basic assumptions

The following procedure is based on asymptotic approximations of the covariance of the estimated parameters. It is applicable to any linear model, $E[Y_i] = X_i\beta + \epsilon_i$, where the data are approximately multivariate normal ($Y_i \sim N(X_i\beta, \Sigma_i)$) and the proposed analysis is maximum likelihood estimation. There is an implied assumption that missing data will be MAR and *ignorable* for the specified model.

If the sample size is sufficiently large, then the distribution of the test statistic $z_\theta = \theta/\sqrt{\sigma_\theta^2/N}$ is well approximated by a univariate standard normal distribution, where $\sqrt{\sigma_\theta^2/N}$ is the standard error of θ and σ_θ^2 is N times the variance of the estimate of θ. That is, $\sigma_\theta = N \operatorname{Var}(\hat{\theta})$.

The general form of the sample size approximation for a two-sided test is

$$N = (z_{\alpha/2} + z_\beta)^2 \frac{\sigma_\theta^2}{\delta_\theta^2}. \qquad (12.16)$$

For any hypothesis of the form $\theta = C\beta$, we can estimate the required sample size if we can determine σ_θ^2 and δ_θ^2.

Equation 12.16 should appear familiar, as there are two well-known univariate sample size formulas that are special cases of this general formula. In the first case, a test of the equality of means from two independent samples of the same size with equal variance corresponds to $N = n_A + n_B$, $\delta_\theta = \mu_A - \mu_B$, $\sigma_\theta^2 = N \times \operatorname{Var}(\mu_A - \mu_B) = N \times 2\sigma_Y^2/n = 4\sigma_Y^2$. Thus, the total sample size is

$$N = (z_{\alpha/2} + z_\beta)^2 \frac{\sigma_\theta^2}{\delta_\theta^2} = (z_{\alpha/2} + z_\beta)^2 \frac{4\sigma_Y^2}{(\mu_A - \mu_B)^2} \qquad (12.17)$$

or the more familiar formula for the number required in each group

$$n = (z_{\alpha/2} + z_\beta)^2 2\sigma_Y^2/(\mu_A - \mu_B)^2.$$

The second special case is the test of equality of means in a paired sample: $N = n$, $\delta_\theta = \mu_A - \mu_B$, $\sigma_\theta^2 = N \times \operatorname{Var}(\mu_A - \mu_B) = N \times 2\sigma_Y^2(1-\rho)/N = 2\sigma_Y^2(1-\rho)$. Thus, the number of pairs is

$$N = (z_{\alpha/2} + z_\beta)^2 \frac{\sigma_\theta^2}{\delta_\theta^2} = (z_{\alpha/2} + z_\beta)^2 \frac{2\sigma_Y^2(1-\rho)}{(\mu_A - \mu_B)^2}. \qquad (12.18)$$

Incomplete designs

We assume that we can reasonably estimate the timing of the assessments (and thus the design matrix for each individual, X_i) and the proportion of individuals who drop out of the study at each assessment, such that there are K patterns of observations,

SAMPLE SIZE AND POWER

Table 12.2. Proportions in each pattern with equal allocation.

Pattern	Group	T1	T2	T3	T4	p_k
1	A	X	X	X	X	0.32
2	A	X	X	X		0.10
3	A	X	X			0.05
4	A	X				0.025
5	A					0.005
6	B	X	X	X	X	0.32
7	B	X	X	X		0.10
8	B	X	X			0.05
9	B	X				0.025
10	B					0.005

X indicates an observed assessment of HRQoL. p_k is the proportion of the total sample with the indicated pattern.

where

n_k = the number of subjects with the design matrix, X_k, for the kth pattern

p_k = the proportion of subjects, $p_k = n_k/N$, with the kth pattern of assessments ($\sum^K p_k = 1$)

Let us assume that dropout is equal in the two groups and that all missing data are due to dropout. The rate of dropout is 1, 5, 10, and 20% at each of the four assessments (T1 to T4). Thus, 64% will complete all assessments. If subjects are equally allocated to both groups, the pattern of observations will appear as displayed in Table 12.2.

In our example, the design matrix (cell means model) for the subjects in group A with all four observations is

$$X_k = \begin{bmatrix} 1 & 0 & 0 & 0 & 0 & 0 & 0 & 0 \\ 0 & 1 & 0 & 0 & 0 & 0 & 0 & 0 \\ 0 & 0 & 1 & 0 & 0 & 0 & 0 & 0 \\ 0 & 0 & 0 & 1 & 0 & 0 & 0 & 0 \end{bmatrix}, \quad p_k = 0.32.$$

The design matrix for the subjects in group A with only the first two observations is

$$X_k = \begin{bmatrix} 1 & 0 & 0 & 0 & 0 & 0 & 0 & 0 \\ 0 & 1 & 0 & 0 & 0 & 0 & 0 & 0 \end{bmatrix}, \quad p_k = 0.05.$$

Finally, it is assumed that the total number of subjects is large and $[\sum_i^N X_i' \hat{\Sigma}_i^{-1} X_i]^{-1}$ is a valid approximation of the covariance of the parameter estimates ($\hat{\beta}$). This variance can be expressed as a function of the total number of subjects, N:

$$\text{Var}[\hat{\beta}] = \left[\sum_{i=1}^{N} X_i' \hat{\Sigma}_i^{-1} X_i\right]^{-1} = \left[\sum_{k=1}^{K} n_k X_k' \hat{\Sigma}_k^{-1} X_k\right]^{-1}$$

$$= \frac{1}{N}\left[\sum_{k=1}^{K} p_k X_k' \hat{\Sigma}_k^{-1} X_k\right]^{-1}. \quad (12.19)$$

The variance of θ is $C \text{ Var}(\hat{\beta})C'$ and

$$\sigma_\theta^2 = N \text{ Var}(\hat{\theta}) = NC \text{ Var}(\hat{\beta})C' = C\left[\sum_{k=1}^{K} p_k X_k' \hat{\Sigma}_k^{-1} X_k\right]^{-1} C'. \quad (12.20)$$

For incomplete designs, the sample size approximation can be written as

$$N = (z_{\alpha/2} + z_\beta)^2 C \left[\sum_{k=1}^{K} p_k X_k' \hat{\Sigma}_k^{-1} X_k\right]^{-1} C'/\delta_\theta^2. \quad (12.21)$$

Example 1: Repeated measures

To use Equation 12.21, we need to define the following: $z_{\alpha/2}$, z_β, p_k, X_k, Σ_k, C, and δ_θ. The first two are familiar critical values associated with the Type I and Type II error rates. For a two-sided test with $\alpha = 0.05$ and 90% power, $z_{\alpha/2} = -1.96$ and $z_\beta = -1.282$.

To determine the remaining parameters, we need to define the dropout pattern, design, covariance of the observations, null hypothesis, and minimum difference of interest under the alternative hypothesis. The dropout pattern was defined above. Let the design be defined as a cell means model: $\beta = [\mu_{A1}, \mu_{A2}, \ldots, \mu_{B4}]'$. For a subject in group A with all four assessments,

$$X_k = \begin{bmatrix} 1 & 0 & 0 & 0 & 0 & 0 & 0 & 0 \\ 0 & 1 & 0 & 0 & 0 & 0 & 0 & 0 \\ 0 & 0 & 1 & 0 & 0 & 0 & 0 & 0 \\ 0 & 0 & 0 & 1 & 0 & 0 & 0 & 0 \end{bmatrix}.$$

For a subject in group B with only the first two assessments,

$$X_k = \begin{bmatrix} 0 & 0 & 0 & 0 & 1 & 0 & 0 & 0 \\ 0 & 0 & 0 & 0 & 0 & 1 & 0 & 0 \end{bmatrix}.$$

Based on the previously stated assumptions, we would expect to see 32 and 5% of the sample with these designs, respectively.

If we have good estimates of the variance of the HRQoL measure over time, we can use them. However, in their absence we will have to assume some covariance structure for the repeated measures. Suppose the variance is constant over time and $\rho = 0.5$. Then, $\Sigma_i = \sigma_Y^2 [(1-\rho)\mathbf{I}_{n_i} + \rho \mathbf{J}_{n_i}]$, where $\mathbf{I}_{n_i}$ is an $n_i \times n_i$ identity matrix and $\mathbf{J}_{n_i}$ is an $n_i \times n_i$ matrix of 1s. If we wish to examine the difference between the baseline assessment and the average of the three follow-up assessments, Equation 12.6 gives $C_1 = [-3\ 1\ 1\ 1\ 3\ -1\ -1\ -1]/3$ and Equation 12.11 gives $\delta_1 = 0.05$.

The SAS program for the estimation of σ_θ^2 for repeated measures design (Example 1) appears as follows:

```
DATA WORK.WORK1;
  INPUT M GROUP TIME p_k Y @@;
  CARDS;
1 1 1 .32   .0   1 1 2 .32   .0   1 1 3 .32   .0   1 1 4 .32   .0
2 1 1 .1    .0   2 1 2 .1    .0   2 1 3 .1    .0
3 1 1 .05   .0   3 1 2 .05   .0
4 1 1 .025  .0
6 2 1 .32   .0   6 2 2 .32   .4   6 2 3 .32   .5   6 2 4 .32   .6
7 2 1 .1    .0   7 2 2 .1    .4   7 2 3 .1    .5
8 2 1 .05   .0   8 2 2 .05   .4
9 2 1 .025  .0
RUN;

PROC MIXED DATA=WORK.WORK1 MAXITER=1 METHOD=ML;
  CLASS M GROUP TIME;
  WEIGHT P_K;
  MODEL Y=GROUP*TIME/NOINT COVB;
  REPEATED TIME/SUBJECT=M TYPE=UN;
  PARMS (1)
        (.5) (1)
        (.5) (.5) (1)
        (.5) (.5) (.5) (1)/NOITER;
  ESTIMATE 'THETA' GROUP*TIME -3 1 1 1  3 -1 -1 -1/DIVISOR=3 E;
RUN;
```

Note that in the generated data set, all four assessments appear only for patterns 1 and 6. The fourth assessment is omitted in patterns 2 and 7, the third and fourth assessments are missing in patterns 3 and 8, all but the initial assessment are missing in patterns 4 and 9, and patterns 5 and 10 are omitted completely.

In theory, the calculations in Equation 12.21 could be performed by hand. However, the inversion of the matrix required for the calculation of σ_θ^2 is very time consuming. The calculations can also be performed using programs that facilitate matrix algebra (e.g., SAS Proc IML). However, the calculation of σ_θ^2 can be performed using analysis software (e.g., SAS Proc Mixed), by limiting the software to one iteration and providing starting values for the covariance parameters. First, a data set is created with one subject for each of the M patterns of observations. The design matrix (X_k) is defined as intended in the analysis, in this case by GROUP and TIME. Weights are equal to the proportion of subjects in the group (p_k). Note that there are two groups of subjects with no assessments that are not included and the total proportion is only 0.99. The outcome $(\mathbf{Y_k})$ can be any numeric value; however, if the values of the alternative hypothesis are used, this procedure will also calculate δ_θ. The MIXED procedure is run with only a single iteration (MAXITER=1 in MODEL statement) and (NOITER in PARMS statement) with the covariance specified (PARMS statement) and fixed (NOITER option).

Note that in the above example, Y and Σ are scaled so that the variance of Y_{ijk} is standard normal ($N(0,1)$) and PARMS specifies the correlation of Y. It is not necessary to convert everything to a standard normal distribution; it is critical that one consistently use either the unstandardized or standardized values of Y (*delta*) and Σ.

Selected SAS output from PROC MIXED for Example 1 appears as follows:

```
Covariance Matrix for Fixed Effects
Effect       GROUP TIME COL1  COL2  COL3  COL4  COL5  COL6  COL7  COL8
GROUP*TIME   1     1    2.02  1.01  1.01  1.01  0.00  0.00  0.00  0.00
GROUP*TIME   1     2    1.01  2.10  1.03  1.03  0.00  0.00  0.00  0.00
GROUP*TIME   1     3    1.01  1.03  2.26  1.07  0.00  0.00  0.00  0.00
GROUP*TIME   1     4    1.01  1.03  1.07  2.73  0.00  0.00  0.00  0.00
GROUP*TIME   2     1    0.00  0.00  0.00  0.00  2.02  1.01  1.01  1.01
GROUP*TIME   2     2    0.00  0.00  0.00  0.00  1.01  2.10  1.03  1.03
GROUP*TIME   2     3    0.00  0.00  0.00  0.00  1.01  1.03  2.26  1.07
GROUP*TIME   2     4    0.00  0.00  0.00  0.00  1.01  1.03  1.07  2.73
ESTIMATE Statement Results
Parameter        Estimate      Std Error
Theta            -0.50000      1.72635534
```

The matrix displayed in the SAS output as the Covariance Matrix for Fixed Effects is $N\operatorname{Var}(\hat{\beta}) = [\sum_{k=1}^{K} p_k X_k' \hat{\Sigma}_k^{-1} X_k]^{-1}$. When the outcome ($Y$) is specified as the expected values under the alternative hypothesis, the ESTIMATE Statement Results contains $\delta_\theta = -0.500$ as the Estimate. The square root of σ_θ^2 is displayed as the Std Error: $\sqrt{\sigma_\theta^2} = 1.726$. We can use these values in the calculation of the sample size N. For a two-sided test with a Type I error of 5% and 90% power, the total required sample is 126 (or 63 subjects per arm):

$$N = (z_{1-\alpha/2} + z_\beta)^2 \frac{\sigma_\theta^2}{\delta_\theta^2} = (1.96 + 1.282)^2 (1.726)^2/(0.5)^2 = 125.3.$$

Example 2: Growth curve model

Consider the same two-group design where the four assessments are assumed to occur at 0, 6, 12, and 26 weeks. The dropout rates are the same. Instead of using a repeated measures design, we plan to use a piecewise linear growth curve model. The model is defined with four parameters per group: β_1 is the intercept, β_2 is the slope for the first 6 weeks, β_3 is the change in the slope after 6 weeks, and β_4 is the change in the slope after 12 weeks. For a subject in group A with all four assessments,

$$X_i = \begin{bmatrix} 1 & 0 & 0 & 0 & 0 & 0 & 0 & 0 \\ 1 & 6 & 0 & 0 & 0 & 0 & 0 & 0 \\ 1 & 12 & 6 & 0 & 0 & 0 & 0 & 0 \\ 1 & 26 & 20 & 14 & 0 & 0 & 0 & 0 \end{bmatrix}.$$

SAMPLE SIZE AND POWER

Let us consider the sample size required for several endpoints. The first three endpoints are the change from baseline to 6, 12, and 26 weeks (Equations 12.3 through 12.5). The fourth endpoint is the trapezoidal approximation of the area under the HRQoL vs. time curve (Equation 12.2). The final endpoint is the same as in the previous example: the averages of the estimates at 6, 12, and 26 weeks minus the baseline assessments. The null hypothesis is that there is no difference between the two groups.

The following SAS program is very similar to that used in Example 1; the major difference is the setup of the variables used to model change over time. We use the same method of defining the covariance structure, noting that the compound symmetry is identical to assuming a random intercept in a mixed-effects model. If there is sufficient information to estimate a more complex variance structure, such as two random effects, then Σ_i should be defined as if the subject would have assessments at 0, 6, 12, and 26 weeks.

```
DATA WORK.WORK1;
  INPUT M GROUP TIME WEIGHT Y @@;
  TIME00=TIME;
  TIME06=MAX(TIME-6,0);
  TIME12=MAX(TIME-12,0);
CARDS;
1 1 0 .32  .0   1 1 6 .32 .0   1 1 12 .32 .0   1 1 26 .32 .0
2 1 0 .10  .0   2 1 6 .1  .0   2 1 12 .1  .0
3 1 0 .05  .0   3 1 6 .05 .0
4 1 0 .025 .0
6 2 0 .32  .0   6 2 6 .32 .4   6 2 12 .32 .5   6 2 26 .32 .6
7 2 0 .10  .0   7 2 6 .10 .4   7 2 12 .10 .5
8 2 0 .05  .0   8 2 6 .05 .4
9 2 0 .025 .0
RUN;

PROC MIXED DATA=WORK.WORK1 MAXITER=1 METHOD=ML;
  CLASS M GROUP TIME;
  WEIGHT WEIGHT;
  MODEL Y=GROUP GROUP*TIME00 GROUP*TIME06 GROUP*TIME12/NOINT COVB;
  REPEATED TIME/SUBJECT=M TYPE=UN;
  PARMS (1)(.5)(1)(.5)(.5)(1)(.5)(.5)(.5)(1)/NOITER;
  ESTIMATE '6 WK'   GROUP*TIME00 6 -6/E;
  ESTIMATE '12 WK'  GROUP*TIME00 12 -12 GROUP*TIME06 6 -6/E;
  ESTIMATE '26 WK'  GROUP*TIME00 26 -26 GROUP*TIME06 20 -20
                    GROUP*TIME12 14 -14/E;
  ESTIMATE 'AUC/26' GROUP 26 -26 GROUP*TIME00 338 -338
                    GROUP*TIME06 200 -200 GROUP*TIME12 98 -98
                    /DIVISOR=26 E;
  ESTIMATE 'MEAN'   GROUP*TIME00 44 -44 GROUP*TIME06 26 -26
                    GROUP*TIME12 14 -14/DIVISOR=3 E;
  MAKE 'ESTIMATE' OUT=WORK.ESTIMATE;
  RUN;

DATA WORK.SSIZE;
  SET WORK.ESTIMATE;
```

```
N=((1.96+1.282)*SE/EST)**2;
RUN;
PROC PRINT DATA=WORK.SSIZE;
 ID PARM;
 VAR N EST SE;
RUN;
```

The results of the estimate statements are output to a data set and the total sample size (N) is calculated in a subsequent DATA Step. The output is displayed below. Note that the estimated sample size varies among the hypotheses.

PARM	N	EST	SE
6 wk	276.0	-0.40000000	2.04977813
12 wk	190.8	-0.50000000	2.13056662
26 wk	159.7	-0.60000000	2.33866920
AUC/26	149.5	-0.44615385	1.68248549
Mean	125.3	-0.50000000	1.72635534

Other considerations

Intermittent missing data patterns and time-varying covariates

In the previous two examples, we assumed that missing data occurred only as a result of dropout. We ignored the possibility of intermittent patterns of missing data. Another problem is that there may be considerable variation in the exact timing of the assessments. Both will have some impact on the power (and sample size estimates). If there is enough information to predict the expected patterns, it is possible to address these problems. One strategy is to consider all patterns of observed data. However, in most cases this is cumbersome. An alternative approach is to obtain an estimate of σ_θ^2 by randomly generating a large (e.g., $N_S = 10000$) number of subjects with their expected pattern of observation (X_i) and corresponding variance (Σ_i). Then estimate $\sigma_\theta^2 = N_S C [\sum^{N_S} X_i' \Sigma_i^{-1} X_i]^{-1} C'$. One can do this again using PROC MIXED (omitting the WEIGHT statement and modifying the SUBJECT= option). The value of SE in the output labeled ESTIMATE Statement Results of PROC MIXED is $\sigma_\theta^2 / \sqrt{N_S}$, so it is necessary to multiply this value by $\sqrt{N_S}$, where N_S is the number of observations used to simulate the pattern of observations.

If we extend Example 2, adding an additional 10% of missing data at each point in time due to reasons other than dropout, we obtain estimates of 2.18, 2.26, 2.47, 1.70, and 1.83 for σ_θ^2 for the five hypotheses and sample size estimates of 312, 214, 178, 153, and 141, respectively. This represents an inflation of 12 to 13% in the sample size requirements for all but the AUC.

Unequal allocations of subjects to treatment groups

Some clinical trial designs specify an unequal allocation of subjects to treatment arms. Because the sample size calculation is specified in terms of the

Table 12.3. Proportions in each pattern with unequal (2:1) allocation.

Pattern	Group	T1	T2	T3	T4	p_k
1	A	X	X	X	X	0.4267
2	A	X	X	X		0.1333
3	A	X	X			0.0667
4	A	X				0.0333
5	A					0.0067
6	B	X	X	X	X	0.2133
7	B	X	X	X		0.0667
8	B	X	X			0.0333
9	B	X				0.0167
10	B					0.0033

X indicates an observed assessment of HRQoL. p_k is the proportion of the total sample with the indicated pattern.

total sample size (N), this requires only an adjustment of the proportions within each pattern of observations (p_k). For example, if subjects were allocated in a 2:1 ratio to treatments A and B, then the pattern would appear as displayed in Table 12.3.

Multivariate tests

Sample size approximations can also be created for multivariate tests. For example, we might wish to test simultaneously for differences in the change from baseline in our example.

$$H_0: (\mu_{B2} - \mu_{B1}) - (\mu_{A2} - \mu_{A1}) = 0,$$
$$(\mu_{B3} - \mu_{B1}) - (\mu_{A3} - \mu_{A1}) = 0,$$
$$(\mu_{B4} - \mu_{B1}) - (\mu_{A4} - \mu_{A1}) = 0.$$

For large samples, one can generalize the univariate z-statistic to a multivariate χ^2-statistic. The null hypothesis is $H_0: \theta = C\beta = G$, where $C_{(\nu \times p)}$ and $G_{(\nu \times 1)}$ are known. The χ^2 test statistic is $\hat{\theta}'(\text{Var}(\theta))^{-1}\hat{\theta}$ and the power of the test is

$$Pr[\chi_\nu^2(\lambda) > \chi_{\nu,\alpha}^2] = 1 - \beta, \qquad (12.22)$$

where $\chi_{\nu,\alpha}^2$ is the critical value for a χ^2 distribution with ν degrees of freedom (α). λ is the noncentrality parameter, such that

$$\lambda = \theta'(\text{Var}(\theta))^{-1}\theta$$
$$= N\theta' \left(C \left[\sum_{k=1}^K p_k X_k' \hat{\Sigma}_k^{-1} X_k \right]^{-1} C' \right)^{-1} \theta, \qquad (12.23)$$

when $\theta = C\beta - G$ is calculated under the alternative hypothesis.

We can again use the output from our SAS program to simplify the calculations. First, we calculate the critical value. In our example, this is $\chi^2_{3,\alpha=0.05} = 7.815$.* Second, we calculate the noncentrality parameter (λ) from Equation 12.23. In our example, $\lambda = 14.17$.** Finally, we obtain the quantity $\theta'(C[\sum_{k=1}^{K} p_k X_k' \hat{\Sigma}_k^{-1} X_k]^{-1} C')^{-1} \theta$ by adding to the Proc MIXED statements.

```
CONTRAST 'Change from Baseline'
   GROUP*TIME00 6 -6,
   GROUP*TIME00 12 -12 GROUP*TIME06 6  -6,
   GROUP*TIME00 26 -26 GROUP*TIME06 20 -20 GROUP*TIME12 14 -14
   /CHISQ;
```

The estimate of the total sample size is $\lambda/\text{CHISQ} = 14.17/0.086 = 163.1$, where CHISQ is obtained from the Proc MIXED output.

Small sample size approximations

For previous sample size calculations, the approximations assume the sample size is sufficiently large that the asymptotic approximation of the covariance of the parameters is appropriate and the loss of degrees of freedom when using t- and F-statistics will not affect the results. When the sample sizes are small, the above procedures can be used to obtain the first estimate of the sample size. The estimation procedure is repeated, using the t- or F-distributions with updated estimates of the degrees of freedom (ν), until the procedure converges.

$$N = (t_{\nu,\alpha/2} + t_{\nu,\beta})^2 \frac{\sigma_\theta^2}{\delta_\theta^2}$$

$$= (t_{\alpha/2} + t_\beta)^2 C \left[\sum_{k=1}^{K} p_k X_k' \hat{\Sigma}_k^{-1} X_k\right]^{-1} C'/\delta_\theta^2. \quad (12.24)$$

Restricted maximum likelihood estimation

Kenward and Rogers [78] provide the details for modifying the estimated covariance of $\hat{\beta}$ for restricted maximum likelihood estimation (REML) and propose an F-distribution approximation for small sample inference.

12.6 Reporting results

All the standard guidelines for reporting clinical trials apply to the reporting of HRQoL studies. Because all readers are not as familiar with some of the issues associated with measurement of HRQoL as they are with other clinical endpoints, some additional guidelines are worth mentioning. Based on a systematic

---

* SAS: c_alpha=cinv(1-0.05,3).
** SAS: lambda=cnonct(c_alpha,3,1-0.9).

Table 12.4. Checklist for reporting requirements for HRQoL trials.

Introduction
- Rational for assessing HRQoL in the particular disease and treatment.
- State specific *a priori* (pretrial) hypotheses.

Methods
- Justification for selection of instruments assessing HRQoL (see Chapter 2). References to instrument and validation studies. Details of psychometric properties if a new instrument. Include copy of instrument in appendix if previously unpublished. Details of any modifications of the questions or formats.
- Details of cross-cultural validation if relevant and previously unpublished.
- Method of administration (self-report, face-to-face, etc.).
- Planned timing of the study assessments.
- Method of scoring, preferably by reference to a published article or scoring manual, with details of any deviations.
- Interpretation of scores. Do higher values indicate better outcomes?
- Methods of analysis. What analyses were specified *a priori* and which were exploratory?
- Which dimensions or items of the HRQoL instruments were selected as endpoints prior to subject accrual?
- What summary measures and multiple-comparison procedures were used? Were they specified *a priori*?

Results
- Timing of assessments and length of follow-up by treatment group.
- Missing data:
  - Proportions with missing data and relevant patterns.
  - How were patients who dropped out of the study handled?
  - How were patients who died handled?
- Results for all scales specified in protocol/analysis plan (negative as well as positive results).
- If general HRQoL benefit reported, summary of all dimensions.
- If no changes were observed, describe evidence of responsiveness to measures in related settings and the lack of floor and ceiling effects in current study.

review of 20 articles reporting HRQoL in cancer trials in 1997, Lee and Chi [85] identify the major deficiencies that should be addressed as (1) the failure to provide a rationale of HRQoL assessment and (2) inadequate description of methodology. In addition to the checklist included here (Table 12.4), the reader is encouraged to read other published guidelines [145].

12.7 Summary

- The analysis plan is driven by explicit research objectives.
- Analyses of HRQoL data are often more complex, because of the longitudinal and multidimensional nature, than the analyses of traditional univariate outcomes.
- The analysis plan should be developed prior to initiation of the study regardless of whether HRQoL is a primary or secondary endpoint.

APPENDIX I

Abbreviations

ABB	approximate Bayesian bootstrap
ACMV	available case missing value
AIC	Akaike's information criterion
ANOVA	analysis of variance
ARMA	autoregressive moving average
AUC	area under the curve
BCQ	Breast Chemotherapy Questionnaire
BIC	Bayesian information criterion
BLUE	best linear unbiased estimate
BLUP	best linear unbiased predictor
BRM	biologic response modifier
CAF	cyclophosphamide, doxirubicin, and 5-flurouracil
CCMV	complete case missing value
13-CRA	13-*cis*-retinoic acid
CRD	completely random dropout
EB	empirical Bayes
EBLUP	empirical best linear unbiased predictor
ECOG PS	Eastern Cooperative Oncology Group scale for performance status
EM	estimation—maximization
FACT-BRM	Functional assessment of cancer-biological response modifiers
FACT-G	Functional assessment of cancer—general questionnaire
FACT-Lung	Functional assessment of cancer—lung questionnaire
FU	follow-up
HRQoL	health-related quality of life
ID	informative dropout
IFNα	interferon alpha-2a
LVCF	last value carried forward
LOCF	last observation carried forward
MANOVA	multivariate analysis of variance
MAR	missing at random
MCAR	missing completely at random
MCMC	multiple chain Monte Carlo
MCS	mental component scale (SF-36)
MI	multiple imputation
ML	maximum likelihood
MLE	maximum likelihood estimation (estimate)

MNAR	missing not at random
NCMV	nearest case missing value
NSCLC	non-small-cell lung cancer
OLS	ordinary least squares
PCS	physical component scale (SF-36)
RD	random dropout
REML	restricted maximum likelihood estimation
S.D.	standard deviation
S.E.	standard error of the mean
SF-36	Medical Outcome Study Short Form–36
TOI	treatment outcome index

APPENDIX II

Notation

β	the vector of fixed-effects parameters
β_h	the vector of fixed-effects parameters for the hth group
β_i	$\beta + d_i$
$\beta^{\{p\}}$	the vector of fixed-effects parameters for subjects in the pth missing data pattern
$\mathcal{B}^*$	the vector of fixed-effects parameters from the imputation model ($Y_i^{*\mathrm{obs}} = X_i^{*\mathrm{obs}} \mathcal{B}^* + \varepsilon_i^*$)
$\hat{\mathcal{B}}^*$	the vector of estimates of the fixed-effects parameters from the imputation model
$\beta^{(m)}$	the vector of fixed-effects parameters used to impute the mth set of missing values
$\hat{\beta}^{(m)}$	the estimates of the fixed-effects parameters from the mth set of imputed data
d_i	the vector of random effects for the ith individual
$\mathcal{D}$	the covariance of the random effects, d_i; the elements of $\mathcal{D}$ are noted by ς_{rc}
ϵ_i	the vector of residual errors for a fixed-effects model ($\epsilon_i = Y_i - X_i \beta$)
$\mathbf{e}_i$	the vector of residual errors for a mixed-effects model ($\mathbf{e}_i = Y_i - X_i \beta - Z_i d_i$)
h	the indicator of the hth group (usually treatment)
i	the indicator of the ith independent unit of observations (usually patient or subject)
j	the indicator of the jth measurement on the ith subject
k	the indicator of the kth endpoint or HRQoL scale
$\mathbf{M}$	a generic term that is associated with the dropout process; may refer to the time of the event associated with dropout, $\mathcal{T}_i^{\mathcal{D}}$, the pattern of missing observations, R_i, or random effects, β_i or d_i
μ_{hj}	the mean of the hth group at the time of the jth observation.
$\pi^{\{p\}}$	the proportion of subjects in the pth missing data pattern
R_i	a vector of indicators of the missing data pattern for the ith individual, where $r_{ij} = 1$ if y_{ij} is observed and $r_{ij} = 0$ if y_{ij} is missing
$\mathcal{R}_i$	the covariance of $\mathbf{e}_i = Y_i - X_i\beta - Z_i d_i$ for mixed-effects models and $\epsilon_i = Y_i - X_i\beta$ for repeated measures models; in most mixed-effects models, the residual errors are uncorrelated, $\mathcal{R}_i = \sigma^2 \mathbf{I}$

Σ_i	the covariance of the *complete data* (Y_i), which is a known function of the vector of unknown variance parameters, τ: $\Sigma_i = f(\tau)$
σ_{rc}	the element in the rth row and cth column of $\mathcal{R}_i$
ς_{RC}	the element in the rth row and cth column of $\mathcal{D}_i$
t_{hij}	the time elapsed from the beginning of the trial until the observation of the Y_{hij} measure
t_{hij}^c	the value t_{hij} raised to the cth power
$t_{hij}^{[c]}$	the time elapsed from $T^{[c]}$ until the observation of the Y_{hij} measure; the brackets distinguish $t_{hij}^{[c]}$ from t_{hij}^c
$T_i^{\mathcal{D}}$	the time to an *event* associated with dropout, such as the time to the last HRQoL assessment; the time to discontinuation of treatment; or the time to death
$\Theta_{[A.B]}$	a vector of mean and variance parameters estimated from the regression of A on B
X_{hi}	the design matrix of fixed covariates corresponding to the *complete data* (Y_{hi}); the design matrix will include the time of measurement relative to the beginning of the study as well as indicators of treatment and other explanatory variables
X_i	the design matrix of fixed covariates corresponding to the *complete data* (Y_i), where the group indicator (h) has been dropped for simplification of notation
$X_i^{*\text{obs}}$	the design matrix corresponding to $Y_i^{*\text{obs}}$ included in the imputation model ($Y_i^{*\text{obs}} = X_i^{*\text{obs}} \mathcal{B}^* + \varepsilon_i^*$)
Y_{hi}	the *complete data* vector of planned observations of the outcome for the ith individual in the hth group, which includes both the observed data Y_{hi}^{obs} and missing Y_{hi}^{mis} observations of HRQoL
Y_i	the *complete data* vector of planned observations of the outcome for the ith individual (the indicator of group (h) has been dropped to simplify notation when it is not necessary for clarification)
Y_i^C	designates the *complete cases* as the set of responses from subjects who completed all possible assessments (e.g., $r_{ij} = 1$ for all possible y_{ij} from the ith subject)
Y_i^I	designates the *incomplete cases* as the set of responses from subjects who did *not* complete all possible assessments (e.g., $r_{ij} \neq 1$ for all possible observations on the ith subject)
Y_{hij}	the jth observation on the ith individual in the hth group
$Y_i^{*\text{obs}}$	the vector of observed data included in the imputation model ($Y_i^{*\text{obs}} = X_i^{*\text{obs}} \mathcal{B}^* + \varepsilon_i^*$)
$(\mathbf{Y}, \mathbf{R})$	the *complete data* of the joint distribution of $\mathbf{Y}$ and $\mathbf{R}$
$(\mathbf{Y}^{\text{obs}}, \mathbf{R})$	the *observed data* of the joint distribution of $\mathbf{Y}$ and $\mathbf{R}$

$f(\mathbf{R} \mid \mathbf{Y}, \mathbf{X}, \mathbf{\Psi})$	the distribution of $\mathbf{R}$ for a given set of outcomes ($\mathbf{Y}$) and covariates ($\mathbf{X}$)
$f(\mathbf{Y}, \mathbf{R} \mid \mathbf{\Theta}, \mathbf{\Psi})$	the joint density function for the complete data
$f(\mathbf{Y}^{\text{obs}}, \mathbf{R} \mid \mathbf{\Theta}, \mathbf{\Psi})$	the joint distribution of the observed data
Z_i	the design matrix corresponding to the random effects (d_i) on the ith individual
$z_\xi^{(m)}$	a vector of random numbers drawn from a standard normal distribution of the same dimension as ξ for the mth imputation

APPENDIX III

Formal Definitions for Missing Data

Let Y_i denote a vector of scores from a series of planned HRQoL assessments, some of which are observed, Y_i^{obs}, and some of which are missing Y_i^{mis}. X_i denotes explanatory variables (or covariates) that include indicators of treatment, time since the beginning of treatment or diagnosis, and other subject characteristics. Let Θ denote the parameters that describe the HRQoL process. M_i denotes a vector of variables representing the missing data process. Often $M_i = R_i$, where R_i denotes a vector of binary indicators of whether a particular HRQoL score was observed ($r_{ij} = 1$) or missing ($r_{ij} = 0$), but it can also denote the time to dropout, an associated event ($T_i^{\mathcal{D}}$), or a random coefficient (β_i). Let Ψ denote the parameters that describe the missing data process.

III.1 Joint distribution of Y and M

Complete data

The *complete data* for both the measurement and the missing data process is the joint distribution of $\mathbf{Y} = (\mathbf{Y}^{\text{obs}}, \mathbf{Y}^{\text{mis}})$ and $\mathbf{M}$:

$$f[\mathbf{Y}, \mathbf{M} \,|\, \mathbf{X}, \Theta, \Psi]. \tag{III.1}$$

There are two ways to factor the density function for the complete data. In the first factorization, $f[\mathbf{Y} \,|\, \mathbf{M}, \mathbf{X}, \Theta]$ is the density function for the measurement process which depends on the missing data pattern ($\mathbf{M}$).

$$f[\mathbf{Y}, \mathbf{M} \,|\, X, \Theta, \Psi] = f[\mathbf{Y} \,|\, \mathbf{M}, \mathbf{X}, \Theta] f[\mathbf{M} \,|\, \mathbf{X}, \Psi]. \tag{III.2}$$

This factorization forms the basis of a family of models referred to as *mixture models*. In this factorization, the model for the missing data mechanism, $f[\mathbf{M} \,|\, \mathbf{X}, \Psi]$, does not depend on the HRQoL measurements. In the second factorization, $f[Y_i \,|\, X_i, \Theta]$ is the density function for the measurement process, which depends only on the covariates and the parameters Θ.

$$f[\mathbf{Y}, \mathbf{M} \,|\, \mathbf{X}, \Theta, \Psi] = f[\mathbf{Y} \,|\, \mathbf{X}, \Theta] f[\mathbf{M} \,|\, \mathbf{Y}, \mathbf{X}, \Psi]. \tag{III.3}$$

The model of the missing-data mechanism, $f[M_i \,|\, Y_i, X_i, \Psi]$, may depend on the covariates, the observed data Y_i^{obs}, and the missing data Y_i^{mis}. This factorization forms the basis of a family of models referred to as *selection models*. In both classes of models, strong assumptions must be made about the missing values (Y^{mis}). The important distinction between the two is whether the assumption is part of the model for missingness (**M**), as in the selection models, or the model for the outcome (**Y**), as in the mixture models.

Observed data

The *observed data* for the measurement and missing data process has the joint distribution of $\mathbf{Y}^{\text{obs}}$ and **M**:

$$\begin{aligned}f(\mathbf{Y}^{\text{obs}}, \mathbf{M} \mid \mathbf{X}, \mathbf{\Theta}, \mathbf{\Psi}) &= \int f(\mathbf{Y}, \mathbf{M} \mid \mathbf{X}, \mathbf{\Theta}, \mathbf{\Psi}) d\mathbf{Y}^{\text{mis}} \\ &= \int f(\mathbf{Y}^{\text{obs}}, \mathbf{Y}^{\text{mis}} \mid \mathbf{X}, \mathbf{\Theta}) \\ &\quad \times f(\mathbf{M} \mid \mathbf{Y}^{\text{obs}}, \mathbf{Y}^{\text{mis}}, \mathbf{X}, \mathbf{\Psi}) d\mathbf{Y}^{\text{mis}}. \end{aligned} \quad \text{(III.4)}$$

III.2 Missing data mechanism

The following taxonomy is based on a model for the missing data mechanism, denoted as in the selection models:

$$f\left[M_i \middle| Y_i^{\text{obs}}, Y_i^{\text{mis}}, X_i, \Psi\right]. \quad \text{(III.5)}$$

Thus, the missing data mechanism is defined by the dependence of missingness on the covariates (X_i), the observed responses (Y_i^{obs}), and the missing responses (Y_i^{mis}).

MCAR: Missing completely at random

The strongest assumption about the missing data mechanism is that the data are *missing completely at random* (MCAR).

$$f\left[M_i \middle| Y_i^{\text{obs}}, Y_i^{\text{mis}}, X_i\right] = f[M_i]. \quad \text{(III.6)}$$

This mechanism assumes that the probability that an observation is missing is independent of observed HRQoL measures (Y_i^{obs}) at other times and the missing HRQoL measure (Y_i^{mis}). Little and Rubin (see Little [92]) distinguish MCAR from *covariate-dependent* missingness.

$$f\left[M_i \middle| Y_i^{\text{obs}}, Y_i^{\text{mis}}, X_i\right] = f[M_i \mid X_i]. \quad \text{(III.7)}$$

This mechanism assumes that the probability that an observation is observed is dependent only on covariates (X_i). Thus, conditional on the covariates, missingness is independent of observed HRQoL measures (Y_i^{obs}) and the missing HRQoL measure (Y_i^{mis}). When the missing data are the result of dropout and have a monotone pattern, this mechanism is sometimes referred to as *covariate-dependent dropout* [92] or *completely random dropout* (CRD) [36].

MAR: Missing at random

The assumptions about the missing data mechanism are relaxed slightly when we assume the data are *missing at random* (MAR).

$$f[M_i|Y_i^{\text{obs}}, Y_i^{\text{mis}}, X_i] = f[M_i|Y_i^{\text{obs}}, X_i]. \qquad (\text{III.8})$$

The probability that an observation is observed may depend on the fixed covariates, X_i, and the observed data, $\mathbf{Y}^{\text{obs}}$, but may not depend on the value of the missing data $\mathbf{Y}^{\text{mis}}$. Note that when this is true, $\mathbf{Y}^{\text{mis}}$ drops out of Equation III.4 and the joint distribution of the *observed data*, $(\mathbf{Y}^{\text{obs}}, \mathbf{M})$, reduces to

$$\begin{aligned}
f(\mathbf{Y}^{\text{obs}}, \mathbf{M} \,|\, \mathbf{X}, \Theta, \Psi) &= \int f(\mathbf{Y}^{\text{obs}}, \mathbf{Y}^{\text{mis}} \,|\, \mathbf{X}, \Theta) \\
&\quad \times f(\mathbf{M} \,|\, \mathbf{Y}^{\text{obs}}, \mathbf{Y}^{\text{mis}}, \mathbf{X}, \Psi) d\mathbf{Y}^{\text{mis}} \\
&= \int f(\mathbf{Y}^{\text{obs}} \,|\, \mathbf{X}, \Theta) f(\mathbf{M} \,|\, \mathbf{Y}^{\text{obs}}, \mathbf{X}, \Psi) d\mathbf{Y}^{\text{mis}} \\
&= f(\mathbf{Y}^{\text{obs}} \,|\, \mathbf{X}, \Theta) f(\mathbf{M} \,|\, \mathbf{Y}^{\text{obs}}, \mathbf{X}, \Psi). \qquad (\text{III.9})
\end{aligned}$$

MAR vs. ignorable

Often we interchange the terms MAR and ignorable. They are not strictly equivalent. If a dropout process is random (MAR or MCAR), then unbiased estimates can be obtained from likelihood-based estimation that ignores the dropout mechanism, provided the parameters describing the measurement process of HRQoL (Θ) are functionally independent of the parameters describing the dropout process (Ψ). This is referred to as the *separability* or *parameter distinctness* condition and is called *ignorable* by Little and Rubin [88]. When the separability condition is satisfied, inference can be based solely on the marginal density of the observed data [32, 75, 154]:

$$L(\Theta \,|\, \mathbf{X}, \mathbf{Y}^{\text{obs}}) \propto f(\mathbf{Y}^{\text{obs}} \,|\, \mathbf{X}, \Theta). \qquad (\text{III.10})$$

This allows straightforward estimation of Θ using procedures such as the EM algorithm [32, 75, 115].

MNAR: Missing not at random

The final mechanism relaxes the remaining assumption.

$$f[M_i|Y_i^{\text{obs}}, Y_i^{\text{mis}}, X_i] = f[M_i|Y_i^{\text{obs}}, Y_i^{\text{mis}}, X_i]. \qquad (\text{III.11})$$

The probability that an observation is missing may depend on the value of the missing data $\mathbf{Y}^{\text{mis}}$.

The terms *outcome-based* and *random-effect dependent* have been used to distinguish between missing data mechanisms dependent on Y_i^{mis} and those dependent on $\beta_i = \beta + d_i$ in mixed-effects models.

References

[1] Aaronson, N.K. et al., The European Organization for Research and Treatment of Cancer QLQ-30: a quality-of-life instrument for use in international clinical trials in oncology, *J. Natl. Cancer Inst.*, 85: 365–376, 1993.

[2] Bacik, J. et al., The Functional Assessment of Cancer Therapy-BRM (FACT-BRM): a new tool for the assessment of quality of life in patients treated with biologic response modifiers, submitted.

[3] Bacik, J. et al., Quality of life analysis for a randomized Phase III trial of interferon alfa-2a versus IFN plus 13-*cis*-retinoic acid in patients with advanced renal cell carcinoma, in *ASCO Proceedings*, New Orleans, 2000.

[4] Barnard, J. and Meng, X.L., Applications of multiple imputation in medical statistics: from AIDS to NHANES. *Stat. Meth. Med. Res.*, 8: 17–36, 1999.

[5] Barnard, J. and Rubin, D.B., Small-sample degrees of freedom with multiple imputation, *Biometrika*, 86: 948–955, 1999.

[6] Bernhard, J. et al., Missing quality of life data in clinical trials: serious problems and challenges, *Stat. Med.*, 17: 517–532, 1998.

[7] Bonomi, P. et al., Comparison of survival and quality of life in advanced non-small-cell lung cancer patients treated with two dose levels of Paclitaxel combined with cisplatin versus etoposide-cisplatin: results of an Eastern Cooperative Group trial, *J. Clin. Oncol.*, 18: 623–31, 2000.

[8] Bouchet, C. et al., Selection of quality-of-life measures for a prevention trial: a psychometric analysis, *Controlled Clin. Trials*, 21: 30–43, 2000.

[9] Brooks, M.M. et al., Quality of life at baseline: is assessment after randomization valid? *Med. Care*, 36: 1515–1519, 1998.

[10] Brown, C.H., Protecting against nonrandomly missing data in longitudinal studies, *Biometrics*, 46: 143–155, 1990.

[11] Buck, S.F., A method of estimation of missing values in multivariate data suitable for use with an electronic computer, *J. R. Stat. Soc. Ser. B*, 22: 302–306, 1960.

[12] Busch, P. et al., Life quality assessment of breast cancer patients receiving adjuvant therapy using incomplete data, *Health Econ.*, 3: 203–220, 1994.

[13] Cella, D.F., Skeel, R.T., and Bonomi, A.E., Policies and Procedures Manual, Eastern Cooperative Oncology Group Quality of Life Subcommittee, unpublished, 1993.

[14] Cella, D.F. et al., The Functional Assessment of Cancer Therapy (FACT) scales: development and validation of the general measure, *J. Clin. Oncol.*, 11: 570–579, 1993.

[15] Cella, D.F. et al., Reliability and validity of the Functional Assessment of Cancer Therapy—Lung (FACT-L) quality of life instrument, *Lung Cancer*, 12: 199–220, 1995.

[16] Cella, D.F., Bonomi, A.E., Measuring quality of life: 1995 update. *Oncology*, 9 11(supplement) 47–60, 1995.

[17] Cella, D.F., Personal communication.

[18] Cohen, J., *Statistical Power Analysis for the Behavioral Sciences*, 2nd ed., Lawrence Erlbaum Associates, Hillsdale, NJ, 1988.

[19] Cook, N.R., An imputation method for nonignorable missing data in studies of blood pressure, *Stat. Med.*, 16: 2713–2728, 1997.

[20] Cox, D.R. et al., Quality-of-life assessment: can we keep it simple? (with discussion), *J. R. Stat. Soc. A*, 155: 353–393, 1992.

[21] Crawford, S.L., Tennstedt, S.L., and McKinlay, J.B., A comparison of analytic methods for non-random missingness of outcome data, *J. Clin. Epidemiol.*, 48: 209–219, 1995.

[22] Curren, D. et al., Summary measures and statistics in the analysis of quality of life data: an example from an EORTC-NCIC-SAKK locally advanced breast cancer study, *Eur. J. Cancer*, 36: 834–844, 2000.

[23] Curren, D., Analysis of Incomplete Longitudinal Quality of Life Data, doctoral disertation, Linburgs Universitair Centrum, June 2000.

[24] Center for Drug Evaluation and Research, Food and Drug Administration, E9 Statistical Principles for Clinical Trials, *Fed. Regis.*, 63: 49584–49598, 1998.

[25] Converse, J.M. and Presser, S., *Survey Questions: Handcrafting the Standardized Questionnaire. Survey Research Methods.*, Sage Publications, Newbury Park, CA, 1986.

[26] Daniels, M.J. and Hogan, J.W., Reparameterizing the pattern mixture model for sensitivity analyses under informative dropout, *Biometrics*, 56: 1241–1248, 2000.

[27] Dawson, J.D. and Lagakos, S.W., Analyzing laboratory marker changes in AIDS clinical trials, *J. Acq. Immune Deficiency Syndr.*, 4: 667–676, 1991.

[28] Dawson, J.D. and Lagakos, S.W., Size and power of two-sample tests of repeated measures data, *Biometrics*, 49: 1022–1032, 1993.

[29] Dawson, J.D., Stratification of summary statistic tests according to missing data patterns, *Stat. Med.*, 13: 1853–1863, 1994.

[30] DeGruttola, V. and Tu, X.M., Modeling progression of CD-4 lymphocyte count and its relationship to survival time, *Biometrics*, 50: 1003–1014, 1994.

[31] DeKlerk, N.H., Repeated warnings re repeated measures, *Aust. N.Z. J. Med.*, 16: 637–638, 1986.

[32] Dempster, A.P., Laird, N.M., and Rubin, D.B., Maximum likelihood estimation from incomplete data via the EM algorithm (with discussion), *J. R. Stat. Soc. Ser. B*, 39: 1–38, 1977.

[33] Devellis, R.F., *Scale Development: Theory and Application,* Sage Publications, Newbury Park, CA, 1991.

[34] Diehr, P. et al., Including deaths when measuring health status over time, *Med. Care*, 33(suppl.): AS164–172, 1995.

[35] Diggle, P.J., Liang, K.Y., and Zeger, S.L., *Analysis of Longitudinal Data,* Oxford Science Publications, Clarendon Press, Oxford, U.K., 1994.

[36] Diggle, P.J. and Kenward, M.G., Informative dropout in longitudinal data analysis (with discussion), *Appl. Stat.*, 43: 49–93, 1994.

[37] Fairclough, D.L. and Cella, D.F., A cooperative group report on quality of life research: lessons learned. Eastern Cooperative Oncology Group (ECOG), *J. Natl. Cancer Inst.*, 40: 73–75, 1996.

[38] Fairclough, D.L. and Cella, D.F., Functional assessment of cancer therapy (FACT-G): non-response to individual questions, *Qual. Life Res.*, 5: 321–329, 1996.

[39] Fairclough, D.L., Summary measures and statistics for comparison of quality of life in a clinical trial of cancer therapy, *Stat. Med.*, 16: 1197–1209, 1997.

[40] Fairclough, D.L., Method of analysis for longitudinal studies of health-related quality of life, in *Quality of Life Assessment in Clinical Trials: Methods and Practice,* Staquet, M.J., Hayes, R.D., and Fayers, P.M., Eds., Oxford University Press, New York, 1998, chap. 13.

[41] Fairclough, D.L., Peterson, H., and Chang, V., Why is missing quality of life data a problem in clinical trials of cancer therapy? *Stat. Med.*, 17: 667–678, 1998.

[42] Fairclough, D.L. et al., Comparison of model based methods dependent of the missing data mechanism in two clinical trials of cancer therapy, *Stat. Med.*, 17: 781–796, 1998.

[43] Fairclough, D.L. et al., For the Eastern Cooperative Oncology Group, Quality of life and quality adjusted survival for breast cancer patients recieving adjuvant therapy, *Qual. Life Res.*, 8: 723–731, 1999.

[44] Fayers, P.M. and Hand, D.J., Factor analysis, causal indicators and quality of life, *Qual. Life Res.*, 6: 139–150, 1997.

[45] Fayers, P.M. and Machin, D., *Quality of Life: Assessment, Analysis and Interpretation,* John Wiley & Sons, New York, 2000.

[46] Feeny, D. et al., A comprehensive multi-attribute system for classifying the health status of survivors of childhood cancer, *J. Clin. Oncol.*, 10: 923–928, 1992.

[47] Fetting, J. et al., CAF vs. a 16-week multidrug regimen as adjuvant therapy for receptor-negative, node positive breast cancer: an intergroup study, *Proc. Am. Soc. Clin. Oncol.*, 114(83), 1995.

[48] Fetting, J.J. et al., A 16-week multidrug regimen versus cyclophosphamide, doxorubicin and 5-flurouracil as adjuvant therapy for

node-positive, receptor negative breast cancer: an intergroup study, *J. Clin. Oncol.*, 16: 2382–2391, 1998.

[49] Fleiss, J.L., *The Design and Analysis of Clinical Experiments*, John Wiley & Sons, New York, 1986.

[50] Floyd, J. and Fowler, J.R., *Survey Research Methods*, Sage Publications, Newbury Park, CA, 1988.

[51] Follman, D. and Wu, M., An approximate generalized linear model with random effects for informative missing data, *Biometrics*, 51: 151–168, 1995.

[52] Frank-Stromborg, M. and Olsen, S., *Instruments for Clinical Health Care Research*, 2nd ed., Jones & Bartlett, Boston, 1997.

[53] Friedman, L.M., Furberg, C.D., and Demets, D., *Fundamentals of Clinical Trials*, 2nd ed., John Wright, Boston, 1985.

[54] Frison, L. and Popcock, S.J., Repeated measures in clinical trials: analysis using mean summary statistics and its implications for design, *Stat. Med.*, 11: 1685–1704, 1992.

[55] Gelber, R.D., Gelman, R.S., and Goldhirsh, A., A quality of life oriented endpoint for comparing therapies, *Biometrics*, 45: 781–795, 1998.

[56] Glasziou, P.P., Simes, R.J., and Gelber, R.D., Quality adjusted survival analysis, *Stat. Med.*, 9: 1259–1276, 1990.

[57] Glynn, R.J., Laird, N.M., and Rubin, D.B., Multiple imputation in mixture models for non-ignorable nonresponse with follow-ups, *J. Am. Stat. Assoc.*, 88: 984–993, 1993.

[58] Goldhirsch, A. et al., Costs and benefits of adjuvant therapy in breast cancer: a quality adjusted survival analysis, *J. Clin. Oncol.*, 7: 36–44, 1989.

[59] Gotay, C.C. et al., Building quality of life assessment into cancer treatment studies, *Oncology*, 6: 25–28, 1992.

[60] Gould, A.L., A new approach to the analysis of clinical drug trials with withdrawals, *Biometrics*, 36: 721–727, 1980.

[61] Guyatt, G.H. et al., A comparison of Likert and visual analogue scales for measuring change in function, *J. Chronic Dis.*, 40: 1129–1133, 1987.

[62] Guyatt, G. et al., Glossary, *Controlled Clin. Trials*, 12: 274S–280S, 1991.

[63] Heitjan, D.A. and Landis, J.R., Assessing secular trends in blood pressure: a multiple imputation approach, *J. Am. Stat. Assoc.*, 89: 750–759, 1994.

[64] Heyting, A., Tolbomm, T.B.M., and Essers, J.G.A., Statistical handling of dropouts in longitudinal clinical trials, *Stat. Med.*, 11: 2043–2061, 1992.

[65] Hicks, J.E. et al., Functional outcome update in patients with soft tissue sarcoma undergoing wide local excision and radiation (Abstr.), *Arch. Phys. Med. Rehabil.*, 66: 542–543, 1985.

[66] Hogan, J.W. and Laird, N.M., Mixture models for the joint distribution of repeated measuress and event times, *Stat. Med.*, 16: 239–257, 1997.

[67] Hogan, J.W. and Laird, N.M., Model-based approaches to analyzing incomplete longitudinal and failure time data, *Stat. Med.*, 16: 259–272, 1997.
[68] Hollen, P.J. et al., A dilemma in analysis: issues in serial measurement of quality of life in patients with advanced lung cancer, *Lung Cancer*, 18: 119–136, 1997.
[69] Holm, S., A simple sequentially rejective multivariate test procedure, *Scan. J. Statis.*, 6: 65–70, 1979.
[70] Hommel, G., Tests of overall hypothesis for arbitrary dependence structures, *Biom. J.*, 25: 423–430, 1983.
[71] Hopwood, P. et al., Survey of the administration of quality of life questionnaires in three multicentre randomised trials in cancer, *Eur. J. Cancer*, 90: 49–57, 1997.
[72] Hürny, C. et al., Quality of life measures for patients receiving adjuvant therapy for breast cancer: an international trial, *Eur. J. Cancer*, 28: 118–124, 1992.
[73] Hürny, C. et al., The perceived adjustment to chronic illness scale (PACIS): a global indicator of coping for operable breast cancer patients in clinical trials, *Supportive Care Cancer*, 1: 200–208, 1993.
[74] Hürny, C. et al., Impact of adjuvant therapy on quality of life in node-positive patients with operable breast cancer, *Lancet*, 347: 1279–1284, 1996.
[75] Jennrich, R. and Schluchter, M., Unbalanced repeated-measures models with structured covariance matrices, *Biometrics*, 42: 805–820, 1986.
[76] Jones, R.H. *Longitudinal Data with Serial Correlation: A State-Space Approach*, Chapman & Hall, London, 1993.
[77] Kaplan, R.M. and Bush, J.W., Health-related quality of life measurement for evaluation research and policy analysis, *Health Psychology*, 1: 61–80, 1982.
[78] Kenward, M.G. and Roger, J.H., Small sample inference for fixed effects from restricted maximum likelihood, *Biometrics*, 53: 983–997, 1997.
[79] Korn, E.L. and O'Fallon, J., Statistical Considerations, Statistics Working Group. Quality of Life Assessment in Cancer Clinical Trials, Report on Workshop on Quality of Life Research in Cancer Clinical Trials, Division of Cancer Prevention and Control, National Cancer Institute, 1990.
[80] Korn, D.L., On estimating the distribution function for quality of life in cancer clinical trials, *Biometrika*, 80: 535–542, 1993.
[81] Kosinski, M. et al., Improving estimates of SF-36 health survey scores for respondents with missing data, *Med. Outcomes Trust Monitor*, 5(1): 8–10, 2000.
[82] Laird, N.M. and Ware, J.H., Random-effects models for longitudinal data, *Biometrics*, 38: 963–974, 1982.
[83] Lauter, J., Exact t and F tests for analyzing studies with multiple endpoints, *Biometrics*, 52: 964–970, 1996.

[84] Lavori, P.W., Dawson, R., and Shera, D., A multiple imputation strategy for clinical trials with truncation of patient data, *Stat. Med.*, 14: 1912–1925, 1995.

[85] Lee, C.W. and Chi, K.N., The standard of report of health-related quality of life in clinical cancer trials, *J. Clin. Epidemiol.*, 53: 451–458, 2000.

[86] Levine, M. et al., Quality of life in stage II breast cancer: an instrument for clinical trials, *J. Clin. Oncol.*, 6: 1798–1810, 1988.

[87] Littel, R.C. et al., *SAS System for Mixed Models*, SAS Institute, Inc., Cary, NC, 1996.

[88] Little, R.J. and Rubin, D.B., *Statistical Analysis with Missing Data*, John Wiley & Sons, New York, 1987.

[89] Little, R.J.A., A test of missing completely at random for multivariate data with missing values, *J. Am. Stat. Assoc.*, 83: 1198–1202, 1988.

[90] Little, R.J.A., Pattern-mixture models for multivariate incomplete data, *J. Am. Stat. Assoc.*, 88: 125–134, 1993.

[91] Little, R.J.A., A class of pattern-mixture models for multivariate incomplete data, *Biometrika*, 81: 471–483, 1994.

[92] Little, R.J.A., Modeling the dropout mechanism in repeated-measures studies, *J. Am. Stat. Assoc.*, 90: 1112–1121, 1995.

[93] Little, R.J.A. and Wang, Y., Pattern-mixture models for multivariate incomplete data with covariates, *Biometrics*, 52: 98–111, 1996.

[94] Little, R. and Yau, L., Intent-to-treat analysis for longitudinal studies with dropouts, *Biometrics*, 52: 1324–1333, 1996.

[95] McDowell, I. and Newell, C., *Measuring Health: A Guide to Rating Scales and Questionnaires*, 2nd ed., Oxford University Press, New York, 1996.

[96] Marcus, R., Peritz, E., and Gabriel, K.R., On closed testing procedures with special reference to ordered analysis of variance, *Biometrika*, 63: 655–660, 1976.

[97] Matthews, J.N.S. et al., Analysis of serial measurements in medical research, *Br. Med. J.*, 300: 230–235, 1990.

[98] McNeil, B.J., Weichselbaum, R., and Pauker, S.G., Tradeoffs between quality and quantity of life in laryngeal cancer, *N. Engl. J. Med.*, 305: 982–987, 1981.

[99] Meinert, C.L., *Clinical Trials: Design, Conduct and Analysis*, Oxford University Press, New York, 1986.

[100] Michiels, B., Molenberghs, G., and Lipsitz, S.R., Selection models and pattern-mixture models for incomplete data with covariates, *Biometrics*, 55: 978–983, 1999.

[101] Miller, G.A., The magic number seven plus or minus two: some limits on our capacity for information processing, *Psychol. Bull.*, 63: 81–97, 1956.

[102] Moinpour, C. et al., Quality of life endpoints in cancer clinical trials: review and recommendations, *J. Natl. Cancer Inst.*, 81: 485–495, 1989.

[103] Mori, M., Woodworth, G.G., and Woolson, R.F., Application of empirical Bayes inference to estimation of rate of change in the presence of informative right censoring, *Stat. Med.*, 11: 621–631, 1992.

REFERENCES

[104] Motzer, R.J. et al., Phase III trial of interferon alfa-2a with or without 13-*cis*-retinoic acid for patients with advanced renal cell carcinoma, *J. Clin. Oncol.,* 18: 2972–2980, 2000.

[105] Murray, G.D. and Findlay, J.G., Correcting for the bias caused by dropouts in hypertension trials, *Stat. Med.,* 7: 941–946, 1988.

[106] Neter, J. and Wasserman, W., *Applied Linear Statistical Models,* Richard Irwin, Homewood, IL, 1974, 313–317.

[107] Norton, N.J. and Lipsitz, S.R., Multiple imputation in practice: comparison of software packages for regression models with missing variables, *Am. Stat.,* 55: 244–254, 2001.

[108] O'Brien, P.C., Procedures for comparing samples with multiple endpoints, *Biometrics,* 40: 1079–1087, 1984.

[109] Smith, D.M., *Oswald: Object-Oriented Software for the Analysis of Longitudinal Data in S.,* 1996, available at http://www.maths.lancs.ac.uk/Software/Oswald.

[110] Omar, P.Z. et al., Analysing repeated measurements data: a practical comparison of methods, *Stat. Med.,* 18: 1587–1608, 1999.

[111] Pater, J. et al., Effects of altering the time of administration and the time frame of quality of life assessments in clinical trials: an example using the EORTC QLQ-C30 in a large anti-emetic trial, *Qual. Life Res.,* 7: 273–778, 1998.

[112] Patrick, D. and Erickson, P., *Health Status and Health Policy: Allocating Resources to Health Care,* Oxford University Press, New York, 1993.

[113] Piantadosi, S., *Clinical Trials: A Methodologic Perspective,* John Wiley & Sons, New York, 1997.

[114] Pledger, G. and Hall, D., Withdrawals from drug trials (letter to editor), *Biometrics,* 38: 276–278, 1982.

[115] SAS Proc Mixed, in *The MIXED Procedure. SAS/STAT Software. Changes and Enhancements* (through Release 6.11), SAS Institute, Cary, NC, 1996, chap. 18.

[116] Bernard, G., et al., Factors associated with noncompliance with self-administered quality of life assessments of node-positive patients receiving adjuvant therapy for operable breast cancer, *Stat. Med.,* 17: 587–603, 1997.

[117] Pocock, S.J., Geller, N.L., and Tsiatis, A.A., The analysis of multiple endpoints in clinical trials, *Biometrics,* 43: 487–498, 1987.

[118] Pocock, S.J., Hughes, M.D., and Lee, R.J., Statistical problems in the reporting of clinical trials, *N. Engl. J. Med.,* 317: 426–432, 1987.

[119] Proschan, M.A. and Waclawiw, M.A., Practical guidelines for multiplicity adjustment in clinical trials, *Controlled Clin. Trials,* 21: 527–539, 2000.

[120] Raboud, J.M. et al., Estimating the effect of treatment on quality of life in the presence of missing data due to dropout and death, *Qual. Life Res.,* 7: 487–494, 1998.

[121] Revicki, D.A. et al., Imputing physical function scores missing owing to mortality: results of a simulation comparing multiple techniquest, *Med. Care*, 29: 61–71, 2000.

[122] Ribaudo, H.J., Thompson, S.G., and Allen-Mersh, T.G., A joint analysis of quality of life and survival using a random-effect selection model, *Stat. Med.*, 19: 3237–3250, 2000.

[123] Reitmeir, J. and Wassmer, G., Resampling-based methods for the analysis of multiple endpoints in clinical trials, *Stat. Med.*, 18: 3455–3462, 1999.

[124] Rosenbaum, P.R. and Rubin, D.B., Reducing bias in observational studies using subclassification in the propensity score, *J. Am. Stat. Assoc.*, 79: 516–524, 1984.

[125] Rubin, D.B. and Schenker, N., Multiple imputation for interval estimation from simple random samples with ignorable nonresponse, *J. Am. Stat. Assoc.*, 81: 366–374, 1986.

[126] Rubin, D.B., *Multiple Imputation for Nonresponse in Surveys*, John Wiley and Sons, New York, 1987.

[127] Rubin, D.B. and Schenker, N., Multiple imputation in health-care data bases: an overview and some applications, *Stat. Med.*, 10: 585–598, 1991.

[128] Rubin, D.B., Multiple imputation after 18+ years, *J. Am. Stat. Assoc.*, 91: 473–489, 1996.

[129] Schafer, J., *Analysis of Incomplete Multivariate Data*, Monograph on Statistics and Applied Probability 72, Chapman & Hall, London, 1997.

[130] Schipper, H. et al., Measuring the quality of life of cancer patients: The Functional Living Index—Cancer: development and validation, *J. Clin. Oncol.*, 2: 472–482, 1984.

[131] Schipper, H., Guidelines and caveats for quality of life measurement in clinical practice and research, *Oncology*, 4: 51–57, 1990.

[132] Schluchter, M.D., 5V: unbalanced repeated measures models with structured covariance matrices, in *BMDP Statistical Software Manual, 2*, Dixon, W.J., Ed., University of California Press, Berkeley, CA, 1990, 1207–1244, 1322–1327.

[133] Schluchter, M.D., Methods for the analysis of informatively censored longitudinal data, *Stat. Med.*, 11: 1861–1870, 1992.

[134] Schluchter, D.M., Green, T., and Beck, G.J., Analysis of change in the presence of informative censoring: application to a longitudinal clinical trial of progressive renal disease, *Stat. Med.*, 20: 989–1007, 2001.

[135] Schumacher, M., Olschewski, M., and Schulgen, G., Assessment of quality of life in clinical trials, *Stat. Med.*, 10: 1915–1930, 1991.

[136] Schwartz, D., Flamant, R., and Lellouch, J., *Clinical Trials*, Academic Press, London, 1980.

[137] Searle, S.R., *Linear Models*, John Wiley & Sons, New York, 1971, 46–47.

[138] Simes, R.J., An improved Bonferroni procedure for multiple tests of significance, *Biometrika*, 73: 751–754, 1986.

[139] Simon, G.E. et al., SF-Summary Scores: are physical and mental health truly distinct, *Med. Care,* 36: 567–572, 1998.

[140] *Solas for Missing Data Analysis 1.0 User Reference,* Statistical Solutions Ltd, Cork, Ireland, 1997.

[141] Spilker, B., *Guide to Clinical Trials,* Lippincott-Williams & Wilkins, Baltimore, MD, 1991.

[142] Spilker, B., Ed., *Quality of Life and Pharmacoeconomics in Clinical Trials,* Lippincott-Raven, Philadelphia, 1996.

[143] Schuman, H. and Presser, S., *Questions and Answers in Attitude Surveys: Experiments on Question Form, Wording and Context,* Academic Press, New York, 1981.

[144] Staquet, M. et al., Editorial: Health-related quality of life research, *Qual. Life Res.,* 1: 3, 1992.

[145] Staquet, M. et al., Guidelines for reporting results of quality of life assessments in clinical trials, *Qual. Life Res.,* 5: 496–502, 1996.

[146] Staquet, M.J., Hayes, R.D., and Fayers, P.M., *Quality of Life Assessment in Clinical Trials: Methods and Practice,* Oxford University Press, New York, 1998.

[147] Streiner, D.L. and Norman, G.R., *Health Measurement Scales—A Practical Guide to Their Development and Use,* 2nd ed., Oxford Medical Publications, Oxford University Press, New York, 1995.

[148] Sugarbaker, P.H. et al., Quality of life assessment of patients in extremity sarcoma clinical trials, *Surgery,* 91: 17–23, 1986.

[149] Tandon, P.K., Applications of global statistics in analyzing quality of life data, *Stat. Med.,* 9: 819–827, 1990.

[150] Torrance, G.W., Thomas, W.H., and Sackett, D.L., A utility maximizing model for evaluation of health care programs, *Health Serv. Res.,* 7: 118–133, 1971.

[151] Troxel, A. et al., The generalized estimating approach when data are not missing completely at random, *J. Am. Stat. Assoc.,* 92: 1320–1329, 1997.

[152] Troxel, A. et al., Statistical analysis of quality of life data in cancer clinical trials, *Stat. Med.,* 17: 653–666, 1997.

[153] VanBuuren, S., Boshuizen, H.C., and Knook, D.L., Multiple imputation of missing blood pressure covariates in survival analysis, *Stat. Med.,* 18: 681–694, 1999.

[154] Verbeke, G. and Molenberghs, G., Eds., *Linear Mixed Models in Practice: A SAS-Orientated Approach,* Lecture Notes in Statistics, Springer, New York, 1997.

[155] Verbeke, G. and Molenberghs, G., *Linear Mixed Models for Longitudinal Data,* Springer, New York, 2000.

[156] Ware, J.E. et al., Choosing measures of health status for individuals in general populations, *Am. J. Public Health,* 71: 620–625, 1981.

[157] Ware, J.E. et al., *SF-36 Health Survey: Manual and Interpretation Guide,* The Health Institute, New England Medical Center, Boston, 1993.

[158] Ware, J., Kosinski, M., and Keller, S.D., SF-36 Physical and Mental Component Summary Scales: A User's Manual, The Health Institute, New England Medical Center, Boston, 1993.

[159] Weeks, J., Quality-of-life assessment: performance status upstaged? *J. Clin. Oncol.*, 10: 1827–1829, 1992.

[160] Wei, L.J. and Johnson, W.E., Combining dependent tests with incomplete repeated measurements, *Biometrika*, 72: 359–364, 1985.

[161] Westfall, P.H. and Young, S.S., p-value adjustment for multiple testing in multivariate bionomial models, *J. Am. Stat. Assoc.*, 84: 780–786, 1989.

[162] Wiklund, I., Dimenäs, E., and Wahl, M., Factor of importance when evaluating quality of life in clinical trials, *Controlled Clin. Trials*, 11: 169–179, 1990.

[163] Wilson, I.B. and Cleary, P.D., Linking clinical variables with health-related quality of life—a conceptual model of patient outcomes, *J. Am. Med. Assoc.*, 273: 59–65, 1995.

[164] World Health Organization, *Constitution of the World Health Organization, Basic Documents*, WHO, Geneva, 1948.

[165] World Health Organization, *The First Ten Years of the World Health Organization*, WHO, Geneva, 1958.

[166] Wu, M.C. and Bailey, K.R., Analyzing changes in the presence of informative right censoring caused by death and withdrawal, *Stat. Med.*, 7: 337–346, 1988.

[167] Wu, M.C. and Bailey, K.R., Estimation and comparison of changes in the presence of informative right censoring: conditional linear model, *Biometrics*, 45: 939–955, 1989.

[168] Wu, M.C. and Carroll, R.J., Estimation and comparison of changes in the presence of informative right censoring by modeling the censoring process, *Biometrics*, 44: 175–188, 1988.

[169] Yabroff, K.R., Linas, B.P., and Schulman, K., Evaluation of quality of life for diverse patient populations, *Breast Cancer Res. Treatment*, 40: 87–104, 1996.

[170] Yao, Q., Wei, L.J., and Hogan, J.W., Analysis of incomplete repeated measurements with dependent censoring times, *Biometrika*, 85: 139–149, 1998.

[171] Young, T. and Maher, J., Collecting quality of life data in EORTC clinical trials—what happens in practice? *Psycho-oncology*, 8: 260–263, 1999.

[172] Zeger, S.L. and Liang, K.Y., An overview of methods for the analysis of longitudinal data, *Stat. Med.*, 11: 1825–1839, 1992.

[173] Zhang, J. et al., Some statistical methods for multiple endpoints in clinical trials, *Controlled Clin. Trials*, 18: 204–221, 1997.

[174] Zwinderman, A.H., The measurement of change of quality of life in clinical trials, *Stat. Med.*, 9: 931–942, 1990.

Index

13-cis-retinoic acid (13-CRA), 15–18

A

Aaronson, N.K., 1
ABB (Approximate Bayesian bootstrap), 142–146; *see also* Covariance structure; Multiple imputation
ACMV restriction, *see* Available case missing value (ACMV) restriction
Adjuvant breast cancer study, 7–10
    appropriateness of, 30
    global tests, 246
    multivariate analyses, 247–248, 248–249
    repeated measures cell means model, 46–47
    selection between models, 42
    timing of, 25
Administration of assessments, 31–32
Age, and missing data, 10, 11, 47, 48, 76, 77, 86
Akaike's Information Criterion (AIC), 46; *see also* Models
Alpha adjustments, 249–253
Analysis plans, 257–274, 260–261; *see also* Multiple endpoints; Summary measures; Summary statistics
    general analysis plan, 258–259
    introduction, 257–258
    models for longitudinal data, 259–260
    multiple comparisons, 244, 261–262
    reporting results, 272–273
    sample size and power, 262–272
        basic assumptions, 264
        growth curve model, 268–272
        incomplete designs, 264–266
        repeated measures example, 266–268
        simple linear combinations of ß, 262–263
    secondary endpoints, 260–261, 263
Analytic models, vs. imputation, 151
Approximate Bayesian bootstrap (ABB), 142–146; *see also* Covariance structure; Multiple imputation
Area under the curve (AUC), 225–227
    with missing data handled by multiple imputation, 250
    and summary statistics across time, 231–235
ARMA (autoregressive moving average), 50
Assessments, *see* Study design and protocol development
AT MEANS option, 107–108
AUC, *see* Area under the curve
Autoregressive covariance structure, 45, 49, 50
Autoregressive error structure, 58, 60
Autoregressive moving average (ARMA), 50
Available case missing value (ACMV) restriction, 164, 167, 169; *see also* Pattern mixture models
Available data, *see* Missing at random (MAR)
Average of ranks, 227
Average rate of change (slopes), 222

B

Bailey, K.R., 183, 184, 185, 186, 192
Barnard, J., 131, 148
Baseline
  adding other covariates, 110–112
  assessment as covariate, 105–108
  change from, 108–110
Bayes estimates, empirical, 112–113, 210–211, 223–224
Bayesian bootstrap, approximate (ABB), 142–146
Bayesian Information Criterion (BIC), 46
BCQ (Breast Chemotherapy Questionnaire), 8, 30, 246
Best linear unbiased estimate (BLUE), 113
Best linear unbiased predictor (BLUP), 113, 141
Between imputation variance, 132, 147, 150
BIC (Bayesian Information Criterion), 46
Biologic response modifiers (BRM), 15–16
Bivariate correlation, 76
Bivariate data, 155–161
  Brown's protective restrictions, 158–160
  complete-case missing variable (CCMV) restriction, 156–158
  non-small-cell lung cancer (NSCLC) study example, 156, 158
  sensitivity analyses with intermediate restrictions, 160–161
BLUE (best linear unbiased estimate), 113
BLUP (best linear unbiased predictor), 113
Bonferroni adjustment, 215, 249–250, 253–254
Bonomi, A.E., 2
Bootstrap procedure, 192, 254
Bouchet, C., 27
Breast cancer study, adjuvant, see Adjuvant breast cancer study
Breast Chemotherapy Questionnaire (BCQ), 8, 30, 246
BRM (biologic response modifiers), 15–16
Brown, C.H., 158–160
Brown's protective estimate, 259

Brown's protective restrictions, 158–160; see also Pattern mixture models
Buck's conditional means, 123
Building models, see Models
Bush, J.W., 2

C

CAF (Cyclophosphamide, doxirubicin, and 5-flurouracil) treatment, 7–10
Cancer, see Adjuvant breast cancer study; Non-small-cell lung cancer (NSCLC)
Carcinoma study, see Renal cell carcinoma study
Carroll, R.J., 210
Casewise deletion, 97
CCMV restriction, see Complete-case missing value (CCMV) restriction
Ceiling effect, see Validity of instruments
Cella, D.F., 2
Cell means model, 46, 52–53; see also Repeated measures
Change points, see Growth curve models
Characteristics of patients, see Covariates
Cholesky decomposition, 134
Cisplatin, treatment with, 10–12
Cleary, P.D., 1–2
Clinical trial endpoints, see Endpoints
Closed tests, 246–248
Closest neighbor and predictive mean matching, 140–142
Complete-case missing value (CCMV) restriction, 179–180; see also Pattern mixture models
  bivariate data, 156–158
  comparison of ACMV, NCMV and, 167, 169
  monotone dropout, 162–167
Complete cases, 73, 97–101
Complete data, use of term, 73
Completely random dropout (CRD), 198, 201, 204
Compound symmetry, 44, 45, 49, 50, 59; see also Covariance structure

INDEX

Conditional linear model, 184, 185–192
  assumptions, 192
  and designing analysis plan, 260
  estimation of the standard errors, 192
  non-small-cell lung cancer (NSCLC) study example, 187–192
  random-coefficient mixture model, 192
  testing MAR vs.MNAR under assumptions of, 187
Conditional predicted values, 123–125
Condition-driven designs, 23
Confirmatory tests, 243–244
Construct validity, 29
CONTRAST statement., 53
Convergent validity, 29
Covariance structure, 57–59; *see also* Repeated measures models
  piecewise linear regression model, 66–67
  polynomial growth curve models, 59–63
Covariates, 46–50
  baseline assessment as, 105–108
  dropout dependent on, 75–76
  time-varying, 270
COVB option, 174
COVTEST option, 195
CRD (completely random dropout), 198, 201, 204
Criterion validity, 29
Cubic terms, 54
Cultures, and instrument appropriateness, 30
Curren, D., 161, 217
Cut-off test statistics, 254
Cyclic therapy, 25
Cyclophosphamide,doxirubicin,and 5-flurouracil (CAF) treatment, 7–10
Cytokine treatment, 15

D

Daniels, M.J., 154, 178
Data collection and management, 32, 34, 35
Dawson, J.D., 228
DeGruttola, V., 184, 194

Delta method, 173–174
Designing analysis plan, *see* Analysis plans
Diggle, P.J., 184, 198, 202, 204, 210, 260
Discontinuation of therapy, assessment after, 27
Disease-specific instruments, 4; *see also* Measures
Divergent validity, 29
Domains, HRQoL, 235–240
Dropout; *see also* Missing data; Monotone dropout; Nonmonotone dropout
  informative, 199, 201, 205, 206–207
  intermittent, 71–72, 146–147
  joint mixed-effects and time to, *see* Joint mixed-effects model
  model for, 208–210
  random, 201, 204, 205
  time of, 185–187
  use of term, 69
Duration of assessments, 26–27

E

EBLUP (empirical best linear unbiased predictors), 123
Economic evaluations, 28
EM algorithm, 140, 178, 283
Empirical Bayes estimates
  of individual subject slopes, for informative dropout, 210–211
  use with ignorable missing data, 112–114
  use with missing data, 223–224
Empirical best linear unbiased predictors (EBLUP), 123
Endpoints; *see also* Multiple endpoints
  checklist for statistical analysis plan, 258
  primary, 260–261
  secondary, 260–261, 263
EORTC QLQ-C30 (European Organization for Research and Treatment of Cancer), 3, 5, 6; *see also* Measures
Erickson, P., 2
Error rates, 245, *see* Type I error rate; Type II error rate

Estimable functions, 113
Etoposide-cisplatin treatment, 10–12
European Organization for Research and Treatment of Cancer (EORTC QLQ-C30), 3, 5, 6; *see also* Measures
Event-driven designs, 23, 259–260
Exclusion, of observations/subjects, 104–105
Experimentwise error rates, 245
Explanatory investigational aims, 21–22
Explicit regression models, 118–125
Explicit univariate regression assumptions, 135–136
  computation of imputed values, 134
  extensions to longitudinal studies, 135
  non-small-cell lung cancer (NSCLC) study, 136–140
Extensions to longitudinal studies, 144

F

Face validity, 29
FACT, *see* Functional Assessment of Cancer Therapy
FACT BRM, *see* Functional Assessment of Cancer Therapy -Biologic Response Modifiers (FACT BRM)
FACT-G (Functional Assessment of Cancer Therapy Version 3), 15–18
FACT-L (Functional Assessment of Cancer Therapy,Lung Cancer Version 2), 12
FACT-Lung Trial Outcome Index (FACT-Lung TOI), 12, 78–80, 85–86
Factor-analytic weights, 36–37, 236–237
FACT-TOI (FACT Trial Outcome Index), 55, 198, 200
Fairclough, D.L., 130
Familywise error rates, 245
Fayers, P.M., 36, 225
Findlay, J.G., 78
Fixed effects, 57; *see also* Mixed-effects models
FLIC (Functional Living Index -Cancer), 3

Floor effect, 30; *see also* Validity of instruments
Follow-up HRQoL assessments, 24
Follow-up procedures, explicit, 34
Frequency of assessments, 25–26
Functional Assessment of Cancer Therapy (FACT), 3
  global index vs. profile of domain-specific measures, 5
  period of recall, 6
  sample questions, 12, 36
Functional Assessment of Cancer Therapy,Lung Cancer Version 2 (FACT-L), 12
Functional Assessment of Cancer Therapy -Biologic Response Modifiers (FACT BRM)
  renal cell carcinoma study, 87, 89, 90, 198, 199
  sample questions from, 16
  standard deviation of baseline, 235
  summary measures, 236
Functional Assessment of Cancer Therapy Version 3 (FACT-G), 15–18
Functional Living Index -Cancer (FLIC), 3

G

General analysis plan, 258–259
Generic instruments, 4, 28
Global index of HRQoL, 4–5
Global tests, 246
Gould, A.L., 128
GROUP parameter, 206
Growth curve models, 54–67; *see also* Mixed-effects models; Piecewise linear regression
  and area under the curve (AUC), 232–233
  covariance structure, 57–59
  and designing analysis plan, 260
  model for means, 54–57
  for non-small-cell lung cancer (NSCLC) study, 43
  for renal cell carcinoma study, 43
  sample size and power, 268–272

SAS example of piecewise linear regression model, 65–67
SAS example of polynomial growth curve model, 59–65
Guttman scale, 38
Guyatt, G., 27

H

Half rule, 37–38
Hall, D., 128
Hand, D.J., 36
Health, defined, 1
Health-related quality of life (HRQoL), use of term, 2
Health status assessment, 2–4
Heckman probit stochastic dropout model, 210
Heterogeneous autoregressive covariance structure, 45, 49, 50
Heterogeneous compound covariance structure, 45, 49, 50
Heterogeneous Toplitz covariance structure, 45, 49, 50
Heyting, A., 128
Higher-order terms, 54
Hogan, J.W., 84, 154, 178, 195
Hommel, G., 252
Hopwood, P., 31, 34–35
Hotelling-Lawley trace, 246
Hypothesis testing
   building growth curve models, 64–65
   building repeated measures models, 52–53
   pattern-mixture model, 177
   polynomial growth curve models, 64–65

I

ID (informative dropout), 199, 201, 205
Ignorable missing data, 93–114; *see also* Imputation; Missing data
   adding other baseline covariates, 110–112
   baseline assessment as a covariate, 105–108
   change from baseline, 108–110
   and designing analysis plan, 259
   empirical Bayes estimates, 112–113
   introduction, 93–94
   multivariate methods, 96–105
      complete case analysis, 97–101
      exclusion of observations, 105
      exclusion of subjects, 104–105
      maximum likelihood estimation with all available data, 101–104
   repeated univariate analyses, 94–96
Imputation, *see* Multiple imputation; Simple imputation
Incomplete cases, *see* Missing data
Individual tests, vs. global, 246
Information criterion, 46, 49, 52
Informative dropout (ID), 199, 201, 205
informative missing data, *see* Missing data
Initial assessments, *see* Analysis plans
Instruments
   defined, 27
   disease-specific instruments, 4
   generic, 4
   scoring, 35–39
   selecting, 27–30
   validity and reliability, 29–30
Intent-to-treat analysis, 22, 257; *see also* Research objectives
Interferon alpha-2·, 15–18
Intermittent dropout, 71–72, 146–147
Intermittent missing data, 210, 270
International assessments, 30
Interpolation, 221
Interviews, for assessments, 31
Inverse correlation, 238–239
Investigation aims, *see* Research objectives
Item-nonresponse, *see* Missing data

J

Joint mixed-effects model, 184, 185, 193–198
   and designing analysis plan, 260

extension to more complex mixed-effects models, 198
initial estimates, 197
non-small-cell lung cancer (NSCLC) study example, 195–197
renal cell carcinoma example, 198
testing MAR vs.MNAR under the assumptions of, 194–195

K

Kaplan, R.M., 2
Kenward, M.G., 184, 198, 202, 204, 210, 260, 272

L

Lagakos, S.W., 228
Laird, N.M., 84, 195
Languages, and instrument appropriateness, 30
Large-sample inferences for μ_2, 160–161
Last observation carried forward (LOCF), 125–128
Last value carried forward (LVCF), 125–128, 223, 224
Lavori, P.W., 144, 145
Likelihood ratio tests, 44–46
Likert scale, 6, 36
Linear minimum variance unbiased estimator (LMVUB), 186
Lipsitz, S.R., 131
Listwise deletion, 97
Little, R., 135
Little, R.J.A., 79, 81, 84, 87, 160, 161, 178, 195
LMVUB (linear minimum variance unbiased estimator), 186
LOCF (last observation carried forward), 125–128
Logistic selection model, 185
Longitudinal studies, models for, *see* Models
LSMEANS option, 111
LSMEANS statement, 107–108

Lung cancer study, *see* Non-small-cell lung cancer (NSCLC)
LVCF (last value carried forward), 125–128, 223, 224

M

Machin, D., 225
Macros, for scoring, 38–39
M analyses, combining, 147–150
MANOVA statement, 98
Marcus, R., 247
Marginal model, 198
Markov Chain Monte Carlo (MCMC) method, 147
Maximization converged message, 210
Maximum likelihood (ML) ratio test, 44
Maximum likelihood estimation (MLE), 97
MCMC (Markov Chain Monte Carlo) method, 147
MCS (Mental component scale), 236–237
Mean value substitution, 117–118
Measures; *see also* Models; Study design and protocol development
Breast Chemotherapy Questionnaire (BCQ), 8, 30, 246
disease-specific instruments, 4
EORTC QLQ-C30 (European Organization for Research and Treatment of Cancer), 3, 5, 6
FACT-Lung Trial Outcome Index (FACT-Lung TOI), 12, 78–80, 85–86
FACT-TOI (FACT Trial Outcome Index), 55, 198, 200
generic instruments, 4, 28
global index vs. profile of domain-specific measures, 4–6
Guttman scale, 38
half rule, 37–38
health status vs. patient preferences, 2–4
Medical Outcomes Study SF-36, 7, 236–237
multi-attribute, 3–4
objective vs. subjective assessments, 4

INDEX   301

period of recall, 6–7
response format, 6
reverse coding, 35
scoring, 35–39, 258
standard gamble utilities, 3
summated ratings, 35–36
time trade-off (TTO), 222
utility, 222
Medical Outcomes Study SF-36, 7, 236–237; see also Measures
Meng, X.L., 131
Mental component scale (MCS), 236–237
Metastatic disease (SX_MET), 188
MI (multiple imputation), 223
Missing at random (MAR)
  analytic methods, 80–81
  identification of dependence on observed data, 78–80
  vs. MCAR, 81–83
  vs. MNAR, 194–195
  overview, 74
Missing completely at random (MCAR), 75–77; see also Missing data
  formal definitions for, 282–283
  vs. MAR, 81–83
  overview, 74
Missing data, 69–91; see also Area under the curve (AUC); Complete-case missing value (CCMV) restriction; Ignorable missing data; Imputation; Missing at random (MAR); Missing completely at random (MCAR); Missing not at random (MNAR)
  acceptable amount, 70–71
  and calculation of summary measures, 220–222
  documentation, 34–35
  formal definitions for, 280–283
  intermittent, 210, 270
  notation, 72–77
  patterns of, 71–72
  preventing, 32–35, 71
  renal cell carcinoma study, 87–90
  similar patterns of dropout among intervention arms, 71
  use of term, 69
  why problematic, 69–70

Missing not at random (MNAR), 74, 84–87; see also Missing data
  formal definitions for, 283
  vs. MAR under assumptions of joint model, 187
Mixed-effects models, 57, 187–188; see also Covariance structure; Pattern mixture models; SAS examples
  fixed effects, 57
  random effects, 57–58, 62, 183, 184
MIXED procedure, 112, 195
  for cell means model, 47–48
  repeated measures model, 51
Mixture models, 84, 183; see also Joint mixed-effects
ML (maximum likelihood) ratio test, 44
MLE (maximum likelihood estimation), 97
Models, 41–68; see also Covariance structure
  analytic models, 43–46
  growth curve models, 54–67
    covariance structure, 57–59
    model for means, 54–57
    for non-small-cell lung cancer (NSCLC) study, 43
    for renal cell carcinoma study, 43
    SAS example of piecewise linear regression model, 65–67
    SAS example of polynomial growth curve model, 59–65
  information criterion, 46, 49, 52
  introduction, 41–43
  likelihood ratio tests, 44–46
  nested, 44–46
  repeated measures models, 46–53
    for adjuvant breast cancer study, 42
    covariance structures, 48–50
    hypothesis testing, 52–53
    mean structure, 46–48
    SAS example of repeated measures model, 50–52
  underidentified, 84
MODEL statement, 48, 89, 188, 189
MODEL statements, 59
Monotone dropout, 71–72, 161–167
  comparison of CCMV, ACMV, and NCMV estimates, 167

complete-case missing value
  restriction, 162–167
non-small-cell lung cancer (NSCLC)
  study example, 162
selection model for, 198–210
  Heckman probit stochastic dropout
    model, 210
  intermittent missing data, 210
  nonparametric analyses, 211
  non-small-cell lung cancer
    (NSCLC) study example,
    201–205
  Oswald program, 206–210
  outcome-dependent selection
    model, 201
Mori, M., 210
Multi-attribute assessment measures,
  3–4
Multi-item scales, scoring, 35–37
Multiple comparisons, 244, 261–262; see
  also Summary measures;
  Summary statistics
  alpha adjustment, 249–253
  Bonferroni adjustment, 215, 249–250,
    253–254
  closed tests, 246–248
  global tests, 246
  post hoc adjustment, 243
  p -value adjustments, 253–254
  Rüger's inequality, 252
  Simes' global test, 252
  Stepdown procedure, 247
Multiple endpoints, 243–255
  background concepts and definitions,
    245–246
  and designing analysis plan, 260–262
  introduction, 243–244
  limiting the number of confirmatory
    tests, 243–244
  multiple comparison procedures, 244
  multivariate statistics, 246–249
  resampling techniques, 254
  summary measures and statistics, 244
  univariate statistics, 249–254
    alpha adjustments for K univariate
      tests, 249–253
    non-small-cell lung cancer
      (NSCLC) study example, 249
    sequential rejective Bonferroni
      procedure, 253–254

Multiple imputation (MI), 131–152, 223,
  230; see also Pattern mixture
  models
analysis of M data sets, 132
approximate Bayesian bootstrap,
  142–146
closest neighbor and predictive mean
  matching, 140–142
combining M analyses, 132, 147–150
explicit univariate regression
  assumptions, 135–136
  computation of imputed values,
    134
  extensions to longitudinal studies,
    135
  identification of imputation model,
    133–134
  non-small-cell lung cancer
    (NSCLC) study, 136–140
generation of M imputed data sets,
  132
implications for design, 152
imputation vs.analytic models, 151
introduction, 131
multivariate procedures for
  nonmonotone missing data,
  146
predictive mean matching, 140–142
propensity scores, 144
selection of procedures, 131–132
sensitivity analyses, 150–151
Multivariate analysis of variance, 97–101
Multivariate logistic regression, 76
Multivariate methods, 96–105
  complete case analysis, 97–101
  exclusion of observations, 105
  exclusion of subjects, 104–105
  maximum likelihood estimation with
    all available data, 101–104
Multivariate model, 48
Multivariate statistics, 246–249
Murray, G.D., 78

N

NCMV (neighboring case missing value)
  restriction, 164–167
Negative quadratic terms, 191

Neighboring case missing value (NCMV) restriction, 164–167, 169; *see also* Pattern mixture models
Nested models, 44–46
Non-ignorable missing data, 145–146, 183–184, 259; *see also* Conditional linear model; Joint mixed-effects; Mixture models
Nonmonotone dropout, 71–72, 146–147
Nonparametric analyses, 178, 211
Nonparametric van der Waerden scores, 228
Non-small-cell lung cancer (NSCLC) study, 10–15
  average rate of change (slopes), 222
  baseline assessment as covariate, 107–108
  complete case analysis (MANOVA), 99–101
  conditional linear model, 187–192
  constructing summary measures, 229–230
  explicit univariate regression, 136–140
  maximum likelihood estimation, 102–104
  missing data, 72, 73, 76, 85–87
  monotone dropout, 162
  multivariate procedures for nonmonotone missing data, 146–147
  pattern mixture models, 154–155, 156, 158
  repeated univariate analyses, 96
  selection between models for assessment, 43
  selection model for monotone dropout, 201–205
  summary measures, 229–230
  underestimation of variance, 129–130
  univariate statistics, 249
  use of imputation, 116–117
Norton, N.J., 131
NSCLC study, *see* Non-small-cell lung cancer; Non-small-cell lung cancer (NSCLC)

O

O'Brien, P C., 238, 239
Objective assessments, 4
Objectives of research, 20–22, 26–27
Observations, exclusion of, 105
ODS statement, 83
Ordinary least squares (OLS), 213–214, 222, 223
Oswald program, 206–210
Outcome-dependent selection models, 184, 201
Overidentified models, 178

P

Paper-and-pencil self-reports, 31
Parametric models, 167–177
  with informative dropout, 206–207
  linear trends, 168–172
  SAS example of pattern-mixture model, 174–177
  variance estimation, 172–174
Patient characteristics, *see* Covariates
Patient preference assessment, 2–4
Patient preferences, 2–4
Patient weights, 237–238
Patrick, D., 2
Pattern mixture models, 84, 153–181, 183, 260
  additional reading, 178
  algebraic details, 178–180
  bivariate data, 155–161
    Brown's protective restrictions, 158–160
    complete-case missing variable (CCMV) restriction, 156–158
    non-small-cell lung cancer (NSCLC) study example, 156, 158
    sensitivity analyses with intermediate restrictions, 160–161
  introduction, 153–155
  monotone dropout, 161–167
    comparison of CCMV, ACMV, and NCMV estimates, 167

complete-case missing value restriction, 162–167
non-small-cell lung cancer (NSCLC) study example, 162
parametric models, 167–177
  linear trends, 168–172
  SAS example of pattern-mixture model, 174–177
  variance estimation, 172–174
SAS example of, 174–177
Pcmid function, 206–207, 208
PCS (physical component scale), 236–237
Period of recall, 6–7
Personnel, see Staff
Physical component scale (PCS), 236–237
Piecewise linear regression, 54–57, 66–67
Pledger, G., 128
Polynomial growth curve models, 54, 55, 56
  SAS example of, 59–65
    covariance structure, 59–63
    estimation, 63–64
    fully parameterized model for the means, 59
    hypothesis testing, 64–65
    model reduction, 63
Pooling estimates, 176–177
Post hoc adjustment, 243
Pragmatic investigational aims, 21–22
Predictable functions, 113
Predictive mean matching, 140–142
Primary endpoints, vs. secondary, 260–261
Probit stochastic dropout model, 210
Propensity scores, 144
Protocol development, see Study design and protocol development
P-value adjustments, 253–254; see also Univariate analysis

Q

Quadratic terms, 54
Quality-adjusted life years, 28
Quality of life, use of term, 2
Questionnaires, see Instruments; Measures

R

Raboud, J.M. et al., 130
Random-coefficient mixture model, 192
Random-coefficient selection models, 184, 195; see also Conditional linear model
Random dropout (RD), 198–199, 201, 204, 205
Random effects, 57–58, 62, 183, 184; see also Mixed-effects models
RANDOM statement, 59, 60, 61, 62
Rating, see Scoring
RCORR option, 51
RD (random dropout), 198–199, 201, 204, 205
Recall, period of, 6–7
Regression models
  explicit, 118–125
    assumptions, 135–136
    computation of imputed values, 134
    extensions to longitudinal studies, 135
    non-small-cell lung cancer (NSCLC) study, 136–140
  univariate, 120–122
Reitmeir, J., 254
Reliability of instruments, 29–30
REML (restricted maximum likelihood) estimates, 97–101, 272
REML (restricted maximum likelihood) ratio test, 44
Renal cell carcinoma study, 15–18
  area under the curve (AUC), 232, 234
  covariance structures tested for, 61
  extension to more complex mixed-effects models, 198
  missing data, 87–90
  piecewise linear model for, 54–57
  selection between models for, 43
  summary measures, 221, 232–233, 234
Repeated measures models, 41–42, 46–53
  for adjuvant breast cancer study, 42
  covariance structures, 48–50
  and designing analysis plan, 259–260
  hypothesis testing, 52–53
  mean structure, 46–48

INDEX 305

SAS example of repeated measures model, 50–52
Repeated univariate analyses, 94–96
Resampling techniques, 254
Research objectives, 20–22, 26–27
Residual errors, variance of, 58
Response format of questionnaires, 6
Restricted maximum likelihood (REML) estimates, 97–101, 272
Restricted maximum likelihood (REML) ratio test, 44
Reverse coding, 35
Roger, J.H.,, 272
R option, 51
Rubin, D.B., 145–146, 148
Rüger's inequality, 252

S

Sampling-based imputation, 142–146
SAS examples
    growth curve models, 59–65
        covariance structure, 59–63
        estimation, 63–64
        fully parameterized model for the means, 59
        hypothesis testing, 64–65
        model reduction, 63
        piecewise linear regression, 65–67
    pattern-mixture model, 174–177
    polynomial growth curve models, 59–65
    repeated measures models, 50–52
    scoring, 38
SAS FREQ procedure, 174
SAS IML procedure, 176
SAS macro variables, 174
Schenker, N., 145–146
Schipper, H., 31
Schluchter, M.D., 183, 184, 194
Scoring
    checklist for statistical analysis plan, 258
    instruments for, 35–39
SD (standard deviation), 129–130
SE (standard error), 129–130
Secondary endpoints, 260–261, 263

Selection models, 84, 184; *see also* Joint mixed-effects
    for monotone dropout, 198–210
        Heckman probit stochastic dropout model, 210
        intermittent missing data, 210
        nonparametric analyses, 211
        non-small-cell lung cancer (NSCLC) study example, 201–205
        Oswald program, 206–210
        outcome-dependent selection model, 201
Selection of subjects, 22–23
Sensitivity analyses, 150–151
Sensitivity analysis, 130, 160–161, 258
Sequential rejective Bonferroni procedure, 253–254
Shared-parameter model, 195
Short-term fluctuations, minimizing, 6
Simes' global test, 252–253
Simes, R.J., 252
Simes procedure, 253
Simon, G.E., 237
Simple imputation, 115–130
    explicit regression models, 118–125
    last value carried forward (LVCF), 125–128
    limitations of, 116
    mean value substitution, 117–118
    non-small-cell lung cancer (NSCLC) study, 116–117
    sensitivity analysis, 130
    underestimation of variance, 128–130
Small sample size approximations, 272
Square root method, 134
Staff, training to avoid missing data, 34–35
Standard deviation (SD), 129–130
Standard error (SE), 129–130
Standard gamble utilities, 3
Statistics guiding model reduction, 44–46
Stepdown procedure, 247
Stratified analysis, of summary measures, 228–229
Structured covariance, 49–50
Study design and protocol development, 19–39; *see also* Models
    avoiding missing data, 32–35
    background and rationale, 19–20

data collection and management, 32
introduction, 19
longitudinal designs, 23–27
mode of administration, 31–32
research objectives, 20–22
scoring instruments, 35–39
selection of a quality of life measure, 27–29
selection of subjects, 22–23
Subjective assessments, 4
Subjects of assessments
    exclusion of, 104–105
    selecting, 22–23
    unequal allocations to treatment groups, 270–271
Subscales, HRQoL, summarizing across, 235–240
Summary measures, 213–241; see also Summary statistics
    addressing multiplicity of endpoints, 213
    area under the curve, 240
    choosing, 215–217
    combining HRQoL and time to event, 240
    constructing, 217–230
        average of ranks, 227
        average rate of change (slopes), 222–227
        non-small-cell lung cancer (NSCLC) study example, 229–230
        notation, 220
        when missing data, 220–222
    and multiple endpoints, 244
    nonparametric procedures, 240
    options for weighting, 235–239
    renal cell carcinoma study, 221, 232–233, 234
    stratified analysis of, 228–229
    strengths and weaknesses, 215
    summarizing across HRQoL domains or subscales, 235–240
    vs. summary statistics, 213–214
    and summary statistics, 213–215
    univariate analysis of, 228
    weighting, 235–239
Summary statistics, 213–215; see also Summary measures
    and multiple endpoints, 244

summarizing across HRQoL domains or subscales, 239–240
Summated ratings, 35–36
SX_MET (metastatic disease), 188

T

Taylor series approximation, 173–174
Terminal dropout, see Monotone dropout
Therapy, assessment after discontinuation of, 27
Time-driven designs, 24, 260
Time-to-event mixture, 183
Time trade-off (TTO), 222
Time trade utilities, 3
Time-varying covariates, 270
Timing, of HRQoL assessments, 8–10
    follow-up, 24–25
    initial, 24
Toplitz covariance structure, 45, 49, 50, 52
Tracking patients in studies, 32
Training research personnel, to avoid missing data, 34
TRANSPOSE procedure, 98
Treatments, assessment after discontinuation of, 27
Trial Outcome Index (FACT-BRM TOI), 16, 236
Trials, see Study design and protocol development
Tu, X.M., 184, 194
Tumor response, 261
Two-sample t-test, 228
Type I error rate
    causes of, 95, 110, 213, 243
    controlling, 246, 248, 261, 266
    and Simes' global test, 252
Type II error rate, 266

U

Underestimation of variance, 128–130
Underidentified models, 84
Unequal allocations of subjects to treatment groups, 270–271

Univariate analysis, 228
Univariate regression, 48, 120–122
    assumptions, 135–136
    computation of imputed values, 134
    extensions to longitudinal studies, 135
    non-small-cell lung cancer (NSCLC) study, 136–140
Univariate statistics, 249–254
    alpha adjustments for K univariate tests, 249–253
    vs. multivariate, 245
    non-small-cell lung cancer (NSCLC) study example, 249
    sequential rejective Bonferroni procedure, 253–254
    use of term, 245
Unstructured covariance, 48–49, 50
Utility measures, 222

V

Validity of instruments, 29–30
VanBuuren, S., 146
Variance estimation, 128–130, 172–174
Variation in responses, 29
Visual analog scale (VAS), 6

W

Wang, Y., 178
Ware, J.E. et al., 28
Wassmer, G., 254
Weighting summary measures, 235–239
Westfall, P.H., 254
WHO (World Health Organization), 1
Wilcoxon Rank Sum test, 128, 228
Wilson, I.B., 1–2
Within imputance variation, *see* Multiple imputation (MI)
World Health Organization (WHO), 1
Wu, M.C., 183, 184, 185, 186, 192, 210

Y

Yao, Q., 178
Yau, L., 135, 211
Young, S.S., 254

Z

Zero, assigning to HRQoL scores, 222